EXPRESSING EMOTION

EMOTIONS AND SOCIAL BEHAVIOR

Series Editor: Peter Salovey, Yale University

EXPRESSING EMOTION

Myths, Realities, and Therapeutic Strategies

EILEEN KENNEDY-MOORE
JEANNE C. WATSON

Series Editor's Note by Peter Salovey
Foreword by Jeremy D. Safran

THE GUILFORD PRESS
New York   London

© 1999 The Guilford Press
A Division of Guilford Publications, Inc.
72 Spring Street, New York, NY 10012
http://www.guilford.com

Printed in the United States of America

This book is printed on acid-free paper.

Last digit is print number: 9 8 7 6 5 4 3 2 1

Library of Congress Cataloging-in-Publication Data
Kennedy-Moore, Eileen.
    Expressing emotion: myths, realities, and therapeutic strategies /
  Eileen Kennedy-Moore, Jeanne C. Watson; foreword by Jeremy D.
  Safran.
       p.   cm.—(Emotions and social behavior)
    Includes bibliographical references and index.
    ISBN 1-57230-473-1
    1. Emotions—Health aspects.   2. Adjustment (Psychology).
  3. Mental health.   I. Watson, Jeanne C.   II. Title.   III. Series.
  RC455.4.E46K46   1999
  616.89—dc21
                                                            99-13223
                                                                CIP

"I Want to Breathe" by James Laughlin, from *Selected Poems 1935–1985*.
Copyright © 1986 by James Laughlin. Reprinted by permission of New
Directions Publishing Corp.

*This book is lovingly dedicated
to the memory of
my mother,
Mary Clark Kennedy (1939–1998),
adventurer, feminist, family-maker*

—E. K. M.

To Jonathan

—J. C. W.

About the Authors

Eileen Kennedy-Moore has a PhD in clinical psychology from the State University of New York at Stony Brook. The recipient of an APA Dissertation Award for her work on causal explanations for daily mood, she has also done research on expression and health, coping, and interpersonal models of depression. Her clients have ranged from veterans with post-traumatic stress disorder to children with divorced parents. Currently, she writes and lectures on coping and emotions.

Jeanne C. Watson, PhD, is an assistant professor in the Department of Adult Education, Community Development and Counselling Psychology at the Ontario Institute for Studies in Education of the University of Toronto. She is coeditor (with Leslie S. Greenberg and Germain Lietaer) of the *Handbook of Experiential Psychotherapy* (Guilford Press, 1998) and has written numerous articles on psychotherapy process and outcome. Dr. Watson has a part-time private practice in Toronto.

Series Editor's Note

I am delighted to introduce *Expressing Emotion* as a volume in the Guilford series Emotions and Social Behavior. Emotions are rarely expressed in a psychological vacuum but, rather, in a social context where they color interpersonal perceptions and motivate behavior. As with the other books in the series, *Expressing Emotion* represents seminal thinking about the social impact of emotional experiences and the role of emotion in social life.

Eileen Kennedy-Moore and Jeanne Watson have gathered in a single volume a wonderful array of the very best scholarship concerned with the adaptive and maladaptive consequences of expressing—or failing to express—emotions. They move from the laboratory of the emotions researcher to the psychotherapist's office to the larger world in order to challenge the myth that the emotional system is like a pressure-filled garden hose that must be vented or it will explode. They describe the conditions under which emotional expression can have positive consequences for physical and mental health and interpersonal relationships, and they explore the situations under which the consequences of emotional expression are less salubrious.

In recent years, the term "emotional intelligence" has been used to describe the modern, though still controversial, view that the emotional system provides useful information to humans, informing us in ways that lead to appropriate social behavior and psychological growth. Emotional expression is fundamental to the competencies thought to comprise emotional intelligence. As one brilliant emotions theorist, Sylvan Tomkins, said, "Out of the marriage of reason with affect there issues clarity with passion. Reason without affect would be impotent, affect without reason would be blind" (1962, p. 112). I know that you, the reader, will enjoy this tour of popular myths concerning emotional expression and the scientific and therapeutic realities that confront these legends. You may never view your feelings the same way again.

PETER SALOVEY, PhD
Professor of Psychology and of Epidemiology and Public Health
Yale University

REFERENCE

Tomkins, S. S. (1962). *Affect, imagery, consciousness* (Vol. 1). New York: Springer.

Foreword

In recent years there has been a good deal of interest in the topic of emotion in both academic and popular psychology. The prevailing view is shifting away from one in which emotions are seen as operating in opposition to reason to one in which they contribute to reason and to adaptive functioning. In parallel to this, the traditional distinction between mind and body is giving way to a more holistic, nondualistic perspective. In this perspective the mind is viewed as arising out of an organism in interaction with the environment. The function of emotions is to safeguard the goals of that organism. Emotion can be conceptualized as a form of action disposition information. It provides information about the readiness of the biological system to act in certain ways. For example, anger provides information regarding the readiness of the system to protect itself in an aggressive fashion. Love provides information regarding the readiness of the system to act in an affiliative fashion.

Psychological problems often arise from a failure to fully process potentially adaptive emotional experience. Emotion can provide people with the conviction that a certain course of action is right for them and with the motivation to pursue that course of action. For example, a person in an abusive relationship may begin the process of ending it when she accesses her feelings of anger. A socially isolated individual may begin to face his anxiety and make social contact when he fully accesses his feelings of sadness and pain. Emotion is also the foundation of meaning. The inability to explore one's emotional experience can leave a person disoriented, puzzled, and confused. At the same time, however, emotions can be disorganizing or can interfere with healthy functioning. Intense recurring anger can be destructive to self and others. Jealousy can be painful and crippling. Fear can be disabling.

One of the more important features of Eileen Kennedy-Moore and Jeanne C. Watson's book is that it does an admirable job of grappling with the complexities and paradoxes of emotional experience and expression without oversimplifying. As the authors point out, our culture holds complex and contradictory attitudes toward the human passions. On the one hand, there is an attitude of stoicism that values emotional self-control and cool reason. On the other hand, there is a tradition of romanticism that celebrates the passions and links them to genuineness and authenticity. Kennedy-Moore and Watson avoid the trap of siding with either of these two poles by exploring complex and differentiated questions about what specific types of emotional experience and expression are adaptive in what specific contexts.

In order to accomplish this objective, they synthesize theory and research from a wide range of diverse areas including social psychology, emotion theory, health psychology, and the psychotherapy literature. I am particularly impressed with their ability to review the relevant theory and research findings without being overly dry and academic and to embed this review within a compelling and dynamic narrative that effortlessly carries the reader along. I am also impressed with the way that they creatively weave together findings from disparate areas into a seamless whole and spell out clinical implications. The result is a lively and accessible exploration of key issues in the area that I believe will contribute substantially to the growing interest in emotion.

JEREMY D. SAFRAN, PhD
Professor of Psychology
New School for Social Research

Acknowledgments

Psychology has become an increasingly specialized and fractionated field. This book is our attempt to speak across disciplines, subspecialties, and orientations, to draw together diverse perspectives on a common focus: the expression and nonexpression of emotion.

Working on this book has given us firsthand experience of both the rewards and the challenges of integrative work. In talking about our ideas for this book, we were inspired by the commonalities that emerged from our different backgrounds. Eileen's emphasis on the difference between emotional expression and emotional experience matches Jeanne's distinction between subjective experience and symbolic representation of that experience. Jeanne's work on clients' explorations of their problematic reactions (i.e., emotional responses that clients are aware of but find puzzling) parallels Eileen's study of people's causal explanations for their moods. Eileen's interest in the social context of expression fits well with Jeanne's focus on the therapeutic relationship.

We were also intrigued by the differences in our perspectives and the new ideas that emerged as we compared our diverse views. Jeanne's qualitative approach, focus on psychotherapy process, and knowledge of experiential and client-centered therapy complements Eileen's quantitative research on stress and coping, interest in social psychology, and primarily cognitive-behavioral clinical orientation. However, we also had to struggle to move beyond our interest-specific jargon and unstated assumptions toward a common understanding. We were surprised sometimes at how difficult it was to explain our ideas in a way that someone outside our specialized subfields could understand.

We believe that what has emerged from our collaboration is something better than either of us could have produced alone. We have gained an integrative understanding of expression and nonexpression, a way of conceptualizing emotional behavior that captures the richness and complexity of this topic yet is directly relevant to day-to-day clinical practice. We hope our readers will find the connections we have drawn as fascinating and useful as we do.

We would like to thank Marv Goldfried for suggesting our collaboration. Marv has been a pioneer in psychotherapy integration, and his emphasis on identifying core conceptual similarities while acknowledging specific technical differences has been a guiding theme in our work together.

We would like to thank our mentors, Arthur Stone and Camille Wortman for Eileen, and Les Greenberg and Laura Rice for Jeanne. These individuals inspired us, guided us, and taught us the art and science of our field. We also thank Jeremy Safran and Howard Friedman for their very useful advice concerning the process of writing and publishing a book.

This book would not have been possible without the efforts of the people at The Guilford Press. We thank Seymour Weingarten, Editor-in-Chief, for his interest in our project. We thank his assistant, Carolyn Graham, for answering innumerable pesky questions. We thank Peter Salovey, our Series Editor, for his insightful comments, for his emphasis on making this book both scholarly and fun to read, and especially for his enthusiasm about our work. His support has been invaluable. We also thank members of the production and marketing teams for polishing and promoting our book.

On a personal level, we'd like to thank our friends and family for their love and support. Eileen thanks the members of the Work In Progress (WIP) group—Julie Abrams, Debbie Chaskin, Sue Frigand, Lucy Harrington, and Pam Reid—whose unfailing support, practical advice, and sense of humor provided some of the best highlights of working on this project. We thank our children for bringing joy to our lives and for putting up with the extra work time we needed to produce this book. Eileen's parents actually read drafts of every one of her chapters—truly an expression of love. Her husband, Tony Moore, was heroic as he hunted down references, willingly listened to half-formed ideas, and generally did whatever was necessary to help her finish this project. Eileen can't imagine a better life partner.

Definitions of Key Terms

Components of emotion: Three primary components: emotional expression, experience, and arousal. One secondary component: emotional reflection.

Emotional arousal: The physiological aspect of emotional responses. One of the three primary components of emotion.

Emotional behavior: Emotional expression *or* nonexpression.

Emotional experience: The subjective, felt sense of emotional responses. One of the three primary components of emotion. Inclusive term for the phenomenological aspects of affect, emotions, and feelings.

Emotional expression: Observable verbal and nonverbal behaviors that communicate and/or symbolize emotional experience. Expression can occur with or without self-awareness, it is at least somewhat controllable, and it can involve varying degrees of deliberate intent. One of the three primary components of emotion.

Emotional reflection: Thoughts about emotional expression, experience, or arousal. A secondary component of emotion.

Nonexpression: Lack of expressive behavior.

Contents

PART IV.
TREATMENT IMPLICATIONS

PART V.
CONCLUSION

PART I

Introduction

I

Expression, Nonexpression, and Well-Being: An Overview

INTRODUCTION

Both popular culture and clinical lore contain a belief that people *must* express their emotions or "bad" things will happen to them, physically or psychologically. On talk shows, over dinner tables, in private diaries, and in psychotherapy offices, emotional expression is commonplace. This venting of emotions is fueled in part by the pervasive belief in our society in the importance of "letting one's feelings out" rather than "bottling them up." In support of this belief, numerous empirical studies have demonstrated mental and physical health benefits associated with emotional expression, as well as psychophysiological costs associated with inhibited expression (see Pennebaker, 1995, for recent examples).

Countering the belief that expressing emotions is healthy is the similarly pervasive belief that *not* expressing emotions is a sign of strength or maturity or even virtue. In the media, romantic heroes still tend to be "the strong, silent type." Moreover, describing someone by saying, "Oh, she is very emotional" is usually not a compliment. It carries the connotation that this person is somehow childish or lacking in self-control (cf. Shields,1987). This belief that nonexpression is preferable to expression also has some empirical support. Expression can intensify distress (Laird, 1974; Lanzetta, Cartwright-Smith, & Kleck, 1976), and it can interfere with active coping efforts (Carver, Scheier, & Weintraub, 1989; cf. Nolen-Hoeksema, 1991). Unrestrained expression can also have a destructive influence on interpersonal relationships (Tavris, 1984, 1989).

Either belief, that expressing emotions is universally adaptive or maladaptive, is a black-and-white view of phenomena with numerous shadings. In this book, we hope to capture the complexity of both expres-

3

sion and nonexpression, in order to clarify when and how they are related to well-being. We draw upon the breadth of theory and research on this topic and present it in the context of a coherent conceptual framework. We describe the role of expression in individual and social functioning, emphasizing its importance in daily life as well as in clinical practice.

Throughout the book we refer to several key terms: *Emotional experience* is the subjective, felt sense of emotional responses. We define *emotional expression* as observable verbal and nonverbal behaviors that communicate and/or symbolize emotional experience. Expression can occur with or without self-awareness, it is at least somewhat controllable, and it can involve varying degrees of deliberate intent. *Nonexpression* is the lack of expression. We use the term *emotional behavior* to refer to *either* expression or nonexpression. Expression and nonexpression are overt manifestations, which may or may not correspond to covert processes, like emotional experience (e.g., Kennedy-Moore & Stone, 1999; Kring, Smith, & Neale, 1994; Gross & Levenson, 1997). So, for example, one person might refrain from expressing even though she is experiencing a great deal of emotion. Another person might express vociferously, while experiencing only a minor degree of emotion.

Emotional expression is the link between internal experience and the outside world. As such, it carries enormous theoretical and practical importance. In daily life, expression is the means by which people communicate experience and influence relationships. In therapy, emotional behavior provides important information about how clients are feeling, how they are managing their feelings, and how they are relating to the therapist (J. C. Watson & Greenberg, 1995; J. C. Watson & Rennie, 1994). However, expression and nonexpression come in many different forms, which can have many different consequences for well-being. In the next section, we describe some of these varieties of emotional behavior.

Varieties of Nonexpression

Whether a particular instance of emotional behavior is adaptive or maladaptive depends on the form and the context of that behavior. Looking first at nonexpression, there are many reasons why people might not express their emotions. For example, they might not recognize their emotions, they might dislike expression, or they might not have the opportunity to express. Different causes of nonexpression can yield different consequences.

Consider the case of a rape survivor who insists that she is "over" the rape and says she wants to have an intimate relationship with a man. However, she is puzzled by the fact that every time she starts to get close to a man, she finds a reason to break off the relationship. This might be an instance of nonexpression due to unrecognized feelings. Perhaps, for this woman, being in a close relationship evokes feelings of fear, vulnerability, or shame. Maybe she is not consciously aware of these feelings, or maybe she just interprets them as dissatisfaction with the man. This kind of nonexpression can be harmful when it entails difficulties in understanding one's own emotional experience and using this understanding to guide behavior in an adaptive way. For example, this woman might be focusing on meeting Mr. Right when her difficulties have more to do with coping with the feelings evoked by staying with Mr. Right. In order to change her pattern of prematurely ending relationships, it might be important for this woman to become aware of and to express (to herself, to her lover, perhaps with the help of a therapist) the feelings that have led her to break off relationships in the past.

On the other hand, consider a recently unemployed man who values self-control and stoicism in the face of adversity. He is acutely aware of his feelings of failure or betrayal but nevertheless believes that the best way to handle these feelings is to bravely march forward. In this case, nonexpression reflects personal beliefs and attitudes that are closely tied to this man's sense of identity. For him, nonexpression might be an adaptive coping strategy. Being able to control his emotional behavior is central to his sense of personal competence, and, for him, it could be an important prerequisite to actively dealing with his unemployment.

Still another example of nonexpression is a lonely teenager who relocates because of his parents' divorce. He is filled with a variety of complicated and conflicting feelings, such as anger and relief, guilt and betrayal, sadness and hope. However, because of the move, he no longer has a close group of friends in whom he can confide. He is far away from his father. He senses that his mother is preoccupied with and more than a bit overwhelmed by the process of setting up a new life for them, so he is reluctant to "burden" her with his feelings. He feels the strain of wanting to express his feelings while believing that he can't. This form of nonexpression, which stems from perceptions of the social environment as prohibiting expression, can compound distress and *may* even compromise physical health (see study by Lepore, Silver, Wortman, & Wayment, 1996; and reviews by Pennebaker, 1992; Tait & Silver, 1989).

All three of these examples involve a lack of overt expressive behavior, but they represent different forms of nonexpression. The rape survivor's nonexpression involves a lack of conscious awareness of her feelings. The unemployed man's nonexpression stems from personal values, and the teenager's nonexpression involves a perceived lack of opportunity to express. Because these different forms of nonexpression involve various degrees of understanding and acceptance of emotional experience, we believe they have different consequences for well-being.

Varieties of Expression

The effects of expressing emotions also vary, depending on what is expressed, to whom, and how. Expression can contribute to self-knowledge, and it is necessary for the development of emotional intimacy, but it is a risky undertaking. Even when they believe expression is important, people may be ambivalent about expressing their feelings (e.g., Coyne, Wortman, & Lehman, 1988; L. A. King & Emmons, 1990) or having someone else express to them (e.g., Coates & Winston, 1987; Gottlieb & Wagner, 1991). For example, Pennebaker (1992) describes how, only 3 weeks after the 1989 earthquake in San Francisco, 80% of area residents said that they wanted to talk about the quake, but less than 60% said they wanted to hear about it. In fact, about 1 month after the quake, T-shirts began appearing saying, "Thank you for not sharing your earthquake experience." When someone expresses emotions, particularly intense, negative emotions, it can be frightening, stressful, or overwhelming for the recipient (see review by Pennebaker, 1993c). If recipients of emotional expression respond negatively, the person expressing might feel rejected, misunderstood, embarrassed, or betrayed.

The complexity of the relationship between expression and well-being is apparent when we consider the example of anger expression within a marriage. Ideally, when couples express anger, they feel better afterward: they resolve their conflict, they gain mutual understanding, and they have a greater sense of satisfaction with the relationship. However, expressing anger can also make couples feel worse (Bradbury & Fincham, 1990; Fruzzetti & Jacobson, 1990; Gottman, 1993b; Gottman & Levenson, 1986). Sometimes anger expression deteriorates into an exchange of increasingly hostile criticisms, aimed at hurting the other partner rather than resolving any issues. Which pattern prevails depends on how the partners express their feelings and the overall relationship context of that expression. Is the level of anger expression moderate or intensely negative? Do the partners couch negative statements within a framework of relationship-building remarks or are they completely hostile? How do they respond to each other's expressions? Do they acknowledge the partner's comments or just counterattack? Do the partners generally have positive or negative views of each other and their relationship? Is anger expression a relatively rare occurrence between them or are they constantly battling each other?

Clinical Applications

This kind of multifaceted understanding of the various forms of expression and nonexpression is critically important in clinical work. Many psychotherapy clients present difficulties that can be understood as problems related to emotional behavior. Some clients have explosive outbursts of expression; others show highly constricted expression; still other clients vacillate between these extremes. Each of these patterns can be maladaptive.

In general, therapists need to help clients find a delicate balance in their emotional expression, so that clients can (1) understand their feelings rather than be overwhelmed by them, (2) harness the energy of their emotions for planning and action rather than be either thoughtlessly driven by it or paralyzed by it, and (3) communicate their emotional experience to others in a way that enhances interpersonal functioning rather than impairs it. This delicate balance entails using expression as a means of gaining self-understanding and relating to others in life-enhancing ways. It involves reflecting upon emotional experience and integrating it with other aspects of the self rather than either acting impulsively or shutting oneself off from experience.

The specific ways in which expression is addressed in therapy depend, of course, on the needs of particular clients. For example, therapists might help clients to use expression as a means of processing and symbolizing their emotional experience. They might help clients recognize patterns in their emotional behavior. They might communicate about the impact of clients' expression or nonexpression on the therapist, which could be important information for understanding the clients' other relationships. Therapists might also facilitate clients' efforts to use new forms of emotional expression.

Summary

In summary, emotional behavior (i.e., expression or nonexpression) plays a key role in individual adjustment, social interaction, and therapeutic process. So far in this chapter we have emphasized a multifaceted view of emotional behavior that takes characteristics of the individual and the psychosocial environment into account. We have suggested that expression or nonexpression can take various forms and can have either positive or negative consequences. What and how people express (or don't express) affects their own emotional experience as well as the nature of their relationships with others.

However, just recognizing that emotional behavior is complicated is not enough. If a multifaceted view of emotional behavior is going to be useful for guiding clinical or empirical understanding, it must to be couched in a coherent framework that provides a systematic way of thinking about the various forms of expression and nonexpression and their various consequences.

Below, we introduce our model of the process of expression and nonexpression. The model serves as the organizing framework for this book. As we describe in later chapters, the model also points to ways of cultivating *balance* in emotional behavior. Our central thesis in this book is that adaptive emotional behavior is characterized by integration, flexibility, and interpersonal coordination. What is important is not how much people do or do not express, but rather the degree to which they are able to integrate their thinking and their feeling, to draw upon their emotional experience without being driven blindly by it, and to consider the interpersonal impact of their emotional behavior without discounting their own experience.

A PROCESS MODEL OF EXPRESSION
AND NONEXPRESSION

Before we can understand the role of emotional behavior in day-to-day life or in clinical problems and interventions, we first need to understand how expression and nonexpression come about. Kennedy-Moore, Greenberg, and Wortman (1991) proposed a model for the process by which covert emotional experience is translated into overt emotional expression. This process involves a series of cognitive-evaluative steps that are driven by affective experience and in turn influence that experience. Disruptions at different points in this process result in different forms of nonexpression.

This model was originally developed in an effort to make sense of conflicting findings concerning the health effects of emotional behavior, by integrating emotion theory with research on emotion-related personality traits. Individual steps in the model, and the theory and research supporting them, are discussed in later chapters. For now, we focus on a descriptive overview of the process of expression and the various forms of nonexpression. To illustrate the model, let's look at a hypothetical example:

> The evidence is there in her hand: a letter from the other woman. Marla found it in the pocket of her husband, Alfred's, raincoat, while she was gathering up clothes to take to the dry cleaners. There is no doubt about it. He has been having an affair—apparently for quite a while: Last week's trip downstate wasn't their first rendezvous.

Now what happens? That depends on what sort of person Marla is and what her circumstances are. First we look at the process of expression, and then we consider ways this process might be disrupted, resulting in nonexpression.

The Process of Expression

Let's say Marla does express her emotions in response to finding the letter. How does this expression come about? The rectangles in Figure 1.1 (adapted from Kennedy-Moore et al., 1991) make up our basic model of the process of expression. Each rectangle illustrates an internal, intermediary step between the occurrence of an emotion-eliciting event and overt expressive behavior.

Step 1: Prereflective Reaction

The first step (top rectangle) in the model involves prereflective reaction to an emotion-eliciting stimulus. This reaction entails perception of the stimulus, preconscious cognitive and emotional processing, and accompanying physiological changes. Marla rapidly and automatically (i.e., without effort or intention) appraises the significance of the letter and reacts with some level of affective arousal. This arousal is a bodily signal that something important is happening that warrants attention and/or action.

Step 2: Conscious Perception of Response

In the next step, Marla becomes aware of her affective reaction—in effect, hearing the bodily signal. She consciously perceives that she is distressed. She might even notice specific bodily signs such as a racing heart or shaking hands.

Step 3: Labeling and Interpretation of Response

The third step of the model involves labeling and interpreting the affective response. The bodily signal entailed in affective experience is fairly crude, so as soon as Marla becomes aware of such a response she begins to process this experience cognitively. Drawing upon internal as well as situational cues, Marla determines that the response is emotional rather than purely physiological. At this point, Marla recognizes (for example) that she feels angry and betrayed. She begins to flesh out the meaning of her experience.

Step 4: Evaluation of Response as Acceptable

In the fourth step of the model, Marla evaluates her emotional experience in terms of her own beliefs and goals. At this point, Marla considers her experience in light of her implicit or explicit beliefs about what is important or typical or desirable and determines that her feelings are valid and acceptable.

Step 5: Perceived Social Context for Expression

Finally, Marla evaluates the match between her experience and her current social context. If she perceives that revealing her feelings is possible or desirable in her interpersonal environment, then, finally, she expresses these feelings.

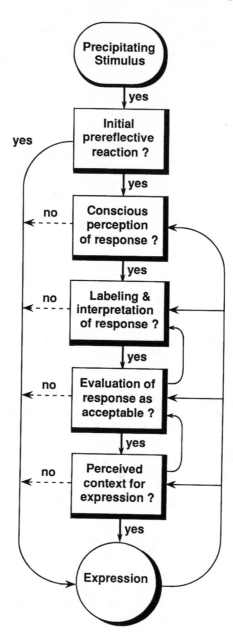

FIGURE 1.1. The process of expression.

The steps in the process model of expression are important not only for determining whether expression occurs, but also for determining the form that it takes. Marla might express her feelings in many ways. She might confront her husband as soon as he walks in the door, angrily flinging the letter at him. She might sob wretchedly by herself. She might call her sister and confide her feelings of betrayal. Specifically what and how she expresses depends on her awareness, interpretation, and evaluation of her experience and her context.

Qualifications to the Basic Model of Expression

The basic model represents expression as the culmination of a series of internal, cognitive-evaluative steps that influence and are influenced by affective experience. However, expression doesn't necessarily occur in such a neat, orderly way. Sometimes people just burst out with an emotional expression without having processed their experience fully or even at all (S. Epstein, 1990; LeDoux, 1989, 1996). Often, expression involves an iterative, reflexive process. People don't usually just process their experience once, express it, and have done with it. More typically, they express repeatedly, reworking and refining their understanding of their emotional experience (e.g., Rimé, Mesquita, Philippot, & Boca, 1991).

The arrows on the left of Figure 1.1 illustrate these important qualifications to the basic model. The first qualification concerns expressive leakage. The downward arrow indicates that some degree of expressive behavior follows directly from the initial prereflective reaction, bypassing the cognitive-evaluative steps. This is particularly the case when the affective reaction is very strong, but subtle expressive signs leak out even with milder reactions (e.g., Ekman & Friesen, 1969; Haggard & Isaacs, 1966; see discussion by Collier, 1985, concerning awareness and control of expression). The dashed sideways arrows feeding into the downward arrow show that expression can leak after each of the steps. This occurs when the magnitude of the reaction exceeds the individual's capacity to contain it or process it further (cf. Gross & Muñoz, 1995). So, for example, Marla might show signs of tension or resentment even if she is not aware of experiencing these. If she is extremely distressed by the letter, she might burst into tears, even if this is the last thing in the world she wants to do. We call this kind of expression *leakage* because it is experienced by the individual as less volitional than the more conscious, more deliberate, step-by-step path to expression represented by the basic model. (We will say more about this point later in this chapter.)

The second qualification to the basic model involves the recursive nature of the process of expression. The upward arrows to the right of the basic model depict feedback loops, in which later steps in the model inform and reelicit earlier steps. Expression is a source of self-knowledge. For example, bursting into tears might prompt Marla to observe that she is more upset about Alfred's affair than she realized. Expression is also a means of eliciting information from others. Marla might tell her best friend about the letter and express feelings of inadequacy. But, hearing her friend remark "I can't believe you're not furious with him" could help Marla recognize and accept her feelings of anger.

This model of expression can be applied to either general dispositions to express or to specific instances of expression, and to either positive or negative emotions. Emotional expression can be thought of as a trait in that there is considerable consistency across time and across situations in the degree to which individuals express their emotions. Some people tend to express a lot, others tend to express less (e.g., Gross & John, 1997; Kring et al., 1994). There is also consistency across emotion domains: In general, people who are very expressive of negative emotions also tend to be expressive of positive emotions (Gross & John, 1997). However, a full understanding of expression requires that we look at both a global, trait level and more specific levels. For example, a particular expressive style may be effective in general but ineffective with respect to a specific situation, such as a traumatic event. A particular instance of expression might carry very different implications for someone who rarely expresses than for someone who frequently expresses. A person who readily expresses positive emotions but has difficulty expressing negative emotions is likely to have a very different social milieu than someone who readily expresses negative emotions and only rarely expresses positive emotions. Laboratory studies suggest that the expression–well-being relationship depends on whether we are looking at between-subject or within-subject variability (Buck, 1980) and whether we are talking about expression of positive or negative emotions (Gross & John, 1997).

So far, we have described our model for the process of emotional expression. We have outlined a series of intervening steps between an emotion-eliciting stimulus and overt emotional expression. We have also suggested that these steps can sometimes be bypassed, resulting in expressive leakage. We now turn to the question of how nonexpression arises.

Disruptions in the Process of Expression

Figure 1.2 (adapted from Kennedy-Moore et al., 1991) illustrates how disruptions at different points in the process of emotional expression result in different forms of nonexpression, which can have different consequences for well-being. The circles in this figure represent various factors associated with nonexpression. These factors can potentially be assessed by clinicians or researchers. They can be either dispositional, meaning they pertain to the individual's enduring personality characteristics, or situational, meaning they involve transitory circumstances.

Disruption at Step 1: Minimal Prereflective Reaction

One form of nonexpression occurs when the precipitating stimulus (top oval) evokes only minimal prereflective reaction (first rectangle). Most people would consider news of a partner's infidelity to be very serious, even alarming, but Marla might not perceive this information as particularly threatening. People differ in the strength of their affective reactions. In laboratory studies, people show marked individual differences in their responsiveness to the same stressor (see reviews by Eisenberg & Fabes, 1992; R. J. Larsen & Zarate, 1991; Rothbart & Posner, 1985). For example, people differ in their thresholds for experiencing pain (A. Petrie, 1967). More broadly, Larsen and his colleagues (R. J. Larsen & Diener, 1987; R. J. Larsen, Diener, & Emmons, 1986) have demonstrated that people differ in the typical intensity or magnitude of their affective experience. Individuals low in affect intensity consistently report milder reactions to both positive and negative events, compared to individuals high in affect intensity. So, perhaps because of her temperament or her cognitive style (R. J. Larsen & Diener, 1987; R. J. Larsen, Diener, & Cropanzano, 1987), Marla might be one of those people who just doesn't tend to get ruffled by life events—no high highs or low lows. She might not react much to finding the letter because, in general, she has a very high distress threshold.

Situational factors could also influence Marla's initial reaction to discovering her husband's affair. If her marriage had been distant and failing for a long time, it is conceivable that Marla might respond to the letter with indifference. If she'd been feeling guilty about her own affair, she might even react with relief.

If Marla truly experiences little or no distress in response to finding the letter, we would not expect her to express any negative affect. Nor would we expect this lack of expression to be detrimental. Clinically, encouraging people with this form of nonexpression to "let their feelings out" makes no sense. They aren't holding their feelings in, they just aren't reacting much. In fact, nonexpression stemming from low reactivity may be a sign of particularly good adjustment (Wortman, Sheedy, Gluhoski, & Kessler, 1992). These individuals may be more serene or content, and their milder emotional reactions may exact less physiological toll than more extreme responses (R. J. Larsen & Diener, 1987).

Disruption at Step 2: Motivated Lack of Awareness

Let's say that Marla *is* distressed by the letter. If Marla finds her experience too threatening, she might block it through motivated lack of awareness. This form of nonexpression entails disruption at the second step in the process of expression, which concerns conscious perception of the affective response. The concrete evidence in the letter means that Marla can't deny the

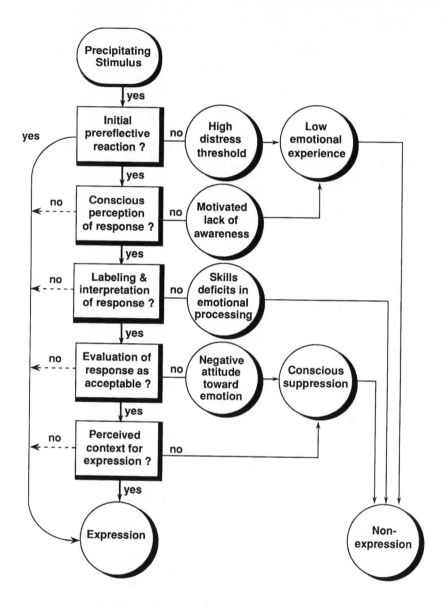

FIGURE 1.2. Disruptions in the process of expression.

existence of the affair, but she *can* deny its impact on her. She might tell herself that she is not really upset, that she feels fine, that the affair is not such a big deal and she is certain she and Alfred will work things out in a reasonable manner. This type of emotional defensiveness could be part of a general disposition to avoid acknowledging unpleasant emotional experience, such as the repressive coping style identified by Weinberger and his colleagues (Weinberger, 1990; see also Bonanno & Singer, 1990; T. L. Newton & Contrada, 1992). Alternatively, it could represent a more specific sensitivity. Marla might be able to acknowledge negative feelings in other areas of her life, but perhaps being happily married is so central to her sense of self that she can't bear to recognize the particular feelings evoked by the letter.

Blocking emotional experience from awareness in this way might have some short-term, "just-getting-through-the-day" kinds of benefits, but the long term is likely to be problematic. The rape survivor described at the beginning of this chapter may be an example of this form of nonexpression. Her behavior suggests that being in a relationship is somehow distressing to her. However, she is not aware of experiencing any distress. Motivated lack of awareness of affective experience means that this experience can't be used to guide behavior in adaptive ways. It's like going through life blindfolded. When nonexpression results from failure to acknowledge emotional distress, particularly intense distress, it is likely to be maladaptive.

Disruption at Step 3: Skill Deficits in Emotional Processing

Even if Marla is aware of her distress, she might not express if she lacks the skill to label or interpret her experience. Marla might know she feels "bad" but be unable to symbolize that experience more completely. This form of nonexpression entails disruption of Step 3 of the model, which concerns the labeling and interpretation of the affective response. Alexithymia (Sifneos, 1972; Taylor, Bagby, & Parker, 1991) is a personality trait that exemplifies this form of nonexpression. It refers to a lack of verbal understanding of emotional experience, and it has been linked to general dysphoria, eating disorders, substance abuse, and somatization.

The problem with an inability to interpret feelings is that it is a dead end. If Marla only knows that she feels bad, this doesn't suggest any ways for her to respond to this feeling. On the other hand, if she is able to symbolize and differentiate her feelings more completely, she might recognize that she feels frightened that Alfred will leave her, that she feels jealous and rejected and wonders what the other woman has that she lacks, that she feels betrayed and questions whether she will ever be able to trust him again, etc. These more comprehensive views of emotional experience make it possible to engage in more targeted and probably more effective coping efforts.

Disruption at Step 4: Negative Attitude toward Emotion

Assuming Marla is aware of her emotional response and able to label and interpret it, she still might not express her feelings if she evaluates her response as unacceptable. This evaluation might stem from a global negative attitude toward emotion (Allen & Hamsher, 1974; Joseph, Williams, Irwing, & Cammock, 1994) or more specific beliefs such as "It is dangerous to express anger" or "People in good marriages don't get mad at each other."

The implications for well-being of this form of value-based nonexpression are not clear cut. Because these individuals are aware of their feelings, they could conceivably deal with them adaptively, even if they don't openly express them. Clinically, we believe it is very important to respect clients' individual values. A conviction concerning the importance of nonexpression may be part of a client's highly valued cultural or personal belief system, like it was for the unemployed man described at the beginning of this chapter. However, sometimes an individual's goals or beliefs concerning emotional behavior can be problematic, such as when they are impossibly difficult or require so much effort that they interfere with functioning in other areas. Expressive goals and beliefs can also be problematic when they are contradictory, creating a distressing sense of ambivalence and inner conflict (King & Emmons, 1990). In these cases, it may be important to help clients reexamine and perhaps alter their beliefs concerning emotional behavior.

Disruption at Step 5: Perceived Lack of Opportunity to Express

Marla might be fully aware of her feelings and consider her experience valid, but she might refrain from expressing if she is afraid other people will respond negatively. Like most of the other potential impediments to expression, this belief can range from being situationally specific (e.g., she expects her mother-in-law to ring the doorbell any minute) to more global (e.g., she is a very lonely person with no close friends or confidants).

Suppressing due to social context is not necessarily a bad thing. Under plenty of circumstances the best thing to do is to refrain from showing any distress: in a meeting with the boss, at a party, on a first date. In fact, the inability to modulate emotional behavior can be problematic. However, having a confidant and social support are critically important to well-being (G. W. Brown & Harris, 1978; Cohen & Wills, 1985; Sarason, Sarason, & Pierce, 1990; Wills, 1990). So, we would expect this type of nonexpression to be maladaptive when it involves not just suppression in a particular context, but a general lack of close relationships that permit emotional sharing, such as the case of the lonely teenager with divorced parents that we described earlier. This type of suppression is especially likely to be troublesome when it is coupled with a strong desire to express (Pennebaker, 1992; Tait & Silver, 1989).

For simplicity, the model presents expression and nonexpression as mutually exclusive alternatives. However, expression and nonexpression are relative rather than absolute terms. There is no such thing as complete expression or complete nonexpression. No one can ever communicate every subtle nuance of his or her emotional experience to another person. This is partly due to limitations of language and other expressive gestures, and partly due to the fact that experience is dynamic. Expressing experience changes that experience (e.g., J. C. Watson & Greenberg, 1996). Similarly, nonexpression is never complete. The different forms of nonexpression described above refer to restricted or attenuated expression rather than a complete absence of overt signs of emotion. For example, the lonely teenager who believes that his context disallows expression might still show subtle nonverbal signs of emotion. Emotional behavior is a continuum, with the degree of expression or nonexpression depending (in some way) on the strength of the precipitating stimulus and the prominence of the various individual and situational factors that can impede expression.

Summary

The model we have presented describes the process of emotional expression and how disruptions in this process can lead to nonexpression. This process begins with an individual's prereflective reaction to an emotionally relevant stimulus. The individual then becomes aware of this reaction, labels it as emotional, and evaluates the response as appropriate with respect to his or her own values and the perceived social context. Then, finally, the covert experience is translated into overt expressive behavior. Each of these steps can be interrupted by characteristics of the individual or the situational context, resulting in different forms of nonexpression. Specifically, nonexpression may stem from minimal reaction, motivated lack of awareness, skill deficits in emotional processing, or deliberate suppression due to personal values or perceptions of the social context.

The model provides a systematic way of thinking about expression and nonexpression that can help clinicians understand their clients' difficulties with emotional behavior and identify ways of addressing these difficulties in therapy. For example, clients whose nonexpression stems from lack of understanding of experience and clients whose nonexpression stems from lack of acceptance of experience would require very different clinical approaches. In the case of lack of understanding, it might be important to help clients focus closely on their experience, so that they can learn to recognize their own bodily and expressive cues and to differentiate and symbolize their feelings (see discussions by Gendlin, 1981; L. S. Greenberg,

Rice, & Elliott, 1993). In the case of lack of acceptance of experience, charging full-speed ahead, dealing directly with emotional experience might be alarming or threatening to clients, so a more gradual approach may be necessary. It may be important to talk about the meaning of expression and experience for that particular client, before he or she can feel safe enough to reveal any feelings to the therapist.

KEY THEMES CONCERNING EMOTIONAL BEHAVIOR

The process model also highlights some important themes concerning emotional expression. Specifically, it illustrates the distinction among the components of emotion, the continuum of expressive awareness and control, the interplay between cognition and emotion, and the importance of the social context. These themes are critical for understanding the relationship between emotional behavior and well-being, and they are emphasized throughout this book. Each of these themes is described below.

Distinction among Components of Emotion

One theme that the model highlights is the distinction among four components of emotion: arousal, experience, reflection, and expression. *Arousal* is the physiological response, which begins in Step 1 of the model, with the initial prereflective reaction. *Experience* is the phenomenological, felt sense, which begins in Step 2, with the conscious perception of response. *Reflection* involves thoughts pertaining to emotion. These thoughts involve monitoring experience, expression, and arousal; making sense of them; and evaluating them (cf. L. S. Greenberg et al., 1993; Kennedy-Moore, 1999; Mayer & Gaschke, 1988; Salovey, Mayer, Goldman, Turvey, & Palfai, 1995; J. C. Watson & Greenberg, 1996a). In the model, reflection is represented by the cognitive-evaluative steps, Steps 3, 4, and 5. Finally, *expression* is the observable behavior component of emotion, which occurs either automatically in response to arousal or more deliberately, after the cognitive processing described by the model.

The four components of emotion do not necessarily correspond. For example, someone might be emotionally aroused without realizing it (high arousal–low experience), express without wanting to (high expression–negative reflection), or exaggerate about a minor degree of experience (high expression–low experience). Assessing all four components of emotion is essential for distinguishing among the different forms of nonexpression, and, more generally, for fully understanding clients' emotional responses. Lack of concordance among the different components can have important clinical implications. For example, Rachman and Hodgson (1974) found that, following treatment, agoraphobics who reported minimal fear on a questionnaire but still reacted physiologically to exposure (low experience–high arousal) were more likely to relapse than those who showed little fear on both questionnaire and physiological measures (low experience–low arousal).

Continuum of Expressive Awareness and Control

Another theme illustrated by the model is the continuum of expressive awareness and control. Expressive behavior ranges from primitive, automatic reactions to deliberate communications. Many theorists have emphasized this distinction between spontaneous and controllable expression, with the former being more innate and the latter being more subject to social learning (e.g., Buck, 1989). In the process model depicted in Figure 1.1, the spontaneous expression is depicted by the downward arrow on the left, stemming from the initial prereflective reaction, whereas the more deliberate expression flows from the various cognitive processing steps. However, the model depicts these two pathways to expression as ending up in the same place, and for the purpose of examining the relationship between expression and well-being, we consider the more primitive and more elaborate forms of expression together. This merging is unconventional. Usually researchers and theorists who talk about the more spontaneous, nonverbal forms of expression don't talk about the deliberate verbal forms and vice versa. Certainly each form has unique characteristics. They also have different neurological underpinnings (e.g., Ekman, 1977; LeDoux, 1989, 1996; Leventhal, 1984; Rinn, 1991). However, we believe linking these forms of expression is important for several reasons.

One reason for addressing these two types of expression together rather than separately is that they are sometimes hard to differentiate. While it is easy to distinguish between extremes such as "I blinked in fear without realizing it" and "I drove over to my friend's house and spent an hour talking over my feelings," many instances of expression are not so easily categorized as controllable or uncontrollable. What about, "I yelled at my daughter when she spilled her oatmeal. I hate doing that, but I couldn't help it. I was tired, and I just lost my cool"? Or how about, "Leslie and I just started laughing in the middle of the meeting. I have no idea why. There wasn't even anything funny. I'm sure everyone thought we were nuts. We just looked at each other, and suddenly we couldn't stop laughing"? Or even, "I wanted to tell him how angry I felt, and what a jerk he had been, but I burst into tears. Inside, I was fuming, but all I did was cry and beg him not to leave"? These examples are instances of expression that occupy some middle ground between completely controllable and completely uncontrollable (cf. Zivin, 1982). In the model, they correspond to the dotted lines coming out of each cognitive-evaluative step. They are more complex expressions than the primitive nonverbal signs accompany-

ing the initial prereflective reaction. Some further degree of cognitive processing has occurred. Yet, none of these is completely volitional, which
suggests that the strength of affective responses can sometimes override
conscious plans concerning expressive behavior.

Another reason for merging these two types of expression is that they
can serve the same functions. For example, one important function of emotional expression is social communication. This function can occur whether
expression is verbal or nonverbal, spontaneous or deliberate. A wife might
recognize and respond to her husband's anger whether he shows it through
narrowed eyes and a tightened jaw or he tells her in words. Another key
function of expression is enhancing self-understanding. Again, this function
can be served through either form of expression. A man might gain insight
into his feelings by noticing that his hands are shaking or by pouring out
his heart in a diary.

Furthermore, clinically, it is important to consider both the more and
the less deliberate forms of expression. Drawing attention to clients' spontaneous expressive signs might be a way of helping them to become more
aware of their feelings or to understand the possible impact of their nonverbal communication on other people. Focusing on the more deliberate forms
of expression can be a direct way of enhancing clients' self-understanding
or interpersonal communication.

Interplay between Cognition and Emotion

The model also illustrates the interplay between cognition and emotion.
Each step in the process of expression represents further cognitive elaboration of affective experience. Emotional experience evolves from raw affect,
to specific emotions, to meaning-laden feelings. This cognitive elaboration
is guided by felt experience and also transforms that experience, in a dialectical process (J. C. Watson & Greenberg, 1996a).

There has been quite a bit of debate concerning whether affect or cognition are primary in emotion (e.g., R. S. Lazarus, 1984; Zajonc, 1984). It
is clear that affect precedes deliberate, conscious thought (i.e., intentional
thought that occurs within awareness). It is less clear whether it precedes
preconscious thought (i.e., nondeliberate thought that occurs very rapidly,
outside awareness). Davidson and Ekman (1994) argue that the general
consensus among emotion theorists is that at least some minimal cognitive
processing, involving very basic sensory information processing, is a prerequisite for the elicitation of most, if not all, affect. Less consensus exists
about whether cognitive appraisals precede affect. Appraisals are judgments about the significance of a particular event or stimulus. They can be
conscious or preconscious. Traditional cognitive theorists (e.g., R. S. Lazarus, 1995) see appraisals as necessary for eliciting emotion, with particular
appraisals corresponding to particular emotions. For example, the ap-

praisal of threat is associated with the experience of fear; the appraisal of loss is associated with the experience of sadness. However, some changes in affective state are difficult to explain in terms of appraisal. For example, what kind of appraisal would be involved when an affective state is induced through music (Ellsworth, 1994)? S. Epstein (1990, 1994) argues that affect can arise through either of two systems: The experiential system processes information rapidly and wholistically. The rational system processes information more slowly, in a more differentiated way. Both systems can operate simultaneously and can influence the other. (See LeDoux, 1994, 1996, for a description of the anatomy underlying cognitive versus emotional information processing and their interconnections.)

In terms of understanding the relationship between expression and well-being, the interplay between affect and cognition is far more important than which component is primary. The model breaks down this interplay into successive stages so that therapists can understand and facilitate combined cognitive-emotional processing.

Importance of the Social Context

The model also points to the importance of the social context of emotional behavior. Interpersonal considerations come into play at three points in the process of expression. First, social interactions may precipitate expression by evoking an emotional reaction. Emotional experiences usually arise in a social context, especially within intimate relationships (M. S. Clark & Reis, 1988; J. C. Schwartz & Shaver, 1987). Second, the social context can determine opportunities for expression (Step 5 of the model). As we described earlier, the availability and quality of interpersonal relationships influences the extent to which people are able to communicate their feelings. Third, responses of other people can be an important consequence of expression. This may involve overt support or rejection of the expresser by other people. Additionally, Fridlund (1992) argues that even emotional expression that takes place in solitude involves implicit or imagined audiences. He sees the self as a role-player in an internalized society, and solitary expression as a means of controlling images projected during imagined social interactions. Clinically, social influences on expression, involving elicitation, opportunity, and consequences, need to be considered in order to get a full understanding of a client's emotional behavior.

OVERVIEW OF THE BOOK

In this chapter, we argued that emotional expression and nonexpression can take many different forms and have many different consequences. We presented our process model as a conceptual framework for understanding the varieties of emotional behavior. We also outlined a number of key themes concerning expression. Our goals for the remainder of the book are to clarify the circumstances under which expression and nonexpression are adaptive or maladaptive, to delineate key mechanisms linking expression or nonexpression to adaptational outcomes, and to spell out the implications of these distinctions for clinical assessment and treatment. The book is divided into three main sections: Intrapersonal Processes, Interpersonal Processes, and Treatment Implications. Each section explains and develops aspects of the process model of emotional expression.

The chapters in the Intrapersonal Processes section trace the beginning stages of the process of emotional expression, as emotional experience is initially evoked, recognized, understood, and evaluated. These chapters point to important functions of expression and nonexpression for an individual. Emotional behavior plays a key role in modulating arousal, providing information about the impact of one's environment, and creating a coherent sense of self. These chapters examine both adaptive and maladaptive instances of emotional behavior.

The chapters in the Interpersonal Processes section concern the social context of emotional expression and nonexpression. They describe patterns of emotional behavior involving reciprocal influence between parent and child and within adult couples. These chapters emphasize the interpersonal functions of emotional behavior, which include developing intimacy and eliciting social support. They also describe ways that emotional behavior can lead to problems in interpersonal relationships.

Chapters in the Treatment Implications section spell out the relationships between emotional behavior, psychopathology, and psychotherapy process. Drawing upon the individual and interpersonal issues concerning emotional behavior identified in the earlier sections, the Treatment Implications chapters examine the role of expression and nonexpression in the development and remediation of several clinical problems: depression, trauma, marital distress, and psychosomatic illness. These particular problems are discussed because difficulties involving emotional behavior are often central to their symptomatology. The Treatment Implications chapters conceptualize these clinical problems in terms of our model, and they point to ways that therapists can facilitate clients' emotional functioning. The overarching theme in this section of the book is cultivating authentic expression of emotion in a way that promotes self-understanding and enhances interpersonal relationships.

PART II

Intrapersonal Processes

2

The Myth of Emotional Venting

INTRODUCTION

The Venting Hypothesis

Hydraulic models of emotion suggest that people are like boiling pots: When negative emotions get hot, it's important to let off some steam, through expression. Otherwise, emotions will spill out in the form of physical or psychological symptoms (see historical reviews by Gross, 1998; Kosmicki & Glickauf-Hughes, 1997; Nichols & Efran, 1985; Straton, 1990). We will refer to the idea that expression diffuses negative emotional experience and/or distress-related physiological arousal as "the venting hypothesis."

The venting hypothesis suggests several corollaries:

1. *The "bigger" the expression of distress the better.* If expression allows one to let off negative emotional steam, then presumably more vigorous or more intense expression lets off more steam, more quickly.
2. *The beneficial effects of distress expression are immediate.* If the function of expression is ventilation, then we should see drops in emotional experience and physiological arousal either during or immediately following expression.
3. *The effects of distress expression are direct.* The venting hypothesis suggests that expression directly influences experience and arousal, rather than operating indirectly through cognitive or interpersonal mechanisms.

The venting hypothesis has inspired a variety of clinical interventions within psychodynamic, experiential, and behavioral therapeutic orientations (see review by Nichols & Efran, 1985). In daily life, this hypothesis leads some couples to justify and even pride themselves on their intense, no-holds-barred arguments. It also leads some parents to encourage their children to yell or beat pillows in order to "get their feelings out of their system."

Unfortunately, it's not that simple.

As we describe below, expression sometimes reflects emotional experience and/or physiological arousal, sometimes changes independently of them, sometimes intensifies them, and sometimes diffuses them. Whereas the venting hypothesis emphasizes the quantity of expression, our review of the literature suggests that it is the quality of expression that determines whether or not it is beneficial. *Expression of negative feelings is adaptive to the extent that it leads to some kind of resolution of distress.*

In this chapter, we consider when and how emotional expression influences emotional experience and physiological arousal. As background to our discussion, we first discuss where expression fits within the rubric of emotional responses by briefly describing the components of emotion. We discuss what we call the paradox of distress expression: that expression of negative feelings is both a sign of distress and a possible means of coping with that distress. We then describe research and theory concerning the impact of expression of negative emotions, focusing on anger expression, crying, and coping with traumatic experiences. We conclude this chapter by outlining some alternatives to the venting hypothesis.

Components of Emotion

Emotion theorists generally agree that emotional responses are not unitary phenomena, but rather are composed of several, partially independent components or response modalities (e.g., Buck, 1988; Leventhal, 1984, 1991). Figure 2.1 depicts our understanding of these components and their interrelationships.[1] The three main components of emotion, represented by circles, are: *expression,* which refers to observable emotional behaviors; *experience,* which refers to subjective, felt responses; and *arousal,* which refers to physiological responses.[2]

There is ample evidence that these three components of emotion do not necessarily correspond (e.g., Izard, 1992; Lacey, 1956; Lang, Levin, Miller, & Kozak, 1983). A particular individual at a particular moment might be reactive with respect to one component but not another. A clinical example of this comes from Rachman and Hodgson's (1974) work showing that phobic clients' physiological responses, fear behaviors, and subjective experience of fear don't necessarily match. These three components also tend to show different patterns of change over time in response to exposure therapy.

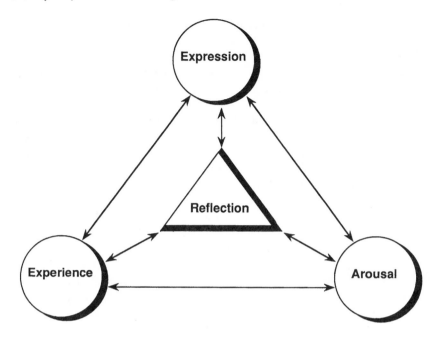

FIGURE 2.1. Components of emotion.

Laboratory studies also provide numerous findings indicating that the components of emotion are not isomorphic. For instance:

A given level of a physiological arousal is associated with different levels of experience for different individuals (arousal–experience discrepancy: Blascovich, 1992; Katkin, 1984).

Facial expressions tend to be more muted when an unfamiliar observer is present than when people are alone (expression–experience discrepancy: Ekman, 1972, see also Matsumoto, 1993).

Some people's emotional experience is more closely linked to their facial expressions, whereas other people's experience is more closely related to their physiological responses (predominance of experience–arousal link vs. experience–expression link: Lang, 1994; Pennebaker & Roberts, 1992).

These findings indicate that both individual and situational characteristics can affect the extent to which expression, experience, and arousal match. Frijda, Ortony, Sonnemans, and Clore (1992) argue that the loose correspondence among the components of emotion suggests that each component has its own particular determinants and that no single component is more fundamental to or representative of emotional responses than any other component.

In addition to the three main components of emotion, a number of theorists add a fourth component that we will call *reflection* (depicted by a triangle in Figure 2.1). Reflection refers to thoughts about one's own emotional responses (see related discussions of "emotional significance" by Frijda, 1993; "meta-emotion" by Gottman, Katz, & Hooven, 1996a, 1996b; "meta-mood" and "meta-experience" by Mayer & Gashke, 1988; Salovey et al., 1995). It involves interpretation and evaluation of expression, experience, and arousal. It includes general beliefs and values, such as "Crying is unmanly" or "It's important to let one's feelings out," as well as situationally specific evaluations, such as "I have every right to feel angry because of what he did" or "I'm overreacting." It also includes beliefs about the causes and controllability of emotional responses (cf. Kennedy-Moore, 1999; Kirsch, Mearns, & Catanzaro, 1990). Reflection can be considered a secondary component of emotion because it comes into play *after* the initial evocation of expression, experience, and/or arousal.[3] Reflection can sometimes heighten distress, leading to emotion about emotion. For example, interpreting one's own expression of anger as dangerous can lead to anxiety. Seeing one's experience of fear as cowardly can evoke shame. Reflection can also diminish distress, such as when intense feelings of sadness are accepted as painful, but understandable and tolerable.

In terms of the components of emotion, the venting hypothesis posits a tradeoff between expression and experience and/or arousal. It does not distinguish clearly between experience and arousal, nor does it recognize different types of arousal. It also makes no mention of the reflection component.

The Paradox of Distress Expression

In emphasizing the importance of "letting out" one's negative feelings, the venting hypothesis overlooks an important paradox: *Expression of negative feelings is both a sign of distress and a possible means of coping with that distress.* The venting hypothesis concerns the role of expression as a coping strategy but ignores its role as a sign of distress. Evidence for the paradox of distress expression comes from research on facial expression, personality and coping, and disclosure in psychotherapy.

Facial Expression

Consistent with the venting hypothesis, Jones (1950, 1960) observed an inverse relationship between people's overt facial expressiveness and their covert autonomic responses. He distinguishes between *internalizers*, who show minimal facial expressions but marked electrodermal responses, and *externalizers,* who are very expressive but show minimal electrodermal response.[4]

Jones speculates that socialization is responsible for creating internalizers and externalizers. He states that infants "naturally" externalize their affective reactions and that they have high thresholds for electrodermal responses compared to older children. Jones argues that as children get older, their overt expressions of distress are apt to elicit disapproval or even punishment rather than succorance, so they learn to "discharge" their emotions along internal channels. He suggests that children who receive especially strong messages to inhibit overt expression become internalizers, whereas those who receive weak socialization along these lines retain the "somewhat infantile pattern" of externalizers (Jones, 1950, p. 163).

Jones's finding of an inverse relationship between facial expression and autonomic responses has been replicated by other investigators looking at a *between-people* level of comparison (e.g., Lanzetta & Kleck, 1970; Notarius & Levenson, 1979): More facially expressive people tend to have autonomic responses that are smaller than those of less facially expressive people. Why this pattern occurs is not clear (see Manstead, 1991, for a discussion of several possible explanations), but these results are consistent with the idea of expression as a coping strategy. Perhaps more expressive people are more comfortable with emotions. Perhaps less expressive people are aroused because of the strain of holding in their feelings. However, Cacioppo and his colleagues (Cacioppo et al., 1992) insist that this inverse association at a between-people level of comparison doesn't necessarily imply the tradeoff between expression and arousal posited by the venting hypothesis. He suggests that different individuals may have differential gain across the different components of emotion. In terms of physical health, the most problematic response pattern involves overly large emotional arousal responses. In this case, Cacioppo et al. suggest it probably makes more sense to deal directly with these individuals' level of physiological responsiveness rather than to urge them to express their feelings.[5]

When we look at a *within-person* level of comparison, laboratory studies reliably find a positive association between facial expression and arousal or experience: When a particular person expresses more distress, he or she also shows higher levels of arousal and greater experience of distress (Buck, 1980; Cacioppo et al., 1992). This directly contradicts the venting hypothesis. Instead, it is consistent with the notion of expression as a sign of distress.

Personality and Coping

Evidence for the paradox of distress expression also comes from research on personality and coping. Gross (1998; Gross & John, 1997) points out that individual differences in expressivity stem from two major determinants: (1) the initial activation of emotional response tendencies and (2) the subsequent modulation of emotional response tendencies. This distinction between emotional activation versus modulation is supported by personality research involving both self-ratings and peer ratings. It suggests that people might be very expressive because they tend to have strong emotional responses to emotional stimuli *or* because they generally express their feelings vigorously. Similarly, people might be very inexpressive because they have a high threshold for distress elicitation *or* because they tend to inhibit their expression.

Personality traits that concern individual differences in emotional modulation emphasize the role of expression as a coping strategy. Examples of these traits include Rationality and Antiemotionality (Grossarth-Maticek, Bastiaans, & Kanazir, 1985; see discussions by Eysenck, 1991a, 1991b), Emotional Control (D. Rogers & Jamieson, 1988; D. Rogers & Nesshoever, 1987), and Self-Concealment (D. Larsen & Chastain, 1990). Consistent with the venting hypothesis, research with these personality traits shows the benefits of expression or the costs of holding in one's feelings.

On the other hand, personality traits that concern individual differences in emotional activation point to the role of expression as a sign of distress. People who express a lot because they have a low threshold for the elicitation of distress tend to be worse off than their more sanguine peers. A key example of this comes from research on Negative Affectivity (NA), which involves a disposition to experience unpleasant emotional states. Daily life experience points to the existence of especially fussy babies and particularly moody adults, and research on temperament and personality bears out this observation. Researchers of infant temperament distinguish between babies who easily become intensely upset compared to more emotionally stable babies who are less distressed by ordinary experiences (e.g., A. H. Buss & Plomin, 1984; Rothbart, 1994). Numerous studies have identified NA as a basic dimension of adult personality involving distress proneness (e.g., Eysenck & Eysenck, 1985; Tellegen, 1985; Costa & McCrae, 1988; Zuckerman, 1995). Although there is some short-term variability in NA, it is generally a stable disposition, even over periods as long as 20 years ($r = .50$; Schuerger, Zarrella, & Hotz, 1989).

High-NA individuals have a propensity to feel a wide variety of negative moods, including anxiety, frustration, sadness, irritability, and anger, even in the absence of obvious stressors (see L. A. Clark & Watson, 1991; D. Watson & Clark, 1984; D. Watson, in press, for reviews). These individuals seem to see the world and themselves through a negative microscope, which heightens their sensitivity to negative information and leads them to perceive situations as stressful, even when other people might not regard these situations as threatening. They are especially sensitive to the ordinary frustrations and irritations of everyday life, and they are more likely than low-NA individuals to respond to these hassles with greater and more enduring distress. High-NA individuals tend to dwell on their personal flaws and failures, as well as negative aspects of other people and the world in general.

Because they tend to experience a great deal of distress, high-NA individuals also tend to express a great deal of distress. Interpersonally, they often behave in hostile and demanding ways, and they report experiencing more social conflict (L. A. Clark & Watson, 1991). Other people find high-NA individuals to be difficult or even unpleasant company. Probably because they are preoccupied with their own distress, high-NA individuals tend to be less attentive and responsive to others (Cegala, Savage, Brunner, & Conrad, 1982). Their propensity to express many negative feelings and few positive or friendly ones tends to evoke negative reactions from others (cf. Segrin, 1998).

In terms of well-being, by definition NA is associated with psychological distress. There is some controversy as to whether or not it is also linked to physical illness (see H. S. Friedman, 1990, 1991; D. Watson & Pennebaker, 1989). Therapeutically, the relevant goal for high-NA clients is not to have them vent their negative feelings (they do plenty of that on their own), but rather to address their propensity to feel distress in the first place.

Gross's distinction between emotional activation versus modulation also suggests that there are two broad categories of strategies for coping with distress (Gross, 1998; Gross & Muñoz, 1995): *Antecedent-focused* strategies address emotion-eliciting cues, in order to influence the extent to which emotional responses are triggered. Such strategies include situation selection (i.e., seeking out or avoiding certain people or circumstances), situation modification, attention deployment, and reappraisal of either the situation or one's coping resources. In general, antecedent-focused strategies involve reducing the occurrence of expression as a sign of distress. *Response-focused* strategies involve modification of emotional response tendencies after the emotion has been generated. These strategies involve intensifying or diminishing ongoing emotional expression, experience, or physiological responding. Antecedent- and response-focused coping strategies may have different consequences. A study by Gross (1998) compared the effects of volunteers' use of cognitive reappraisal versus emotional suppression while watching a disgusting film. Compared to a neutral condition, both coping strategies led to reduced expressive behavior, but they had different effects on the other components of emotion: Reappraisal, which is an antecedent-focused strategy, was associated with reduced experience of disgust, whereas suppression, which is a response-focused strategy, was associated with increased sympathetic activation (as measured by skin conductance, finger temperature, and finger pulse amplitude).

In the context of Gross's model of emotion regulation, it is clear that the venting hypothesis says nothing at all about antecedent-focused strategies and provides a very narrow perspective on response-focused strategies (i.e., that expression is always good and more expression is better).

Disclosure in Psychotherapy

A third line of evidence for the paradox of distress disclosure comes from clinical research. Stiles (1987, 1995) describes a "fever model" of disclosure in psychotherapy. He defines disclosure as first-person statements concerning subjective information (e.g., "I think ...," "I feel ... "). By this definition, disclosure includes verbal forms of expression, but also includes other statements, such as thoughts or wishes. Stiles argues that, like a fever in physical illness, disclosure is associated with both illness and recovery. On the one hand, Stiles cites a number of correlational studies showing that people who are experiencing a great deal of distress, such as anxious or depressed clients, tend to disclose a great deal. On the other hand, he notes that therapists tend to rate high levels of client disclosure as evidence of good therapeutic process. Stiles argues that psychotherapy outcome studies do not show clear benefits of disclosure because process–outcome correlations muddle disclosure as a sign of distress versus disclosure as a means of recovery. More distressed clients disclose more. More distressed clients, on average, have worse psychotherapy outcomes. Yet, by disclosing, clients may be using therapy effectively to process and assimilate their experience. Stiles suggests that disclosure may positively predict movement toward health, rather than absolute levels of well-being.

Thus, research on facial expression, personality and coping, and psychotherapy all point to the fact that expression of negative feelings is both a sign of distress and a possible means of coping with distress. The issue is, when and how does expression help to alleviate distress?

We turn now to three specific instances of distress expression that have been linked to the venting hypothesis: expression of anger, crying, and expression of trauma-related feelings. Research and theory in these areas not only refute a simplistic view of the universal benefits of venting emotions, they also point to some alternative views concerning how expression can be useful in resolving distress. These views consider qualitative as well as quantitative aspects of distress expression, and they place expression within an intrapersonal and interpersonal context.

EXPRESSION OF ANGER

Albert glanced at his watch. He was late for his appointment. The driver in front of him was driving 5 miles below the speed limit and slowing down at each intersection to look for street signs. "Come on! Come on!" Albert muttered. He gritted his teeth and flashed the headlights. The driver in front ignored him. It was a wide road, but a steady stream of oncoming traffic prevented Albert from passing. "Pull over, you idiot!" Albert snarled. He pounded on the horn. The driver in front glanced in the rearview mirror, but did not speed up or pull over. Finally, there was a break in the oncoming traffic. Albert roared past the other driver, giving him the finger.

In the scenario above, Albert is clearly furious at the slow-moving driver. He expresses his anger vividly through his words and his actions. The venting hypothesis predicts that such expression should allow Albert to get his anger "out of his system." Yet, this expression doesn't seem to help. Albert doesn't just express his anger once and then drop it. Instead his expression escalates as he becomes increasingly enraged. Even in this simple anecdote, it is apparent that expression of anger doesn't always bring relief.

Intuitively, the ability to express anger clearly to offending others seems like an important life skill. Anger expression entails a basic "Don't tread on me" message. As Tice and Baumeister (1993) point out, people who fail to express their anger may find that their problems recur. With no information concerning the problem, offenders are likely to repeat the provoking action. The offended parties become increasingly angry, not because their anger builds up, but because they accumulate a list of grievances with each repeated offense. They may end up having a strong outburst of anger expression in response to multiple provocations, whereas the offenders may perceive this as overreacting to a single incident (Baumeister, Stillwell, & Wotman, 1990). It seems plausible that a constructive expression of anger early on might prevent this escalation of anger.

Beliefs in the benefits of anger expression are widespread. In a survey of a random sample of American families, Steinmetz (1977) found that, consistent with the venting hypothesis, many people believe that "letting out" anger is beneficial. They believe that siblings should "fight it out" and that screaming matches between spouses or between parent and child are normal and healthy. Many clinicians also believe that clients' expression of intense anger is therapeutic, especially if that anger has "built up" over time (Biaggio, 1987; E. J. Murray, 1985).

However, research on anger expression has been hard-pressed to find any positive effects of venting anger. For instance, Berkowitz (1970, 1983) showed through a series of laboratory studies that intense verbal and physical expression of anger, rather than "draining" anger, actually reduces the threshold for subsequent aggression. Similarly, Tavris (1984, 1989) argues on the basis of her literature review that frequent and intense expression of anger tends to create an angry habit, rile up one's opposition, and in many cases make people more angry rather than less angry. She notes that research consistently shows that in sports, child rearing, marital arguments, and tantrums (by children or adults), intense expression of anger does *not* drain emotion but rather intensifies and perpetuates it and stimulates both the expresser and the target of expression to continued aggression. Zilbergeld (cited in Tavris, 1984) speculates that after a vicious quarrel, what some couples believe is the catharsis of anger may be just a temporary lull due to exhaustion. Their concerns remain unresolved and their battle is likely to erupt again the next day or the next week, with similar or even greater intensity.

Below, we take a closer look at some of the studies on anger expression. We look at the effects of anger expression on experience, arousal, and interpersonal relationships, in order to infer some guidelines about when and how anger expression is adaptive or maladaptive.

Effects of Anger Expression on Experience

A survey by Tice (1990) suggests that expression may not be the best way to alleviate anger experience and in fact may intensify angry feelings. She asked people about their strategies for controlling or altering their emotional states. Among the strategies mentioned specifically for anger reduction were trying to understand the offenders' actions and motives and reframing the provocation as accidental or justifiable. These anger-reducing strategies all involve antecedent-focused coping, in that they address anger-eliciting cues (cf. Gross, 1998). Albert, the angry driver described earlier, might have benefited from these sorts of strategies. Telling himself, "It's just a meeting. The world won't end if I'm 5 minutes late," or "The driver in front seems to be looking for a particular street. He can't help it if he doesn't know exactly where it is" might have helped Albert to lessen his experience of anger in a way that snarling and pounding on his horn didn't. Interestingly, one of the key strategies that Tice's respondents reported using to sustain their anger was rehearsing their feelings and their perceived cause, especially in the presence of a sympathetic other. This involves using expression as a means of intensifying and prolonging angry feelings.

Consistent with Tice's findings, a classic study by Ebbesen, Duncan, and Konecni (1975) vividly illustrates the role of expression in shaping anger experience. These investigators interviewed laid-off engineers and technicians about their angry feelings. The interviewer subtly directed the focus of the workers' anger expression in one of three directions: toward the company, toward their supervisors, or toward themselves. This was done by asking leading questions, such as "In what ways has the company not been fair with you?", "What action might your supervisor have taken to prevent you from being laid off?", or "Are there things about yourself that led your supervisor not to give you a higher performance review?" To provide a basis of comparison, the investigators also asked some of the laid-off workers neutral, unemotional questions. Results showed that anger expression in the interview did not dissipate feelings of anger. Instead, expressing anger toward the company or toward supervisors *increased* anger toward the specific target discussed, but not toward other targets. Fortunately, expressing anger toward the self did not change anger toward the self or toward the other targets. These results suggest that talking about anger does not get rid of it, but rather identifies it and rehearses it.

However, other research suggests that under some circumstances expression can in fact lead to a reduction in angry feelings. E. J. Murray (1985) describes a series of laboratory experiments showing that the combination of emotional ventilation and cognitive reinterpretation was more effective in reducing subsequent anger and aggression than either ventilation alone or cognitive reinterpretation alone. In one of these studies (Green & Murray, 1975), college students were angered by receiving a derogatory personal critique of themselves that was supposedly written by another student they had just met. Unbeknownst to study participants, this other student was actually the experimenter's assistant. After reading the derogatory critique, study participants received one of three different interventions, involving different anger-coping strategies: In the *expression* condition, the experimenter got participants to express their resentment concerning the derogatory critique. In the *reinterpretation* condition, the experimenter explained that the other student had misunderstood the instructions. He thought he was supposed to write a nasty critique, but he didn't really mean what he said. In the *combination* condition, participants first expressed their feelings and then heard the "it was just a misunderstanding" explanation. In addition to these three intervention conditions, there were also two comparison conditions, one involving no induction of hostility and one involving hostility induction but no intervention. Results showed that only the combination of expression and reinterpretation was effective in reducing later aggression toward the other student. The combination condition also prompted a significantly greater shift to positive feelings toward the experimenter's assistant than the two single-component intervention conditions. In this study, reinterpretation alone was not a very powerful way to reduce aggression or angry feelings. The expression-alone condition also did not appreciably decrease aggression, and it left participants feeling even more negative toward the experimenter's assistant than the no-intervention condition.

The anger-provoking incident in Murray's studies is somewhat contrived, but another series of studies by Bohart, involving naturally occurring anger-arousing incidents, also suggests that anger expression is not helpful in and of itself, but it can be adaptive when it leads to or is accompanied by cognitive changes (see Bohart, 1980, for a review). For instance, Bohart (1977) asked college students to recall and mentally rehearse an anger-arousing incident, in order to induce feelings of anger. Study participants were then given one of four sets of instructions: *Intellectual-Analysis* participants were told to "coldly and rationally analyze" events, motives, and feelings pertaining to the event; *Discharge* participants were told to verbally express their angry feelings as if the person who angered them was in the room; *Role-Play* participants were told to switch chairs as they conducted a dialogue expressing both their own feelings and the feelings of the person who angered them; and, to provide a comparison for the other groups, *Detail* participants were asked to recall physical details of the incident. Self-report measures of angry feelings were taken before and after the intervention. Additionally, as a measure of behavioral aggression, participants were told to choose a level of aversive noise with which to "punish" a person in another room who supposedly made errors on a learning task.

These interventions lasted only a few minutes, but they produced notable group difference. Discharge participants showed *increases* in anger and hostile attitudes. Thus, rather than venting angry feelings, the discharge condition actually intensified it. In contrast, Role-Play participants showed reductions in anger, hostile attitudes, and behavioral aggression. On the basis of this and other similar analogue studies, Bohart (1980) argues that the combination of emotional expression and insight is more helpful than simple venting of emotion. He suggests that anger expression merely sets the stage for resolving a conflict situation. He argues that anger expression is helpful only if it leads to positive cognitive or interpersonal changes such as compromise, reinterpretation, or restoration of self-esteem.

Both Murray's and Bohart's studies can be criticized because they involved students rather than therapy clients and because the interventions were brief. However, similar results were obtained in a clinical study of processes and outcomes in encounter groups by Lieberman, Yalom, and Miles (1973). Seventeen groups, based on a variety of therapeutic approaches, each met for 30 hours. Outcome measures included ratings by participants themselves, other group members, group leaders, and friends of group members. Many of the groups in this study emphasized the therapeutic importance of venting intense emotions, including anger. Results suggested that expression of emotion alone was not therapeutic, but expression accompanied by some cognitive process was helpful. The groups focusing on expression of intense emotions were *not* more successful than other groups. To the investigators' surprise, higher levels of anger expression in the encounter groups were associated with *poorer* outcomes.

As we mentioned in our discussion of the components of emotion, expression, experience, and arousal don't necessarily correspond in terms of either absolute level or patterns of change. So, we can't assume that strategies that reduce anger experience also reduce anger-related arousal or vice versa (cf. Gross, 1998; Gross & Levenson, 1993, 1997). We turn now to look at the effects of anger expression on physiological arousal.

Effects of Anger Expression on Arousal

Research by Siegman and his colleagues shows that expression of anger can produce heightened levels of systolic and diastolic blood pressure—sometimes even to a dangerous extent (see Siegman, 1994, for a review). He and his colleagues note that anger is expressed verbally through loud, rapid, interruptive speech. Siegman's work focuses on the relationship between the expressive quality of speech and cardiovascular reactivity.

In one study, Siegman and his colleagues (Siegman, Anderson, & Berger, 1990) asked undergraduate students to describe neutral and anger-arousing events, using each of three qualitatively different voices: a loud, rapid, angry voice; a normal voice; and a soft, slow, nonangry voice. Comparing descriptions of anger-arousing versus neutral events showed, as expected, that descriptions of anger-arousing events were associated with greater experience of anger and greater cardiovascular reactivity than descriptions of neutral events. However, the cardiovascular differences between descriptions of anger events and neutral events were large when study participants used an angry voice, but trivial when they used a soft, slow, nonangry voice.

Comparing across the three types of description of anger-arousing events, self-ratings of anger experience were highest when study participants used an angry voice, intermediate for a neutral voice, and lowest for a nonangry voice. Physiological responses showed the same pattern: The angry-voice condition for anger events produced the highest levels of heart rate (HR), systolic blood pressure (SBP), and diastolic blood pressure (DBP). The neutral-voice condition produced an intermediate level of cardiovascular reactivity, and the nonangry-voice condition yielded the lowest level of reactivity. The magnitude of these differences was substantial. The angry-voice condition for anger events was associated with levels of reactivity that Siegman et al. (1990) believe are sufficient to be potential risk factors for coronary disease. For instance, discussing anger-related events in an angry voice yielded an average blood pressure reading of 138/79 in these young, healthy undergraduates, whereas the neutral-voice condition yielded an average reading of 126/72, and the nonangry-voice condition yielded an average reading of only 120/65. Some participants showed blood pressure elevations as high as 25 millimeters of mercury (mm Hg) in SBP and 30 mm Hg in DBP between the neutral- and the angry-voice descriptions of anger-arousing events.

The study by Siegman et al. (1990) involved college students, but comparable results emerged in intervention studies involving clinical populations. Two studies with patients with coronary heart disease and patients in an intensive cardiac care unit indicate that teaching patients to speak softly and slowly when they are angry reduces their level of cardiovascular reactivity as well as their feelings of distress (Siegman, 1992, 1993).

On the basis of these studies, Siegman (1994) concludes that only the *expression* of anger, not the mere *experience* of anger, is associated with meaningful elevations in blood pressure and intensified experience of anger. He considers talking about angry feelings in an angry voice to involve both expression and experience whereas talking about angry feelings in a normal or soft voice involves experience of anger without expression.

However, another way of interpreting Siegman's findings is to consider that talking about angry feelings in *any* voice is expression. In that case, rather than concluding that the expression of anger elevates blood pressure and intensifies experience, we would conclude that *different forms of anger expression have different consequences*: Very intense anger expression (i.e., the angry-voice condition) intensifies arousal and experience; moderated anger expression (i.e., the nonangry-voice condition) produces milder arousal and experience than either intense or normal expression. Unfortunately, because Siegman's studies contain no control condition in which participants think about anger-arousing events without expressing in any way, we can't tell whether moderated expression results in greater or lesser experience and arousal than nonexpression.

Effects of Anger Experience and Arousal on Expression

We've been talking about the impact of anger expression on experience and arousal, but it is essential to recognize that these relationships are bidirectional. Not only does anger expression influence experience and arousal, but the intensity of anger experience and arousal influences the ability to modulate expressive behavior. At high levels of anger experience and arousal, people may find it difficult to control when and how they express their feelings. They may find themselves blurting out angry statements they later regret or expressing their anger in ways or at times that they would otherwise consider inappropriate. In terms of the process model of expression presented in Chapter 1, this type of expression entails emotional leakage.

D. G. Gilbert (1991) points out that effective communication and conflict resolution are most likely to occur when participants are at intermediate levels of arousal. At high levels of physiological arousal, people can't think straight. They are less able to effectively process external stimuli, because they are focused on their own experience. Their behavior tends to be impulsive and extreme, focused on immediate relief rather than long-term consequences. Zillmann (1993) notes that anger-reducing cognitive strategies, such as reappraisal, only work at moderate levels of anger experience and arousal. Once people become enraged, laboratory studies show that they are apt to ignore or dismiss mitigating information. Drawing upon LeDoux's physiological research with rats (e.g., LeDoux, 1989, 1996), Goleman (1995) coined the term *emotional hijacking* to refer to times when the emotional (limbic) brain takes over control of behavior from the thinking (neocortex) brain. Similarly, Gottman (1993a) talks about *emotional flooding*, which he defines as occurring when heart rate jumps 10 or more beats per minute above a person's resting rate. While flooded, people feel overwhelmed by intense and subjectively uncontrollable feelings of anger and distress. They are unable to organize their thoughts, communicate clearly, or consider another person's point or view. Jacobson and Holtzworth-Monroe (1986) found that even if individuals know effective communication skills, when they are extremely angry, they don't feel like using these skills. All of these researchers and theorists suggest that when people are in the throes of high levels of anger experience and arousal they are more likely to lash out through extreme, impulsive, and maladaptive forms of anger expression.

This may explain why strategies such as counting to 10 or "sleeping on it" before expressing anger can be useful: These strategies allow bodily arousal to decrease and give the individual time to reappraise the anger-arousing situation, perhaps lessening the intensity of the anger experience, thereby enabling the individual to implement effective forms of expression. Along these lines, Harburg, Blakelock, and Roeper (1979) found that across a variety of hypothetical anger-arousing incidents, the coping strategy associated with the lowest blood pressure was neither expression nor suppression, but an intermediate strategy involving cool, delayed expression, in which participants allowed themselves and the other person time to calm down before they discussed matters. Clinically, behavioral anger-management techniques emphasize helping clients to recognize their early signs of anger experience and arousal and working to diffuse these (e.g., through relaxation, distraction, or soothing self-talk) *before* they escalate into rage (e.g., Zillmann, 1993). D. G. Gilbert (1991) also points out that sustaining active attention to something other than one's grievances and focusing on one's partner are effective strategies for reducing physiological arousal. Marital therapists who focus on active listening as an important part of conflict resolution often encourage using this strategy. Active listening may also help diffuse anger by eliciting positive emotional responses such as empathy.

Anger Expression and Interpersonal Relationships

So far we have talked only about the intrapersonal consequences of anger expression. However, the interpersonal consequences are also important in determining when and how anger expression is adaptive. Part of the reason why Albert the angry driver's expression did not diffuse his feelings of anger is that all of his grimacing and snarling and honking was not effective in changing the behavior of the driver in front of him. On the other hand, Albert was lucky that the other driver didn't reciprocate his expression of anger in a more violent way.

As we noted earlier, being able to express anger constructively seems like a necessary skill in negotiating relationships and resolving conflicts. However, sometimes the most adaptive strategy involves refraining from expressing anger toward a partner. Accumulated resentments can be poison to a relationship, but so can constant bickering. Particularly when the anger trigger involves a minor transgression or an isolated incident or when there are mitigating circumstances, the best coping strategy may be to refrain from expressing anger, in the name of love and/or civility. Zilbergeld (quoted in Tavris, 1984, p. 187) remarks, "My clients [in therapy] do not need to learn how to express anger. They need to learn how to shut up. They're ready to express every little irritation and disagreement, but not to express happiness."

When people do express anger toward another person, they are most likely to elicit positive responses when they express their feelings in a way that the other person can accept and understand. Usually, this involves expressing anger in a moderate, rather than an intense, way. Expression makes emotion contagious. In dyadic interactions, partners tend to match each other's loudness level and speech rate (Feldstein & Welkowitz, 1987). So, as Siegman (1994) points out, when one partner starts yelling, the other partner is likely to reciprocate, intensifying both partners' arousal and experience of anger.

However, it is easy to imagine scenarios that might call for more vigorous anger expression. Such scenarios include abusive situations or situations in which multiple polite discussions have proved ineffectual. (See also Tavris, 1984, 1989, regarding cultural differences in anger expression.) We suspect that in terms of interpersonal impact, no one level of intensity of anger expression is universally adaptive. Rather, it is important to be able to adjust one's level of anger expression flexibly according to the interpersonal circumstances.

In addition to intensity, the frequency of anger expression is an important determinant of whether anger expression is effective in an interpersonal context. One correlational study (Keinan, Ben-zur, Zilka, & Carel, 1992) found that the most adaptive anger expression style involved clear but infrequent anger expression. People who constantly "blow their top" are likely to have other people dismiss their angry outbursts, thinking or saying, "There she goes again!" Parents who scream at their children all the time usually find that their children tune them out (Tavris, 1989).

The content of anger expression is also important in determining whether the message gets across. Behaviorally oriented marital therapists teach clients to make anger expressions more palatable to targets by "sandwiching" negative remarks with positive ones, using "I statements," and focusing on specific problematic behaviors rather than general personal inadequacy (e.g., "I feel irritated when you leave your dirty socks in the middle of the floor" rather than "You are a disgusting and completely inconsiderate jerk!").

Based on her review of the literature, Tavris (1984, 1989) suggests a number of conditions under which anger expression can reduce arousal and dissipate feelings of anger. Several of these conditions point to the importance of the interpersonal impact of anger expression:

1. *Anger expression is most likely to be beneficial when it is directed at the appropriate target.* Indirect strategies like punching pillows, kicking the dog, or snarling at an innocent and unsuspecting spouse are not likely to dissipate anger because they do nothing to alter the source of anger.

2. *Anger expression is most likely to be beneficial when it does not lead to further retaliation by the target.* Tavris points out that this condition is rarely met in everyday life because most people don't just stand there when they are the target of angry tirades. Instead, they defend themselves and even counterattack. However, writing an angry letter that is torn up rather than mailed or expressing anger to an absent but imagined target during the gestalt "empty-chair" technique may be useful ways of expressing intense anger toward a relevant target without eliciting retaliation.

3. *Anger expression is most likely to be beneficial when it results in changes in the perceptions of the expresser or the behavior of the target.* Anger expression is helpful when it resolves the source of anger. This occurs when expression results in the clarification of anger-arousing misunderstandings or misperceptions (e.g., "You thought I was ignoring you? I was so preoccupied, I didn't even see you!" or "It was an accident. I would never do that to you deliberately."). Anger expression is also effective when it produces a desired change in the target's behavior ("I had no idea that bothered you so much. I'm so sorry. I'll try very hard not to do that again.").

Summary

To summarize, research on the effects of anger expression does not support the venting hypothesis. In general, more intense anger expression is associated with greater anger experience and arousal. When anger expression helps, it involves some kind of resolution, in the form of new understanding or changes in other people's behavior. In the next section, we look at another form of distress expression that has been linked to the venting hypothesis: crying.

CRYING

They hadn't seen each other in 2 months, but tonight Christopher and Sophie were sitting together at a table in the little corner restaurant where they had gone for their first date. Christopher couldn't remember a specific incident marking the breakup of their relationship. Six months ago, such a long separation would have been unimaginable.

They had been soul mates. But then there had been too much overtime work and too many out-of-town trips, and somehow they had become disconnected. When they saw each other, they were somehow out of sync. Their conversation was too cheery, too stilted, too irrelevant. They accidently interrupted each other then had silly alternations of "No, you go ahead." Christopher felt confused by the new awkwardness between them and helpless to do anything about it. Gradually, they had seen each other less and less. Tonight's dinner was the result of a chance meeting on the street—just two friends getting together for old times' sake. They talked about everything and nothing: her new job, his peculiar neighbor, the latest movies. The words came easily and they found themselves laughing together. Now, they sat in silence. Sophie pushed some rice around on her plate. Christopher looked out the window. When he turned back to face Sophie, his eyes brimmed with unshed tears. "I've missed you," he said.

Will Christopher feel better because he cried? The venting hypothesis predicts that crying is always beneficial. However, Christopher's subtle unshed tears may not be intense enough to fully drain his negative feelings. The venting hypothesis suggests that Christopher would be better off if he cried more vigorously, perhaps with heaving sobs and tears streaming down his face.

The venting hypothesis sees Christopher's tears as an end in themselves, whereas we see them as a possible beginning. The tears are a sign that Christopher is actively experiencing his feelings of loss or loneliness, which he now has an opportunity to examine and process. The tears are also a means of communicating his feelings to Sophie.

From our perspective, the intensity of Christopher's crying is less important to predicting outcomes than the intrapersonal and interpersonal context in which it occurs. How does Christopher feel about his tears? Does he see them as a normal and understandable expression of his feelings or is he ashamed of them?

How does Sophie respond to Christopher's tears? Ideally, Sophie is touched by them and responds warmly. Maybe she smiles softly and reaches over to hold his hand. Maybe she tells Christopher, "I didn't know you cared" or "I've missed you, too." These positive responses are likely to result in Christopher feeling better after crying.

But what if Sophie responds negatively? Maybe she feels embarrassed by the fact that he is crying in a public restaurant and mutters, "Christopher! Pull yourself together! People are staring." What if Sophie interprets his tears as an attempt to pressure her into a more serious relationship than she wants? She might snarl at him, "Oh, cut the melodrama! I knew it was a mistake to agree to this dinner. This is exactly why we broke up in the first place: Every time things seem to be going well between us, you try to pressure me into getting more involved. Go play your manipulative little emotional games with somebody else! I'm not sticking around for this!" She might storm out of the restaurant before Christopher has a chance to say another word. A negative response from Sophie makes it likely that Christopher will feel worse after crying.

Research shows that there is considerable variability in the form, frequency, and emotional content of crying. Observational studies indicate that crying behavior comes in a variety of forms, including tears in eyes, tears down the face, sobbing, blinking back tears, and wiping eyes (e.g., Labott, Ahleman, Wolever, & Martin, 1990). There is also a great deal of variability in the frequency with which people cry. Some people never shed a tear, even under the most trying circumstances. Other people cry upon viewing commercials for long-distance telephone companies. In terms of emotional content, one study (Frey, Hoffman-Ahern, Johnson, Lykken, & Tuason, 1983) showed that the most frequent elicitors of tears are relationship conflict (40% of crying incidents) and media-related triggers, such as movies (27%). Another study points to death, loneliness, separation, and pain as common precipitants of crying (Kraemer & Hastrup, 1986). For women, about half of crying incidents primarily reflect feelings of sadness, but another third of crying incidents involve feelings of happiness or anger (Frey et al., 1983).

It seems likely that this variability in the form, frequency, and emotional tone of crying translates into different consequences. The anecdote about Christopher points to the role of crying as both a sign of distress and a possible means of coping with that distress. Research, theory, and daily life experience corroborate this duality: On the one hand, frequent crying is associated with self-reports of consistently high levels of distress or Negative Affectivity (NA; in this case measured as trait neuroticism) (Vingerhoets, Van Den Berg, Kortekaas, Van Heck, & Croon, 1993). Crying is also a symptom of a variety of psychological and neurological disorders, including depression (Patel, 1993). On the other hand, more frequent crying is associated with higher self-esteem (Vingerhoets et al., 1993). Some clinicians point to crying as an important component of cathartic expression (Nichols & Zax, 1977). Scheff (1979) describes crying as a "biological necessity" and a curative agent in depression. Most laypeople believe that "having a good cry" allows one to release pent-up negative feelings (Frijda, 1986).

We turn now to a closer look at research and theory on the consequences of crying.

Effects of Crying on Arousal

One theory concerning the physiological benefits of crying suggests that tears are a means of releasing toxins. Based on their observation that emotional tears, produced by watching a sad movie, contain higher concentrations of protein than irritant tears, produced by chopping onions, Frey and his colleagues (Frey, 1985; Frey, DeSota-Johnson, Hoffman, & McCall, 1981) speculate that emotional tears are a means of excreting toxic substances that accumulate during stress. However, Gross, Fredrickson, and Levenson (1994) state that Frey's theory involves "a large inferential leap" (p. 641). They argue that evidence of chemical differences between emotional and nonemotional tears doesn't necessarily mean that emotional tears release toxins.

Other research suggests that crying is associated with poorer physical health. A large survey looking at the relationship between crying and physical health showed that adults who report more frequent crying also report more frequent physical disorders with increasing age (Labott & Martin, 1990). Furthermore, crying may impair immune function. Labott et al. (1990) had college students watch a sad movie with the instructions to either express or inhibit overt signs of their feelings. Participants who cried had lower levels of S-IgA (an antibody found in saliva that protects against respiratory and gastrointestinal infections) than those who did not cry while viewing the same sad movie.

Another theory about the physiological benefits of crying suggests that crying represents a shift in the autonomic nervous system from arousal to recovery (e.g., Efran & Spangler, 1979; Frijda, 1986). According to this view, intense emotions evoke sympathetic activation, which is then followed by opposing parasympathetic activation, to bring about homeostasis. Crying results when the parasympathetic nervous system rebounds and temporarily overcompensates for previous sympathetic hyperactivity.

Contrary to this view of crying as facilitating physiological homeostasis, laboratory studies consistently show that crying is associated with *increased* physiological arousal. For instance, Kraemer and Hastrup (1988) had high- and low-frequency criers watch a sad movie. They expected to see arousal reductions due to crying, but their comparison of criers to noncriers showed that the onset of crying was associated with significant increases in heart rate and skin conductance fluctuations. In another study that did not specifically select high- and low-frequency criers, Gross et al. (1994) found that volunteers who spontaneously cried while viewing a sad movie showed increased responses while crying on four out of five physiological variables reflecting a mixture of sympathetic and parasympathetic arousal.

On the other hand, refraining from crying when one feels like doing so is physiologically stressful. Labott and Teleha (1996) had women watch a sad movie and instructed them either to try to express their feelings fully or to strongly inhibit overt signs of their feelings. Viewing the movie increased the skin conductance level (SCL, an indicator of how sweaty one's palms are) for all study participants, but the inhibition instructions yielded significantly higher SCL than the expression instructions. This difference in SCL was not due to differences in emotional experience, because both the expression and the inhibition participants reported feeling similarly sad. These results suggest that deliberately refraining from crying when one feels like doing so is physiologically taxing, at least in the short term. This finding is consistent with other work pointing to the physiological costs of emotional suppression (Gross & Levenson, 1993).

Effects of Crying on Experience

Anecdotal evidence from clinicians and laypeople suggests that crying can alleviate negative feelings, increase positive feelings, or both (e.g., Beck, Rush, Shaw, & Emery, 1979; Frey, 1985; Kraemer & Hastrup, 1988). Roughly 85% of women and 73% of men say they generally feel better after crying (Frey, 1985). Yet, findings from laboratory studies looking at the effects of crying on emotional experience seem most consistent with the interpretation that crying is a sign of distress rather than a means of alleviating it. For instance, Labott and Martin (1988) found that volunteers who cried while viewing a sad film felt more distressed during the film than those who did not cry, whereas the two groups showed similar levels of distress 2 hours later. Similar results were reported by Choti, Marston, Holston, and Hart (1987) and Gross et al. (1994). Martin and Labott (1991) also showed no mood improvements following crying, whereas presentation of a humorous film was effective in reducing movie-induced sadness. Based on data from natural settings as well as laboratory studies, Kraemer and Hastrup (1986; 1988) argue that distress dissipates over time, usually within an hour or two, regardless of whether or not people cry. Thus, people's belief that they feel better after crying may simply reflect the passage of time.

However, the effects of crying on experience may vary for different people, depending on the meaning that crying carries for them. Labott and Teleha (1996) had women who were either high or low in self-reported crying frequency watch a sad movie with instructions to either try to express their feelings fully or to strongly inhibit overt signs of their feelings. They observed a significant interaction between weeping propensity and expression instructions: Women who typically cried frequently felt most comfortable crying and least comfortable inhibiting their tears, whereas women who rarely cried preferred to inhibit their tears and felt stressed when asked to openly express their emotions. In other words, participants reported feeling least stressed when the experimental instructions matched their usual crying propensity, and they felt most stressed when instructions were contrary to their usual behavior. Labott and Teleha (1996) interpret these findings to mean that "there may be more than one answer to the question of how much expression is 'best' " (p. 282).

The Social Context of Crying

Crying has strong social implications. Several theorists have suggested that crying serves a help-seeking function by acting as a signal to others that the individual is no longer able to manage the situation alone (e.g., Averill, 1968; Labott, Martin, Eason, & Berkey, 1991; Sadoff, 1966). It may be precisely because crying is arousing and unpleasant for both the crier and the observer that it is useful. According to this view, crying serves as a signal that motivates the self and others to alter the situation.

Consistent with this view, Cornelius (1984) had volunteers provide detailed descriptions of a time when they had cried in the presence of another person. Although study participants insisted that their tears were involuntary rather than deliberately manipulative, they perceived crying to be quite effective in changing the interpersonal context in a positive direction, from conflict toward support. Crying got the attention of the other individual and frequently elicited attempts to comfort the crier (especially a female crier).

Other research suggests that the social consequences of crying depend on who is doing the crying. In particular, crying may have more positive consequences for women than for men.

Frey and his colleagues (Frey, 1985; Frey et al., 1983) note a number of interesting facts about gender differences in crying: Before puberty, boys and girls cry at about the same rates, but by age 18, women cry substantially more frequently and intensely than do men. On average, women report crying 5.3 times per month, which is about four times more often than the average crying frequency reported by men. However, the frequency with which individual women cry varies widely, ranging from 0 to 31 times per month. Women also tend to cry more intensely than men. Typically, men just have tears brimming in their eyes rather than streaming down their faces.

These gender differences in crying frequency and intensity are usually explained as a reflection of different socialization experiences for boys and girls. Consistent with this explanation, Crester, Lombardo, Lombardo, and Mathis (1982) found that most of the people they questioned believe crying is more socially acceptable for women, and that it is generally seen as a sign of weakness for men.

However, crying may be becoming more socially acceptable for men (Labott et al., 1991; Ross & Mirowsky, 1984). In 1972, when presidential hopeful Edmund Muskie publicly shed a tear over an unflattering news report concerning his wife, he was widely criticized, and this incident may have cost him his party's nomination. In contrast, in the 1996 presidential race, the sight of teary eyes in Bill Clinton or Bob Dole was so common that *The Wall Street Journal* called it the "weepiest" campaign on record. Ross Perot was the only presidential candidate in this race who did not publicly cry. (See Glaser & Salovey, 1998, for a fascinating discussion of the effects of emotional expression by politicians.) Labott et al. (1991) recently found that student volunteers rated males who cried while watching a sad movie as more likable than males who did not cry. On the other hand, volunteers liked females more when they did *not* cry. This suggests that at least mild levels of male crying (e.g., sniffing and dabbing at eyes) are sometimes perceived as attractive.

The social context in which crying occurs is also critically important to determining its interpersonal consequences. Both men and women say they are more likely to cry in the presence of women than men (Jesser, 1982). Perhaps this is because women are generally more comfortable than men with other people's tears, and they tend to respond more positively. With respect to both general attitudes and specific incidents, women report being more accepting, helpful, empathic, and generally supportive in response to others' crying, whereas men say they are more likely to feel confused or irritated by someone else's tears and to ignore the weeper (Crester et al., 1982; Jesser, 1982). Also, crying is generally more acceptable in intimate settings than more public settings. Crying in a work setting can elicit embarrassment, confusion, and even anger for both the crier and the observer (Hoover-Dempsey, Plas, & Strudler Wallston, 1986).

Crying and Distress Resolution

In parallel to our discussion of expression of negative emotions as both a sign of distress and a possible means of coping with that distress, Bohart (1980) argues that crying does not automatically lead to resolution of distress. Crying is a sign that one is acutely experiencing sad feelings, but it doesn't necessarily make one feel better. Actively experiencing sadness, pain, or loss provides an opportunity to acknowledge, accept, tolerate, or understand these feelings and thereby move on. What is important is assimilating and accommodating the loss experience that triggered tears. However, crying in and of itself is neither necessary nor sufficient for resolution. Along these same lines, Efran and Spangler (1979) note that it is the recovery from tears rather than tears themselves that clients experience as therapeutic.

In his book *The Language of Tears,* Kottler (1996) argues that crying is most likely to be beneficial if it is accompanied by verbal elaboration. Kottler is a strong advocate of giving oneself permission to cry and actively experiencing one's feelings rather than cutting them off. However, he sees this as only the beginning of a process of constructive change rather than an end in itself. He notes that depressed people cry a great deal and feel worse because they are immobilized. He suggests that endlessly staying "mired in the muck, feeling sorry for yourself, helpless to do anything" is not productive (p. 177). Instead, intense emotional experience and expression need to be balanced by efforts to understand these responses, decode their significance, and form meaningful connections with other experiences. Kottler emphasizes the importance of following through after accessing and interpreting one's tearful feelings, by talking to others about these feelings and taking action based on one's insights. Kottler suggests that such action may involve "dealing with unfinished business, feeling greater self-acceptance, and committing yourself to respond in more constructive ways to those around you" (p. 183).

The role of crying as a means of facilitating constructive change, rather than an end in itself, is vividly illustrated in a case study by Labott and her colleagues (Labott, Elliot, & Eason, 1992). These investigators tracked the events surrounding a weeping episode of a psychotherapy client. The client talked about her feelings of pain and anger and felt heard and understood by her therapist. The therapist offered some support and reassurance and commented on links between the client's current feelings and past losses. The client began to sob as she spoke about her experiences of neglect. The client's emotional responses reached a peak as the therapist encouraged her to experience her feelings of hurt and anger. The client's emotional responses then noticeably settled as the therapist encouraged her to make sense of what was happening.

Summary

Laboratory and diary studies routinely find that crying is associated with more intense experience of distress and greater physiological arousal. On the other hand, some people are definitely more comfortable crying and therefore are more likely to benefit from crying than other people. Deliberately refraining from crying when one wants to do so is physiologically taxing.

Crying can be a starting point in a process of distress resolution. Crying is a sign that individuals are actively experiencing their emotions. It indicates an opportunity for people to understand and process their feelings. Crying can sometimes elicit responses from others that are helpful in resolving distress. Kottler (1996) writes that when it comes to crying, "emotional arousal and expression as an end in itself may not only be useless but may even be harmful. Unless people are helped to complete the arousal cycle to a point of returned deactivation, emotions that have been turned on may continue to spin out of control. . . . Helping people to feel comfortable crying is indeed important, but not without also helping them to dry their eyes and make sense of the experience" (pp. 194–195).

EXPRESSION OF TRAUMA-RELATED FEELINGS

Teresa felt exhausted. It had taken her almost 20 years to build up the courage to confront her father, but today she had done it. This time, she was in control. She had decided where and when they would meet. She had cut off his talk about the new furnace and her cousin's upcoming wedding and brought up the incest. Before today, she had rehearsed this conversation in her mind a thousand times. She had imagined that her father would deny sexually abusing her, and she was ready to shout at him if he did. Part of her even hoped he would try denying it, just so she could blast him with her accusations. But he didn't. She had also imagined her father begging for her forgiveness, which she would coldly refuse. But he didn't do that either. He just listened as she explained how desperately she had needed him to care for her after her mother died and how devastated she had been by his betrayal of her trust. "You were all I had," she said, "and you used me." She told him how frightened she had been; how she resented him for stealing her childhood and her sense of safety in her own home. She told him how difficult and painful it was for her even now, as an adult, trying to relate to men. When she had imagined confronting her father, she had pictured herself challenging a ferocious monster. But her father hadn't seemed like a monster today. He seemed old and defeated. He told her that the memory of what he had done to her had eaten at him all these years. He hadn't offered any excuses. He said he would understand if she didn't want anything to do with him. He didn't expect her ever to be able to forgive him. Teresa didn't want to think about forgiveness now. At this point, she wasn't sure what kind of relationship she wanted with her father, if any. For now, she was just relieved that the pretense between them was over. She was exhausted, but she felt an ember of pride glowing inside her—she had faced her worst nightmare and survived.

Teresa clearly feels better after telling her father about her trauma-related feelings. Is this a case of emotional venting? We don't think so. The benefits of Teresa's expression are mediated by cognitive and interpersonal changes (cf. Kelly & McKillop, 1996). Cognitively, expressing her feelings to her father enabled Teresa to see herself in a new light. Teresa planned and initiated this confrontation, which gave her a sense of control in her relationship with her father, to counter her earlier sense of helplessness. Because she was able to confront her father, Teresa now sees herself as a survivor, rather than a victim. There is also a hint that this encounter gave her a new perspective on her father, making her see him as a defeated old man, rather than a monster.

Interpersonally, Teresa's expression elicited positive responses from her father, who acknowledged and respected her feelings. Their relationship has definitely changed because of this confrontation. It is not yet clear how this change will manifest itself, but Teresa is relieved that they no longer have to pretend that everything is "fine" between them. We doubt that Teresa's expression would have had so positive an outcome if her father had dismissed her feelings somehow. He might have done this by refusing to listen, denying the incest, blaming Teresa for being seductive, or ridiculing her for clinging to the past.

As was the case with Cristopher's crying, Teresa's trauma-related expression represents a beginning rather than an endpoint. Teresa did not "get rid" of her distress once and for all by confronting her father. Instead, she acknowledged it, communicated it, and began a process of transforming it. How will Teresa follow through on her new sense of self? What kind of relationship will she build with her father? In sorting out these issues, Teresa may need to talk more about her feelings, either with her father or with someone she trusts.

Pennebaker and his colleagues have conducted a series of studies indicating that talking or writing about feelings related to traumatic events is physically and psychologically beneficial. In the first of these studies, Pennebaker and Beall (1986) had college students write for 15 minutes on 4 consecutive days about either trivial topics (e.g., a description of their shoes) or about the most upsetting and traumatic experiences of their entire lives. Participants who wrote about their traumatic experiences were given one of three sets of instructions: to write only about the facts of the traumatic event (trauma–fact group); to write only about their feelings surrounding the trauma but not the actual event (trauma–emotion group); or to write about both the facts and their feelings surrounding the trauma (trauma–combination group). Although participants in this study were students, Pennebaker states that the trauma essays were, for the most part, quite poignant, addressing topics such as death of a loved one, physical or sexual abuse, and intense family conflict.

Compared to the group who wrote about trivial topics and the trauma–fact group, the trauma–emotion and the trauma–combination groups showed higher blood pressure and more negative mood immediately following each writing episode, but at a 4-month follow-up assessment these groups reported fewer physical health problems. Additionally, the trauma–combination group had fewer student health center visits in the 6 months following the intervention than the other groups. Writing about only the facts surrounding traumatic events was neither upsetting nor physiologically arousing, nor did it have any beneficial health effects.

Thus, Pennebaker and Beall's (1986) findings point to the beneficial effects of emotional expression, but contrary to the venting hypothesis, these benefits appeared only after some time. Immediately after expressing, participants actually felt worse and were more physiologically aroused.

Pennebaker and Beall's results have been replicated and extended in a number of other studies by Pennebaker and his colleagues (Francis & Pennebaker, 1992; Pennebaker, Colder, & Sharp, 1990) as well as studies by other investigators (M. A. Greenberg & Stone, 1992; M. A. Greenberg, Wortman, & Stone, 1996; Mendolia & Kleck, 1993). Several studies have documented short-term positive changes in immune responses as a result of disclosing feelings about traumatic experiences (Esterling, Antoni, Fletcher, Margulies, & Schneiderman, 1994; Lutgendorf, Antoni, Kumar, &

Schneiderman, 1994; Pennebaker, Kiecolt-Glaser, & Glaser, 1988; K. J. Petrie, Booth, Pennebaker, Davison, & Thomas, 1995). Some studies have failed to replicate the health benefits of written or verbal disclosure of traumatic feelings but have documented psychological benefits (Donnelly & Murray, 1991; E. J. Murray, Lamnin, & Carver, 1989). A recent statistical review of studies involving written expression of trauma-related feelings (Smyth, 1998) concludes that the magnitude of improvements associated with the writing intervention (across various measures of well-being) is similar to or larger than those produced by other psychological interventions.

All of these studies point to the benefits of expressing trauma-related feelings. However, detailed content analyses of participants' essays or discussions from several of Pennebaker's experiments show conflicting findings concerning what sort of emotional expression is most beneficial. Pennebaker (1993b) found improved physical and psychological well-being among participants who used more negative emotion words and fewer positive emotion words. Pennebaker and Francis (1996) suggest that expressing both negative and positive emotions is important for health, and they note that in this study use of positive emotion words was a stronger predictor of improved health than use of negative words. Most recently, Pennebaker, Mayne, and Francis (1997, Study 1), found that using fewer negative emotion words and more positive emotion words in trauma essays was associated with improved outcomes in the months after writing. However, exploratory analyses suggested that the relationship between use of negative emotion words and well-being may actually be curvilinear: Participants who used a moderate number of negative emotion words had better outcomes than those who used either very high or very low numbers of negative emotion words.

Other investigators have found that the process of shifting from negative mood to positive mood over the course of written or verbal disclosure in linked to improvements is self-esteem, cognition, and behavior (Donnelly & Murray, 1991; E. J. Murray et al., 1989). In psychotherapy, a shift from negative to positive emotions is often an indication of significant emotional processing (L. S. Greenberg & Safran, 1987).

To us, these findings suggest that expression of trauma-related feelings in and of itself is not necessarily beneficial. Instead, as we noted in the sections on anger and crying, trauma-related expression is adaptive to the extent that it leads to some kind of resolution of distress. This resolution may be marked or facilitated by increases in the experience and expression of positive feelings, but it also requires accessing and processing negative feelings.

Research and theory by Pennebaker and others points to three important mechanisms by which expression of trauma-related feelings can lead to resolution of distress and enhanced well-being. These mechanisms, which we describe in detail below, involve decreasing the physiological work of inhibition, increasing self-understanding, and enhancing positive reflection (the fourth component of emotion). In addition to these three intrapersonal mechanisms, as Teresa's story suggests, the effects of trauma-related expression also depend on the responses of others.

Decreasing the Physiological Work of Inhibition

One possible explanation for the benefits of trauma-related expression is that it undoes the cumulative physiological stress of inhibition. Trauma survivors often deliberately refrain from expressing their feelings because they find these feelings too threatening or too shameful. The story about Teresa alludes to the strain of pretending and effortfully refraining from expressing negative feelings. Pennebaker (e.g., 1985; Pennebaker & Susman, 1988) argues that deliberately inhibiting thoughts, feelings, and actions requires physiological work. Fowles's (1980) experimental work indicates that behavioral activation (i.e., doing something) is associated with increased cardiovascular response, whereas behavioral inhibition (i.e., trying not to do something) is linked to increased SCL. Thus deliberately refraining from talking about one's feelings is likely to be associated with transient increases in SCL. Laboratory experiments also show that deliberately inhibited thoughts and feelings tend to rebound as more frequent or more distressing intrusive rumination (e.g., Wegner & Gold, 1995; Wegner, Schneider, Carter, & White, 1987; Wegner & Zanakos, 1994), requiring renewed efforts at inhibition. It is plausible that over time, the work of inhibition may entail a chronic physiological strain that compromises resistance to disease. Having the opportunity to express previously inhibited feelings may alleviate this strain.

The idea that expression can undo the physiological work of inhibition is consistent with the findings of Pennebaker, Hughes, and O'Heeron (1987, Experiment 1). They asked college students to talk into a tape recorder about their most stressful experiences and also about their plans for the day. Participants who said that they had not previously talked much about their stressful experience showed the largest drops in SCL during the stressful discussion period.

However, not everyone derives arousal-reducing benefits from the opportunity to express trauma-related feelings. Based on judges' ratings of how personal and stressful the discussions were, Pennebaker et al. (1987) classified participants as either high or low disclosers. High and low disclosers did not differ on initial baseline physiological measures obtained while participants relaxed. Both high and low disclosers showed elevations in heart rate and blood pressure *while* talking about stressful topics compared to trivial topics. Only high disclosers showed a substantial drop in SBP below baseline levels *after* talking about stressful topics. Moreover, high disclosers showed *lower* SCL while talking about profound topics rather than trivial ones, whereas low disclosers showed the opposite pattern of much *higher* SCL while talking about profound topics rather than trivial ones. In other words, high disclosers were able to disclose about their stressful experiences and showed the disinhibition effect of reduced SCL. Low disclosers who had the same opportunity to disclose about their stressful experiences, but did so only to a limited extent, showed increased SCL, perhaps reflecting their efforts to inhibit their expression or their discomfort with the task. Similar results were obtained by Pennebaker, Barger, and Tiebout (1989), in a study involving interviews of Holocaust survivors. Those survivors who used more emotional words when describing their traumatic experiences and who showed lower SCL during the interview reported fewer physical symptoms and made fewer physician visits in the year following the interview.

To summarize, Pennebaker's findings indicate that in terms of cardiovascular arousal, expressing trauma-related feelings is physiologically stressful. However, for some people, trauma-related expression is associated with concurrent reductions in SCL-related arousal as well as subsequent reductions in SBP, presumably reflecting a decrease in their efforts to inhibit expression.

Increasing Self-Understanding

Another mechanism by which expression of trauma-related feelings can resolve distress is by enhancing self-understanding. Pennebaker (1993a) notes that across the various studies conducted by his research group, over 75% of the trauma-expression participants mentioned that their writing yielded long-term benefits involving insight. During debriefing, these participants made statements such as "It made me think things out," "It helped me look at myself from the outside," "It was a chance to sort out my thoughts" (p. 110). Only about 10% of trauma-expression participants believed that their writing was beneficial because it involved emotional venting: "I purged some of my feelings" (p. 110). In fact, those participants who did mention venting rarely showed improvements in their health as a result of the intervention.

Content analyses of the trauma-expression essays or discussions support participants' beliefs that expression of traumatic feelings is helpful when it fosters self-understanding (Pennebaker, 1993b; Pennebaker & Francis, 1996; Pennebaker, Mayne, & Francis, 1997). For instance, Pennebaker (1993b) combined the data from trauma-expression participants in several of his studies and selected the top and bottom third of participants based on a composite outcome measure. The bottom-third participants had composite outcomes that were comparable to control participants. Computer linguistic analysis showed that the essays of the top-third participants, who had the most positive outcomes following the intervention, had two distinctive insight-related characteristics compared to the essays of the bottom-third participants:

1. The top-third participants used words reflecting insight (e.g., realize, understand, thought, knew) and causal reasoning (e.g., because, why, reason) at *increasing rates* across the 3 or 4 days of the study. They started out with very low rates of these words on the first day of writing and ended up with very high rates of these words by the last day of the study, suggesting that they acquired insight over the course of writing. In contrast, the bottom-third participants, while showing the same overall rate of insight words, used these words at consistent rates over time.

2. The top-third participants' essays became more focused over time. They showed a decrease over time in the percentage of different words in each essay, indicating that they started out with more scattered content and increasingly focused on a single topic.

Judges' ratings of the essays corroborate these computer analysis findings concerning expression-related increases in self-understanding (Pennebaker, 1993b). Ratings by college student judges showed no differences in the overall extent to which the top-third and bottom-third participants accepted the events described in their essays, nor in the overall organization or "storiness" of the two groups' essays. However, these ratings indicate striking differences in changes over time. The essays of the top-third participants showed increasing organization, acceptance, and optimism. In contrast, the essays of the bottom-third participants started out with relatively clearly organized stories and gradually deteriorated. These results are consistent with theoretical perspectives emphasizing the importance of constructing narratives about experience (e.g., Meichenbaum & Fong, 1993). It seems that the process of creating such narratives is more important than simply having a narrative.

Expression-related increases in self-understanding are not the product of either coldhearted analysis of the situation or simple venting. Instead, this kind of self-understanding stems from a combination of emotional and cognitive processing of the experience. Recall that Pennebaker and Beall (1986) found that writing only about the facts of a traumatic experience was not helpful. In another study, Krantz and Pennebaker (1996) compared verbal and nonverbal expression of traumatic feelings. They found that expressive movement alone did not yield health benefits, but expressive movement combined with written expression did. Thus, accessing feelings, putting them into words, and building a coherent cognitive story are all important components of Pennebaker's interventions.

This emphasis on expression-related self-understanding reflecting a combination of cognitive and emotional processing is echoed by other investigators in both clinical and laboratory settings. Several studies show that being able to structure thoughts and feelings about past traumatic experiences is associated with better adjustment in a variety of clinical populations (e.g., Burgess & Holmstrom, 1979; Fairbank, Hansen, & Fitterling, 1991; Silver, Boon, & Stones, 1983).

Sappington and Russell (1979; Sappington, 1990) also point to the importance of combined cognitive and emotional processing. They distinguish between *intellectually based beliefs,* which are subjectively perceived as rational and based on facts, and *emotionally based beliefs,* which are subjectively perceived as nonrational and supported only by feelings or intuitions rather than facts.[6] Laboratory experiments show that intellectually based beliefs can be altered by obtaining more information. In contrast, emotionally based beliefs are not affected by objective information, but can change under conditions of increased levels of emotional experience and arousal. Clients often note the distinction between intellectually and emotionally based beliefs. They may make remarks such as "Rationally I know X, but I feel as if Y." Writing or talking about traumatic experiences enables people to access and perhaps revise their emotionally based beliefs.

Enhancing Positive Reflection

A third mechanism by which expression can resolve distress and enhance well-being is by eliciting more positive emotional reflection. Expression of trauma-related feelings can enable individuals to perceive their distress as acceptable, or at least tolerable, and perhaps controllable (cf. L. S. Greenberg & Safran, 1987; M. A. Greenberg et al., 1996).

Clinically, clients who have survived traumatic events are often afraid of their emotional experience (e.g., Krystal, 1978). They see their feelings as dangerous and fear falling apart or being utterly overwhelmed if they allow themselves to express their feelings. They may also interpret their intense emotional reactions as a sign that something is wrong with them (Thoits, 1985).

Researchers and theorists of all orientations have noted that expression can be a useful means of helping clients to revise their fearful beliefs concerning their trauma-related emotional experience as well as their sense of helplessness with respect to these feelings. Scheff (1979), a proponent of catharsis theory, argues that, in order to be therapeutic, emotional expression must occur at an optimum psychological distance in order to be therapeutic: Individuals must vividly experience their feelings while in a context of present safety. Neither being completely overwhelmed by intense feelings nor being completely cut off from affective experience is productive. Rather, it is a combination of emotional immersion plus control that fosters a sense of mastery over distressing feelings. Horowitz (1986) also points to the importance of combining distressing material with comforting cues as a means of "dosing" emotional confrontation. Bohart (1980) notes that in therapeutic grief work, clients often start by working through more peripheral material and gradually work up to assimilating the most painful aspects of their experience. Foa and Kozak (1986) invoke similar explanations for the fear-reducing benefits of prolonged exposure to threatening stimuli. As clients stay in the presence of the feared object, the intensity of their physiological response gradually dissipates. This physiological habituation provides new information to clients, which they can use to revise catastrophic beliefs regarding their experience of fear. By extension, when trauma survivors are able to "stay with" their feelings by expressing them rather than avoiding them, it gives them the opportunity to revise their view of these feelings, seeing them as tolerable and manageable rather than dangerous (see related findings and discussions by Creamer, Burgess, & Pattison, 1992, and Lepore et al., 1996). With exposure interventions clients do not "stay with" their painful feelings continuously or indefinitely, but only under controlled circumstances (e.g., during a therapy session) and for periods long enough to have the intensity of their emotional experience and arousal decrease. These theoretical accounts emphasizing the benefits of expression involving emotional immersion plus control are consistent with empirical findings that although writing about trauma-related feelings causes increases in short-term distress, experiencing relatively more short-term distress while writing does *not* lead to greater improvement (Smyth, 1998).

Responses of Others to Expression of Trauma-Related Feelings

Pennebaker's work focuses primarily on intrapersonal processes related to expression of traumatic feelings. However, other researchers and theorists point to the importance of interpersonal processes in this area. How others respond when trauma survivors express their feelings influences not only whether they continue to express, but also whether they benefit from expression (e.g., Albrecht, Burleson, & Goldsmith, 1994; Burleson & Goldsmith, 1998; Kelley & McKillop, 1996; Tait & Silver, 1989). The mechanisms we described above concerning how trauma-related expression can enhance well-being can operate at an interpersonal level as well as an individual level. When another person responds with acceptance, trauma survivors have less need to deliberately conceal their feelings, so, presumably, they are less likely to engage in long-term, physiologically stressful inhibition. When another person responds with empathy and affection, it can help trauma survivors to view their feelings in a more benign light, involving enhanced positive emotional reflection. Another person can also help trauma survivors gain new understanding of their own feelings or the traumatic event.

A study by Donnelly and Murray (1991) offers a comparison of individual versus interpersonal expression of traumatic feelings. These investigators compared the effects of writing essays with talking in therapeutic interviews about traumatic events. In the therapy condition, clinical psychology graduate student therapists reflected and reframed the emotional content of trauma descriptions in a warm and empathic manner. Participants were college students, and the interventions took place over 4 consecutive days. Content analyses showed that, compared to participants who wrote about trivial topics, those who wrote or talked about their traumatic experiences expressed more feelings, both positive and negative. In both trauma-expression groups, positive emotion, self-esteem, and cognitive and behavioral change increased across the 4 days of the study, whereas negative emotion decreased. Both of these groups also felt more positive about their topics and themselves at the end of the experiment, although there were no long-term effects of either intervention on mental or physical health.

The most interesting results of this study were the differences in mood between the writing and the talking groups immediately following each day of the intervention: Participants who wrote essays about their traumatic experiences showed increases in negative mood and decreases in positive mood after each session, whereas participants who talked about their traumatic experiences in therapeutic interviews showed no increase in negative mood and sometimes a decrease. The therapy participants also maintained their levels of positive mood after the first day. Donnelly and Murray interpret these findings to mean that expressing feelings about traumatic events is an aversive task, but that having a therapist respond empathically somehow ameliorates this aversiveness.

Donnelly and Murray also noted individual differences in comfort with different forms of expression. Females and individuals who typically pay a great deal of attention to their inner experience (i.e., those high in a trait called Private Self-Consciousness) reported worse mood following the psychotherapy intervention, whereas males and individuals who typically do not attend to their inner experience reported worse mood following the writing intervention. Perhaps people who are less "in touch" with their feelings have a greater need for support from an empathic other as they struggle to express their trauma-related feelings.

Summary

The short-term effects of expressing feelings related to traumatic experiences are psychologically painful and physiologically arousing. However, the long-term effects may be improved psychological and physical health. The studies we described in this section suggest that these positive long-term outcomes are not the result of simple venting. Rather, they stem from three possible mechanisms: decreased work of inhibition, increased self-understanding, and enhanced positive reflection. These three mechanisms are interrelated. For instance, more positive reflection (i.e., perceiving feelings as more acceptable and tolerable) may enable clients to gain self-understanding and decrease their efforts to inhibit their feelings. Alternatively, decreasing inhibition may provide the opportunity for increased self-understanding, which may lead to more positive reflection.

On the other hand, as we discuss in greater detail in Chapters 4 and 10, expression is not the only means of coping with trauma-related feelings, nor is it necessarily the best coping strategy for all people (e.g., Bonanno, Keltner, Holen, & Horowitz, 1995; Rosenthal, 1993; Shuchter & Zisook, 1993). In a longitudinal study of coping with midlife conjugal bereavement, Bonanno and his colleagues (Bonanno et al., 1995) observed that emotional avoidance, measured as low self-rated experience of distress coupled with heightened cardiovascular arousal during an interview about grieving 6 months after the loss, was associated with *minimal* grief symptoms 8 months later. Although emotional avoidance was linked to initially high levels of self-reported physical symptoms, by 14 months it was associated with low levels of physical symptoms. Bonanno and his colleagues interpret these findings as an indication that emotional avoidance can sometimes serve adaptive functions. Emotional avoidance may enable individuals to regulate their emotional pain or to cope effectively with personal or professional responsibilities. Bonanno et al. speculate that different forms of emotional avoidance (e.g., lack of conscious awareness vs. short-term distraction vs. effortful suppression) may have different consequences for well-being. Like Pennebaker, they suggest that effortful preoccupation with avoiding subjectively unbearable feelings may be detrimental.

ALTERNATIVES TO THE VENTING HYPOTHESIS

We began this chapter with a discussion of the venting hypothesis, which refers to the idea that expression of distress is a universally beneficial means of diffusing negative emotional experience and/or distress-related physiological arousal. The venting hypothesis suggests (1) that the bigger the expression the better, (2) that the beneficial effects of expression are immediate, and (3) that the effects of expression are direct and automatic.

At this point, it should be clear that the venting hypothesis and its corollaries are myths. Whether or not expression of distress is beneficial depends on what is expressed, to whom, and how. Our review of the literature concerning anger expression, crying, and expression of trauma-related feelings points to the following conclusions:

1. *"Bigger" expression of distress is not necessarily better.* We found no evidence that more intense expression of distress is more beneficial than

less intense expression. In fact, the findings we reviewed pointed to the benefits of moderate levels of expression, in which people have access to their emotional experience but are not overwhelmed by it nor driven impulsively by it. Scheff (1979) argues that beneficial catharsis occurs when one is able to participate in and also observe one's own distress. Empirically, compared to more intense forms of expression, more moderate forms of expression are linked to lower physiological arousal, improved cognitive processing, and generally more positive responses from others.

The venting hypothesis makes no mention of the reflection component of emotion. Yet, research on individual and cultural differences suggests that expression can carry very different meanings for different people (e.g., Kitayama & Markus, 1996; Mesquita & Frijda, 1992; R. E. Porter & Samovar, 1998; see Chapter 4 in this volume for an extensive discussion of expressive goals and values). The studies we described by Labott and Teleha (1996) and Pennebaker et al. (1987) suggest that people who feel comfortable with expression are more likely to benefit from it. Similar results were obtained by Stanton, Danoff-Burg, Cameron, and Ellis (1994) in their longitudinal study of "emotional approach coping" with stressful events. Emotional approach coping involves active attempts to understand and express emotions. Stanton et al. (1994) found that college women who used emotional approach coping became less depressed and more satisfied with their lives over time, whereas men who used this type of coping became more depressed and less satisfied. In a laboratory study, Engebretson, Matthews, and Scheier (1989) also found that people's preferred expressive strategy tends to be their most adaptive strategy. Taken together, these findings suggest that the answer to what sort of expression is "best" varies for different people. Seen in this context, the venting hypothesis's insistence that everyone benefits from expressing their feelings as much as possible is not only inaccurate, it's disrespectful.

The venting hypothesis focuses only on distress, but current conceptions of psychological well-being emphasize both the absence of distress and the presence of positive affect. A number of the studies we described in this chapter point to the importance of experiencing and expressing positive feelings along with negative feelings: Empathy can diffuse anger; love and humor can diminish sadness; hope and acceptance can make trauma-related feelings more bearable. Expression of positive feelings along with negative feelings can also make distress expression more palatable to recipients.

2. *The benefits of distress expression often emerge over time.* In all of the studies we reviewed the immediate consequences of expression were *increased* arousal and intensified experience of distress. However, this short-term expression-related exacerbation of emotional responses may be worth it if expression leads to some kind of resolution of distress (see below).

3. *The benefits of distress expression are typically mediated by cogni-*

tive or interpersonal processes. Our review suggests that resolution of distress does not follow directly or automatically from expression. Expression of negative feelings is not an adaptive goal in and of itself, but it can serve as a means of enhancing self-understanding or improving social relationships.

In terms of self-understanding, many of the studies we described emphasized that expression can be a means of processing the information entailed in emotional responses and drawing out its implications. (We discuss the role of expression in fostering emotional insight in detail in Chapter 3.)

Whereas the venting hypothesis suggests that expression is a passive process that involves just "letting out" distress, a perspective that emphasizes the role of expression in fostering self-understanding focuses on expression as an active process. In a thoughtful article on catharsis in psychotherapy, Kosmicki and Glickauf-Hughes (1997) state, "The therapeutic aspect of catharsis is . . . not the expulsion of affect but the retrieval of experiences and ego mediation of associated emotional content. The goal is ultimately self-acceptance and integration of formerly repressed or inaccessible affective experiences" (p. 158). According to this view, expression is adaptive when it fosters an integration of cognitive and experiential processing. The work we described by Bohart (1980), Kottler (1996), and Pennebaker et al. (1997) all point to the benefits of this type of integration. These theorists argue for the importance of expression as a means of accessing emotional experience, putting it into words, and creating meaning.

In terms of social relationships, expression is adaptive when it leads to clarification of interpersonal misunderstandings or elicits desired responses from others. Kosmicki and Glickauf-Hughes (1997) emphasize that expression of distress is most likely to be beneficial when the receiver responds with empathy, acceptance, and containment. Burleson and Goldsmith (1998) also note that recipients of distress expression can be helpful in fostering new appraisals of either feelings or circumstances.

CONCLUSION

The paradox of distress expression is that expression of negative feelings is both a sign of distress and a possible means of coping with that distress. Throughout this chapter, we have argued that expression of negative feelings is adaptive to the extent that it leads to some kind of resolution of distress.

The venting hypothesis views negative emotions as "things to be gotten rid of" and expression as always desirable and beneficial. In contrast, our perspective is that emotions are a source of information about the relationship between the self and the environment. Expression is a means of processing and communicating this information, but it can be done in adaptive or maladaptive ways.

When it is adaptive, expression of distress can lead to enhanced acceptance of feelings ("These feelings are unpleasant, but not unbearable") or increased self-understanding ("This is something that really matters to me" or "I've felt guilty about this for years, but it wasn't my fault"). It can also clarify interpersonal misunderstandings or even directly alter another person's behavior in a desired way. When it is maladaptive, expression exacerbates distress by leading to feelings of guilt or shame ("I really lost it!"), rehearsing rather than resolving grievances, or impairing social relationships.

NOTES

1. Whereas the process model of expression presented in the previous chapter as Figure 1.1 describes the sequential unfolding of influences among the components of emotion, the model of the components of emotion presented in Figure 2.1 is an aggregate summary of the interconnections among these components.

2. Researchers have noted a number of difficulties in trying to operationalize physiological arousal (e.g., Eysenck, 1987; Lacey, 1967): Different measures of arousal such as heart rate, electroencephalogram (EEG), and skin conductance show only modest intercorrelations. Sometimes these measures even show opposite patterns of response, with one measure indicating increased arousal and others indicating decreased arousal. Moreover, the pattern of relationships among different measures of physiological arousal varies across different individuals and across stimuli of different types and intensities. For the purposes of this chapter, we merely note the type of physiological responses investigators have observed in research relevant to the venting hypothesis and, when possible, state how investigators have interpreted their measures of arousal. Readers interested in more detailed discussions of the psychological meaning of physiological responses should see Cacioppo and Tassinary (1990) and Strelau (1987).

3. See Ekman's (1977, 1994) distinction between automatic and extended appraisals. Automatic appraisals occur within milliseconds of an event, often without awareness; extended appraisals involve more deliberate evaluation and consideration. Reflection is like extended appraisals, only the target of reflection is one's own emotional responses rather than an external event.

4. Jones (1950, 1960) also identified a third group of individuals, labeled *generalizers*, who show strong responses in both facial expression and skin conductance, but this group has not received much research attention.

5. Cacioppo et al. (1992) also note two other problems with Jones's internalizer–externalizer distinction: First, very few people can reliably be categorized as either internalizers or externalizers. Second, socialization is not the only cause of individual differences in expressiveness. Innate temperament also plays a part, because individual differences in emotional expression have been observed in newborn babies (e.g., Field, 1982).

6. Sappington and Russell's distinction between intellectually and emotionally based beliefs is similar to Freud's (1921) distinction between intellectual and emotional insight, Zajonc's (1980) distinction between "hot" and "cold" cognitions (the former having a strong emotional component) and S. Epstein's (e.g., 1994) distinction between the rational and experiential information processing systems. Sappington (1990) notes that emotionally based beliefs are not the same as emotional experience: Emotionally based beliefs are derived from emotional experience but they can influence behavior even when a person is not currently experiencing emotion.

3

Blind Spots and Epiphanies: Expression, Nonexpression, and Emotional Insight

INTRODUCTION

"How do I feel?" This simple question is not always easy to answer. It has to do with *emotional insight*: the ability, through self-reflection, to recognize, accurately label, and understand one's own emotional experience. Emotionally insightful people are vividly in touch with the felt flow of their inner experience, and they are able to interpret the subjective meaning of their emotional responses. In other words, they generally know what they are feeling and why.

Fostering emotional insight is usually a basic and central goal in psychotherapy. Therapists often seek to help clients understand and interpret their emotional experience (Kennedy-Moore, 1999). The specific insight-generating techniques vary widely across orientations, ranging from the focused introspection of systematic evocative unfolding used by experiential therapists (e.g., J. C. Watson & Rennie, 1994), to the directive confrontations used by rational-emotive therapists (e.g., Ellis, 1991), to the specific identification of affect-related contingencies used by cognitive-behavioral therapists (e.g., Beck, 1988; Lewinsohn, 1974), to the more subtle interpretations of psychodynamic therapists (e.g., Kernberg, 1993). However, the underlying principle guiding all of these interventions is the belief that if clients understand their feelings and the causes of those feelings, they will be better able to respond adaptively to these feelings.

In this chapter, we focus on the relationships between emotional expression, emotional insight, and adaptational outcomes. We note the possible benefits of emotional insight and describe how such insight (or its lack) can be recognized. We then look at the process of acquiring emotional insight. We discuss three prerequisites of emotional insight and some possible problems associated with these prerequisites that can interfere with the acquisition of emotional insight. In terms of the process model of emotional expression presented in Chapter 1, this chapter addresses the steps involving conscious perception of affective responses and labeling and interpretation of those responses. It also focuses on the distinctions between nonexpression due to a high threshold for distress, nonexpression due to motivated lack of awareness of emotional responses, and nonexpression due to skill deficits in emotional processing. This chapter points to the role of emotional expression as both a sign of emotional insight and a means of fostering this insight.

BENEFITS OF EMOTIONAL INSIGHT

Why do people need emotional insight? What does it matter if clients label their emotional states as "I'm feeling kind of down" versus "I feel guilty and dejected but also slightly hopeful"? To understand what we mean by emotional insight, and why it is important, let's first consider an extreme example of its lack.

> This morning, one of Larry's coworkers noticed that he was having trouble concentrating and asked if anything was wrong. Larry said no, and he assured his coworker that everything was fine. But now, sitting in his too-quiet apartment, Larry realizes that he has been feeling out-of-sorts for the past week and a half—ever since Isabel moved out. The breakup came as a surprise to Larry. Although Isabel had talked before about not feeling close to him, Larry had no idea that she was so unhappy that she would want to end their relationship.
>
> Larry feels restless. He decides he must be hungry and walks to the kitchen to look for something to eat. He reminds himself that he will have to go out to get milk and bread later that evening. Usually Isabel did the grocery shopping. He feels vaguely uncomfortable. Maybe he should change out of his work clothes before eating, he thinks to himself.

In the anecdote above, Larry is strikingly lacking in both expression and emotional understanding. Most people would find the breakup of a relationship to be a very emotional event. Anger, betrayal, loss, relief, exhilaration, guilt, fear, or loneliness are just a few of the feelings and emotions someone might experience under these circumstances. Larry, however, overtly expresses no emotion. Moreover, his private emotional experience consists of only a vague sense of discomfort and confusion. His thoughts about his feelings are hypothetical, extremely concrete, and largely unrelated to the highly emotional events that just occurred: Maybe he is hungry; maybe his clothes are too tight. Larry's emotional obtuseness carries over to his interpersonal relationships. Not only is he unable to understand or articulate his own feelings, but he is unable to understand or respond to Isabel's expression of emotion.

In contrast to Larry, people who are able to understand and interpret their emotional experience have access to a rich and vital source of knowledge that can guide their thoughts and behavior. Emotional experience provides individuals with information about themselves and their environment, as they interact with it and adapt to it (Safran & Greenberg, 1986, 1989; Schwarz, 1990). All forms of emotional experience, from crude affects to focused emotions to highly elaborated feelings, carry subjective meaning (e.g., L. S. Greenberg, Rice, & Elliott, 1993): *Affect* involves a generic sense of arousal or activation that can be either emotional or physiological. The intensity of affect is a signal indicating the perceived importance an individual attaches to environmental events. *Emotions* involve more specific responses that arise from rapid appraisals of the significance of particular environmental events. Perceiving a threat evokes fear, perceiving a loss leads to sadness, etc. These basic emotions carry information about action dispositions that help motivate potentially adaptive behaviors, such as flight with fear or withdrawal with sadness. *Moods* are more enduring but diffuse forms of emotional experience that can color perception, judgment, memory retrieval, and information processing. Finally, *feelings* involve complex, symbolic reactions. Feelings are the most cognitively elaborated form of emotional experience. They incorporate information about beliefs, memories, desires, and expectations and contain information about the personal meaning of environmental circumstances. Emotional insight makes it possible for people to adaptively use all of this information entailed in their emotional experience.

Emotional insight is associated with better individual and interpersonal functioning. At an individual level, recognizing and accurately expressing one's own emotional experience is a prerequisite to being able to draw upon it to guide one's thoughts and actions (Mayer & Salovey, 1997; Salovey, Hsee, & Mayer, 1993; Salovey & Mayer, 1990; J. C. Watson & Greenberg, 1996a). People who understand their feelings can use this information to develop a coherent sense of self and to create meaning from their experiences (J. C. Watson & Greenberg, 1996a). Emotional insight is also necessary for regulation or change of negative affect (Kennedy-Moore, 1999; Mayer & Gaschke, 1988; Mayer & Salovey, 1997; Mayer, Salovey, Gomberg-Kaufman, & Blainey, 1991; Salovey et al., 1993). If people understand their emotional experience, they are in a better position to know how they need to respond to environmental demands. Bringing their feelings and action dispositions to consciousness enables people to reflect upon the appropriateness of these feelings in the current context and to determine whether their expression will be helpful or harmful (J. C. Watson & Greenberg, 1996a). In other words, the better people understand their emotional experience, the better they are able to cope with it.

At an interpersonal level, emotional insight contributes to better relationships. Understanding their emotional experience helps people to communicate and develop intimacy with others (Buck, 1989, 1991). To the extent that they clearly understand and can draw upon their knowledge of their own feelings, they will be better able to empathize with others (J. C. Watson & Greenberg, 1996a). Moreover, being able to differentiate between their own and others' feelings allows people to respond flexibly and adaptively in interpersonal interactions (R. D. Lane & Schwartz, 1992; Salovey & Mayer, 1990).

Emotional insight is critical to healthy human functioning. Understanding one's own emotional experience in a meaningful way makes it possible to know oneself, to regulate one's behavior, and to connect with others. In the next section we discuss how emotional insight or lack of insight can be recognized.

IDENTIFYING EMOTIONAL INSIGHT AND ITS LACK

What are the signs of emotional insight? If therapists want to facilitate emotional insight, they first have to be able to identify its presence or lack. At the start of this chapter, we defined emotional insight as the ability to recognize, label, and interpret emotional experience. However, the acquisition of insight is a covert process. No one can know directly the level of self-understanding that another person experiences. Emotional insight or its lack can only be inferred, indirectly, from a person's verbal or symbolic communication. Nevertheless, it is clear that some individuals have greater awareness and understanding of their emotional experience than others.

Expression as a Sign of Emotional Insight

How people express their emotions can provide an important clue to their level of emotional insight: More insightful people present clearer and better articulated descriptions of their emotional lives. R. D. Lane and Schwartz (1987, 1992; R. D. Lane, Quinlan, Schwartz, Walker, & Zeitlin, 1990) distinguish between five levels of emotional awareness. Each level shows increasing complexity in the cognitive representation of emotional experience. The levels correspond to recognition of (1) physiological sensations, such as "I feel tired" or "I feel a tightness in my gut"; (2) bodily action tendencies or undifferentiated affect, such as "I feel like punching the wall" or "I feel bad"; (3) a single differentiated emotion, such as "I feel happy" or "I feel sad"; (4) combinations of differentiated emotions, such as

"I feel angry and sad"; and (5) differentiated feelings of oneself and another person, such as "I feel disappointed that I didn't win, but glad that my friend did. My friend feels happy and proud but worried that my feelings might be hurt." These levels of emotional awareness involve differences in the ability to be aware of and describe one's own internal experience of emotion. At the lowest levels, individuals have only a crude recognition of global arousal, whereas at the highest levels, individuals have complex, highly elaborated representations of the quality and intensity of their feelings. According to Lane and Schwartz's categorization, Larry, in the anecdote presented earlier in this chapter, showed only the lowest level of emotional awareness. He knew he felt "bad" but was unable to distinguish between feelings of personal loss, hunger, and clothing-related discomfort.

Emotional insight is usually discussed as a between-person variable: Some people are more or less insightful than others. However, it can also be viewed as a within-person variable: A particular person may be more or less insightful at different times (Horowitz et al., 1993; R. D. Lane & Schwartz, 1992; Mayer & Gaschke, 1988).

One kind of within-person variation in emotional insight involves "emotional blind spots." Even people who generally show a great deal of emotional insight regarding some topics may show minimal recognition or understanding of their feelings regarding other topics. Emotional blind spots usually correspond to very threatening feelings that are painful to acknowledge or examine. For instance, a therapist may be generally very aware of her feelings but may have difficulty recognizing or acknowledging that she feels sexually attracted to a particular client. A man who prides himself on being a dutiful son may be very aware of his feelings of love for his elderly father as well as his sense of loss at his father's increasing debility. However, he may not be able to acknowledge his resentment concerning his father's constant demands and lack of appreciation for his efforts. This unacknowledged resentment may leak out in subtle signs such as a sharp voice here, a bit of procrastination there.

At the other end of the continuum, another kind of within-person variation in emotional insight involves emotional epiphanies, which are striking moments of affective insight (Kuiken, Carey, & Nielsen, 1987). Such moments are often described as pivotal events in literature, existential philosophy, and psychotherapy. They are most likely to occur during intensive self-reflection and involve a profoundly felt shift in self-understanding. During moments of affective insight, initially vague feelings are suddenly felt with clarity and certainty. There is a sense that the feelings were always there but are only now recognized and fully acknowledged. The individual experiences a sense of newly emerged self-knowledge and vitality, accompanied by a perception of an increased capacity for self-direction.

Thus, emotional insight can be recognized by the vividness, comprehensiveness, and clarity with which individuals represent and express their emotional experience. But, what about the other end of the continuum? Perhaps even more important than being able to recognize instances of emotional insight is being able to identify the *lack* of emotional insight. As the anecdote about Larry at the beginning of this chapter suggests, individuals with limited understanding of their emotional experience are at risk for difficulties in intrapersonal and interpersonal functioning, and they may require clinical intervention.

Distinguishing between Lack of Emotional Experience and Lack of Awareness of That Experience

Recognizing the lack of emotional insight is more difficult than recognizing its presence. When a client describes her feelings in a lucid and meaningful way, a therapist can conclude, "My, this person certainly understands and has reflected upon her feelings," because communicating a richly elaborated description of one's emotional experience requires emotional insight. However, when someone says, "I'm not experiencing any negative emotions," this could mean a number of different things: (1) She may truly not be experiencing any negative emotions; (2) she may be deliberately trying to hide her distress or "fake good"; or (3) she may be unaware of her actual negative feelings (cf. Gur & Sackeim, 1979; Sackeim & Gur, 1979; Schedler, Mayman, & Manis, 1993). All three of these circumstances involve nonexpression, but only the third instance would qualify as lack of emotional insight.

Let's assume that deliberate deception is not an issue. How, then, can a therapist distinguish between *lack of negative emotional experience* and *lack of awareness* of this experience? This distinction is critically important because these two circumstances carry very different implications for well-being (see discussion of varieties of nonexpression in Chapter 1). People who are truly not experiencing any negative emotions are doing just fine. They don't need any help. On the other hand, people who are "tuned out" to their emotional experience are unable to draw upon their experiential knowledge for effective coping. When there is a problem, they don't realize it, so they can't fix it. It's like they are navigating through life without being able to use their internal compass. A number of strategies have been used in both clinical and research settings to identify signs of unacknowledged emotional experience. We briefly describe four of these strategies below. Because all of these strategies represent indirect assessments of covert processes, they all have limitations.

Emotional Memories

One strategy for identifying lack of insight is to inquire about memories of situations evoking specific emotions. This approach assumes, for example, that if individuals can't clearly remember or describe times when they felt angry, they probably wouldn't recognize when they experienced anger in their day-to-day life. So, according to this strategy, someone who says, "I am not angry now, and I don't remember getting angry much in the past," would be considered to lack emotional insight. Asking about emotional memories is a highly questionable strategy for distinguishing between lack of emotional experience and lack of awareness of that experience. Few emotional memories might be related to a lack of emotional insight, but it could also stem from a poor memory, a high threshold for labeling a memory or situation as emotional, or maybe just a dull life. Furthermore, responses to general inquiries about memories of emotional experience may or may not translate to awareness of actually occurring emotional experience.

Situational Context

Another strategy for identifying lack of insight involves making inferences about emotional experience from the situational context. Some events or circumstances, such as the death of a spouse, are particularly likely to elicit emotional reactions. According to this strategy, individuals whose current life context involves what most people would view as emotional events, but who don't report much negative emotion, are assumed to lack emotional insight. The situational context strategy is more valid than the emotional memory strategy, because it focuses on current experience. The problem with this strategy is that one person's perception of an emotion-eliciting context may not match another's. Even normatively severe stressors, such as the death of a spouse, may have different meanings and different impact for different individuals, depending on personal or situational factors such as whether the marriage was happy, whether the widowed individual has other close friends, whether the death was expected, etc.

Signs of Emotional Blocking

A third strategy for identifying lack of emotional insight is to look for indicators of blocking when discussing feelings. The most obvious example of this would be direct statements such as "I know I'm feeling something, but I don't know what." Content-related cues could also indicate emotional blocking, as when physical sensations or concrete details are discussed obsessively. More subtle signs of emotional blocking involve linguistic cues suggesting defense, such as pausing before responding, taking back a response ("I didn't mean that!"), or simply avoiding a response (e.g., Horowitz et al., 1993; Mandler, Mandler, Kremen, & Sholiton, 1961). This strategy entails an assumption that blocking behavior indicates the presence of some emotional experience to be blocked. It is possible that some of the more subtle behaviors, such as response latency, could be caused by other factors, such as limited verbal skills.

Covert Indicators of Emotional Experience

The fourth and final strategy for identifying lack of emotional insight is to look for covert signs of emotional experience. These signs might include nonverbal expressive behaviors or, in a laboratory setting, physiological responses. For example, an individual who reports feeling no emotion but shows changes in heart rate or blood pressure or whose facial, vocal, or postural expression indicates signs of emotion in response to some emotion-eliciting cue would be seen as lacking emotional awareness. The problem in using this strategy lies in accurately identifying and interpreting these sometimes subtle signs of emotion.

Undoubtedly the best way to assess the lack of emotional insight is to use multiple indicators of the presence of emotional response coupled with reports of lack of conscious awareness of that response. In a research context this may be done explicitly. In a clinical context, this information may be summarized implicitly in clinical judgment. An experienced clinician can draw upon a variety of sources of information to infer the presence of unrecognized emotion, including information about normative responses, as well as observation of emotional blocking behaviors and nonverbal signs of emotion.

Clinical Judgment

Schedler et al. (1993) recently discussed the unique benefits of subjective clinical judgment in assessment. They argue that clinical judgment is the only "measurement instrument" capable of going beyond manifest content and registering the complex, psychologically important meanings entailed in human communication. In other words, they suggest, it takes a person to really know another person. Schedler et al.'s key point is a criticism of blind reliance on self-report questionnaires. We agree with this criticism, but we also urge caution in reliance upon clinical judgment, particularly in the area of emotional insight. (See Dawes, 1996, and Salovey & Turk, 1991, for extensive discussions of problems with clinical judgment.)

Excessive reliance on clinical judgment concerning emotional experience carries the risk of dictating how another person *should* feel. In the manner of a self-fulfilling prophesy, clients may be forced to conform their emotional experience to therapists' implicit expectations or explicit demands. For example, in the area of bereavement, pervasive beliefs about what constitutes "appropriate" coping can become "requirements" of mourning, even though empirical data show considerable individual variability in response to major losses (see Bonanno et al., 1995; Silver & Wortman, 1980; Wortman & Silver, 1987, 1989, for reviews). These beliefs may lead therapists (or well-meaning friends and family members) to insist that the person experiencing loss express the "right" emotions, in the "right" way, for the "right" amount of time. The prominence of various stage theories, such as the one proposed by Kübler-Ross in her book *On Death an Dying* (1969), led one investigator (Pattison, 1977) to observe, "Dying persons who did not follow these stages were labeled 'deviant,' 'neurotic,' or 'pathological' diers. Clinical personnel became angry at patients who did not move from one stage to the next. . . . I began to observe professional personnel demand that the dying person 'die in the right way' " (p. 242). Consistent with these observations is the exhortation of one theorist (Nemiah, 1957), discussing adjustment to spinal cord injury, who writes, "It is often necessary to confront the patient gently but firmly with the reality of his situation, and to force him into a period of depression while he works out his acceptance of his loss" (p. 146).

It is inherently difficult to discern what is going on inside another person (C. E. Hill, Helms, Spiegel, & Tichenor, 1988; J. Martin, Martin, Mayer, & Sleman, 1986). An individual's feelings are the product of his or her unique constellation of perceptions, beliefs, and experience. Certainly, the observations of a trained therapist are often valuable and can be the basis of important feedback for clients. However, we believe these observations must be tempered by recognition of and respect for each client's perspective. In other words, the idea that a particular client lacks emotional insight should be a lightly held hypothesis. If clinicians see signs of unacknowledged feelings, they should view these as tentative areas for exploration, rather than definite proof of lack of insight. In psychotherapy, the goal is to facilitate clients' self-understanding, rather than to impose therapists' views. The vast majority of the time, when someone says, for example, "I am not feeling angry," that is exactly what it means. Ultimately, each individual is the only possible expert on his or her own emotional experience (cf. Safran & Segal, 1990).

Summary

The examples that we have mentioned in this section have drawn on signs of emotional expression to infer the presence or absence of emotional insight. Clearer, more comprehensive expression indicates greater emotional insight. Lack of expression, particularly coupled with circumstances, behaviors, or involuntary responses indicating the presence of emotional experience, suggests the lack of emotional insight. However, emotional expression is not simply a passive indicator of emotional insight. It can also play a key role in fostering insight.

In the next section, we shift from simply describing emotional insight or its lack to examining the process of acquiring insight. We focus on the role of expression as a means of fostering emotional insight.

THE ROLE OF EXPRESSION IN FOSTERING EMOTIONAL INSIGHT

The way that emotional insight influences expression is obvious: Some degree of insight is usually a necessary precondition for expression. There are exceptions: Some kinds of acting and automatic, script-based behavior (e.g., a flight attendant saying, "I hope you enjoyed your flight") involve expression but don't require recognition of one's true feelings (Hochschild, 1983). Also, biologically based, spontaneous emotional communication is unintentional (Buck, 1989) and can occur without conscious awareness of emotional experience (LeDoux, 1989; 1996). An example of this type of expression without insight is tensing one's body in fear during a car accident, but realizing only afterward that one felt frightened. Fleeting, micro-momentary facial expressions may also constitute instances of expression without insight (e.g., Haggard & Isaacs, 1966). However, deliberate, symbolic, and especially verbal emotional communication usually requires some degree of awareness of one's emotional state (Buck, 1989). This is the basis of the usefulness of expression as a sign of emotional insight, as we described in the previous section.

The reverse causal relationship, the way that expression influences emotional insight, is more complex. Three mechanisms underlie the impact of expression on insight. These are self-observation, verbalization, and social feedback. These three means of gaining insight through expression occur frequently in day-to-day life, and they are also used systematically in a therapeutic context.

Self-Observation

Expression can foster emotional insight through self-perception (Bem, 1972; Laird & Bresler, 1992). Just as observing other people's expression provides information about how they are feeling, observing one's own overt emotional behavior can lead to inferences about one's own emotional states. For example, a young man who notices that he always grins foolishly and drops things when he sees the woman next door may infer that he is attracted to that neighbor. A woman who observes that every day this week she has spent an extended period of time fidgeting and rearranging files on her desk before starting work may realize that her current project makes her feel bored or anxious. Particularly when emotional states are weak or ambiguous, self-observation of one's own emotional behavior can be an important source of information concerning emotional experience.

In a clinical context, therapists sometimes ask clients who are having difficulty identifying their emotional states to notice their nonverbal expressive cues. For example, a client might observe that his jaw is clenched and his hands are tightly gripping the chair while he talks about his wife. These observations might prompt him to revise his assessment that he feels "fine" about his impending divorce. In addition to focusing on current expressive behavior, noticing patterns in expressive behavior across time can also be useful. For instance, a client who is working in therapy on controlling her angry outbursts might find it helpful to look for patterns in the circumstances under which she expresses extreme anger. If she observes that her outbursts occur mostly when her elderly mother refuses her help, she might conclude that these outbursts reflect her feelings of helplessness or fear for her mother's well-being. In this case, therapy needs to address these feelings rather than (or perhaps in addition to) focusing on managing the expression of anger.

Verbalization

Another way in which expression can contribute to emotional insight is through verbalization of feelings. Translating emotions into language changes the way they are experienced. Talking or writing about one's feelings involves bringing them from prereflective to reflective awareness (Collier, 1985): Individuals transform their emotional experience by labeling it, cognitively structuring it, calling attention to certain details rather than others, drawing connections, and actively constructing the meaning of that experience (cf. Harvey, Weber, Galvin, Huszti, & Garnick, 1986; Meichenbaum & Fong, 1993; Pennebaker, 1993b; Weber, Harvey, & Stanley, 1987). Representing emotional experience symbolically, in words, creates a new awareness or understanding of that experience.

Experiential therapists describe a dialectical process between emotional expression and experience: Initially vague emotional experience guides the choice of words used to represent that experience, and the verbal expression of experience, in turn, shapes and gives fuller form to emotional experience (J. C. Watson & Greenberg, 1996). For example, whether a client describes her experience as being "revealed" or being "exposed" carries very different implications for understanding those feelings. The term *revealed* connotes openness and a desire for connection; the term *exposed* connotes threat and a desire for withdrawal.

Social Feedback

A third way in which expression can contribute to emotional insight is by eliciting social feedback. Buck's developmental-interactionist theory (e.g., Buck, 1989, 1991) emphasizes the role of emotional expression in fostering emotional competence. Buck argues that among young children, those who are spontaneously more expressive create an emotionally enriched environment. Their expressivity elicits emotional expression from others, giving them opportunity to observe and learn about emotions from social models. Moreover, their emotional expression elicits "social biofeedback." The caregiver observes the child's expressive behavior and responds to it, thereby helping the child to label and understand her internal emotional experience. To use Buck's example, in response to a child's expression of anger, a caregiver might say, "You're angry. You must be frustrated. Everybody gets frustrated sometimes, but you shouldn't throw blocks at people." This feedback teaches the child that the emotional state she is experiencing is called anger, that it is associated with frustration, that it is a common experience, and that throwing things is not an acceptable expression of anger. More expressive children elicit more of such feedback and thus have more opportunities for emotional education.

Caregivers provide the best opportunity for the development of emotional insight when they accurately label a child's emotional states and recognize and respond appropriately to a child's emotional needs (Stern, 1985). On the other hand, sometimes emotional education is impaired because of inappropriate social feedback. A child whose expression of anger is met with a slap and a "Bad girl!" scolding will be less able to deal with such feelings in the future. She will associate the experience of anger with being "bad" and may feel anxious or guilty when this state is aroused.

Buck's theory focuses on the role of social responses to expression in fostering emotional insight in children, but it is easy to think of examples of the continued relevance of this process in adults: A stranger on the street returns a smile that a woman didn't realize was on her face. A surly clerk reciprocates a man's expression of irritation, thus intensifying and drawing his attention to this annoyance. A coworker, hearing an officemate whistle, comments, "Gee, you're in a good mood this morning!" A husband, after listening to his wife's long, convoluted narrative, perceptively observes, "I think you're jealous." Because of their external perspective, people in the social environment are sometimes better able to observe an individual's expression than that individual is (cf. Kennedy-Moore & Stone, 1999). Having others point out and respond to one's emotional expression, particularly expression of which one is not aware, is an important means of gaining understanding of one's feelings.

The therapeutic relationship provides a unique context for expression-related feedback that can be helpful in acquiring emotional insight (e.g., Safran & Muran, 1995; Safran, 1990a, 1990b). As a participant–observer in the relationship, the therapist can use his or her own feelings and observations to help identify clients' significant or problematic emotional communications and to explore their emotional implications. For example, a therapist might notice and inquire about a client's laughter that seems incongruous with the content of what the client is saying. This inquiry might prompt the client to become aware of feelings of anxiety. Moreover, a therapist's empathic attunement and ability to refrain from responding in a complementary manner to emotional expressions can provide clients with a safe context for expressing and examining their emotional experience. For instance, when a client's expression of anger at the therapist is met with openness and empathic reflection rather than withdrawal or counterattack, the client has an opportunity to elaborate on and understand these feelings.

Summary

In summary, expression can contribute to emotional insight by providing information for self-observation, by verbally creating and transforming the meaning of emotional experience, and by eliciting social feedback. These processes all involve the use of emotional expression as a means of gaining information about one's own emotional experience. They occur in day-to-day life, and they can also be useful in a therapeutic setting.

However, these expression-related processes do not always occur, and they do not always result in the acquisition of emotional insight. People sometimes cry without knowing why, are unable to find words for their feelings, or are oblivious to social feedback. We turn now to a discussion of the conditions required for fostering emotional insight.

PREREQUISITES OF EMOTIONAL INSIGHT

Emotional insight has several necessary prerequisites. First, attention must be focused on internal emotional experience in order to recognize its occurrence. Second, some degree of skill in emotional processing is required to label and appropriately interpret emotional experience. Third, the perception and interpretation of emotional experience must not be blocked or distorted by defensiveness. In this section, we consider these three prerequisites of emotional insight and possible related problems, and we examine their relationship to physical and mental health outcomes. As we describe below, emotional behavior is often a sign of the extent to which these three prerequisites of emotional insight are met.

Attention to Inner Experience

One prerequisite of emotional insight is that attention be focused inward, on oneself. Before one can fully understand one's feelings one has to perceive them when they occur. Focusing attention on one's emotional experience provides the opportunity to notice and reflect upon that experience. However, when inwardly directed attention is rigid or excessive, it can interfere with the ability to respond adaptively to other people or the environment. Because introspection plays a key role in many forms of psychotherapy, it is important to understand when and how it is helpful or harmful. As we describe below, personality research highlights both the benefits and the risks of inwardly directed attention.

Private self-consciousness (PSC) is a personality trait that refers to the tendency to engage in self-focused attention. It involves a propensity to be aware of and reflect upon covert aspects of oneself, such as one's thoughts, feelings, and motives (Fenigstein, Scheier, & Buss, 1975). Sample items assessing PSC are "I'm generally attentive to my inner feelings" and "I'm always trying to figure myself out."

The Benefits of Self-Focused Attention

Individuals high in PSC know themselves well. They give more detailed, accurate, and reliable self-descriptions (e.g., Franzoi, 1983; Nasby, 1989; Turner, 1978) and they place a high value on accurate self-knowledge (Franzoi, Davis, & Markwiese, 1990). Perhaps because they are more experienced or more comfortable with self-reflection, they are also more likely to experience epiphanies or moments of affective insight (Kuiken et al., 1987).

Interpersonally, high-PSC individuals tend to be expressive in that they are more willing to disclose private information to intimate others (M. H. Davis & Franzoi, 1987). Interestingly, a 1-year longitudinal study shows that PSC produces greater self-disclosure, but not the reverse: Greater disclosure did not result in higher levels of PSC (M. H. Davis & Franzoi, 1986). To the extent to which high-PSC individuals self-disclose more, they also report more satisfying intimate relationships. In other words, PSC is associated with greater self-disclosure and greater self-disclosure predicts better relationship satisfaction, but PSC in and of itself is not related to relationship satisfaction (Franzoi, Davis, & Young, 1985).

PSC has also been found to buffer the relationship between stressful life events and illness in two short-term (several weeks) longitudinal studies (Mullen & Suls, 1982; Suls & Fletcher, 1985). One possible explanation for these findings is that high PSC individuals, being more aware of their internal reactions to stressful life events, are more likely to take appropriate corrective action.

The Costs of Self-Focused Attention

In contrast to this picture of high-PSC individuals as paragons of self-understanding and positive adaptation is the very large body of research showing the detrimental effects of chronic self-focused attention (e.g., Ingram, 1990; Nolen-Hoeksema, 1991; Wood, Saltzberg, Neale, Stone, &

Rachmiel, 1990). Focusing on one's negative feelings has the immediate effect of intensifying distress. Studies show that ruminating about one's depressed or angry mood causes these moods to be more severe and/or more prolonged (e.g., Nolen-Hoeksema & Morrow, 1993; Nolen-Hoeksema, Morrow, & Fredrickson, 1993; Rusting & Nolen-Hoeksema, 1998). Chronically focusing on one's distress is also associated with poorer functioning. People whose attention is consumed with how miserable they are feeling don't have the cognitive resources to solve problems, to react flexibly to changes in environmental circumstances, or to recognize and respond sensitively to other people's feelings. High PSC, which entails an enduring tendency to focus on inner experience, including emotional experience, has been implicated in virtually all clinical disorders (Ingram, 1990).

Reconciling the Costs and Benefits of Self-Focused Attention

How can these two contradictory views of the effects of attending to one's feelings be reconciled? On the one hand, some degree of self-focused attention is necessary for self-understanding and adaptive responding to stress. One has to know something is wrong, and know what is wrong, before one can change it (cf. G. E. Schwartz, 1983). On the other hand, focusing attention inward can interfere with perception and adaptive responding to external events. Ingram (1990) argues that self-focused attention is detrimental when it is excessive, sustained, and inflexible. He uses the term *self-absorption* to refer to this type of rigid self-focus that interferes with adaptive coping efforts. Thus PSC is maladaptive when it entails an inability to shift attention from inner experiences to outward circumstances in response to situational demands.

This distinction between flexible and rigid self-focused attention makes intuitive sense, but it doesn't address why certain individuals are unable to shift their attention when necessary. We argue that self-focused attention is adaptive only to the extent that it is associated with emotional insight, because self-focus without insight is likely to be perseverative and distressing. Furthermore, self-focused attention that is accompanied by emotional expression (rather than nonexpression) is more likely to result in emotional insight. We discuss each of these hypotheses below.

Our first premise, that *self-focused attention is only helpful when it produces insight,* is based on our belief that focusing on one's feelings without understanding them is likely to result in perseveration of that inward attention and an increase of distress. Similar to the Zeigarnik effect (Zeigarnik, 1927), in which an unfinished task is hard to put out of one's mind, distressed individuals with only a vague understanding of what they are feeling, or why, are likely to continue to think about this distress, in an effort to figure it out.

Evidence that perceiving one's feelings with less clarity is associated with more enduring preoccupation with distress comes from a study by Salovey et al. (1995). In this study, volunteers were shown a distressing movie about victims of drunk driving. They then listed their thoughts at 30-second intervals in a supposedly unrelated experiment. Those people who had previously indicated that they tend to experience their moods clearly recovered more quickly from the film and listed fewer distressing ruminations. One explanation for these findings is that being able to clearly understand one's feelings (i.e., having greater emotional insight) enhances one's ability to regulate these feelings. In contrast, poor understanding of one's feelings increases the chances of being caught in an aversive ruminative process, trying to figure out one's internal state.

Further evidence for this lack-of-insight/rumination/distress hypothesis comes from studies examining components of private self-consciousness. Two factors have been identified composing PSC (Mittal & Balasubramanian, 1987): *Internal State Awareness,* which refers to being aware of and attentiveness to one's own thoughts and feelings, and *Self-Reflectiveness,* which involves attempts to clarify or understand one's thoughts and feelings. Greater dysphoria and poorer self-esteem are associated with more Self-Reflectiveness, but not more Internal State Awareness (Conway & Giannopoulos, 1993; Conway, Giannopoulos, Csank, & Mendelson, 1993). In other words, being aware of one's feelings is not distressing, but chronically trying to figure out one's feelings is distressing.

Other studies show that a less certain sense of self is linked to neuroticism and low self-esteem (e.g., Campbell, 1990; Eysenck, 1973). Schwarz and Clore (1988) found that not knowing the cause for one's negative mood makes it more likely that that mood will negatively affect one's self-evaluation. Interestingly, most instances of depression do not have a clear precipitating event (Lloyd, 1980), and many clinical interventions involve providing clients with a plausible and controllable causal explanation for their emotional states (Kennedy-Moore, 1999). All of these studies are consistent with the idea that when self-focused attention stems from a lack of self-understanding, it tends to be perseverative, and it compounds distress.

Our second premise, that *self-focused attention accompanied by expression is more likely to result in emotional insight,* is based on our belief that emotional expression, particularly in a social context, clarifies feelings and limits rumination. When merely thinking about one's feelings, it is possible to go around in obsessive mental circles or jump sporadically from one thought to another loosely related thought. In contrast, talking to someone or writing about one's feelings inherently involves structuring and organizing one's thoughts about these feelings. These thoughts become more orderly and less perseverative. The process of trying to explain one's feelings to someone else necessarily involves clarifying these feelings in one's own mind. Numerous studies have found that having the opportunity to talk or write about one's feelings leads to less rumination and fewer intrusive thoughts about those feelings (see M. A. Greenberg, 1995, for a review).

Expression can help limit rumination, when it involves moving from lower to higher levels of emotional awareness, thereby fostering greater emotional understanding. Expression that persists at the lowest levels of emotional awareness, that is merely a symptom of perseverative attention to distress, is not likely to be helpful. It may even be harmful because it focuses attention on the distress and interferes with functioning. In other words, no amount of saying "I feel bad" is likely to help, but saying and realizing "I feel lonely and unfulfilled in this relationship" could translate directly into adaptive coping efforts.

Thus, attention to inner experience is a necessary but not sufficient condition for emotional insight. To understand one's feelings, one has to notice their occurrence. But, just noticing feelings is not enough. Some degree of skill in comprehending these feelings is also needed in order to gain emotional insight.

Skill in Emotional Processing

A second prerequisite of emotional insight is skill in emotional processing. To fully understand one's feelings, one must have the ability to label and interpret these feelings accurately. Like introspection, efforts to label and verbalize feelings are often an important part of psychotherapy. However, some clients find it very difficult to describe their feelings.

Alexithymia is an extreme instance of the inability to articulate feelings. This trait, which literally means "no words for feelings," refers to a cognitive-affective style involving (1) difficulty identifying feelings and distinguishing between feelings and bodily sensations, (2) difficulty communicating subjective feelings, and (3) concrete, externally oriented, bluntly reality-based thinking, associated with impoverished imagination and a general lack of dreams or fantasies (e.g., Taylor, Ryan, & Bagby, 1985). Larry, from the anecdote at the beginning of this chapter, is an example of an alexithymic individual. He is aware that he feels "bad," but he is at a complete loss in terms of understanding more precisely what he feels or why. It seems likely that his distress is related to his recent relationship breakup, but Larry does not make this connection. Instead, he feels vaguely confused by his distress and focuses only on possible causes that are very concrete and immediate (i.e., lack of food, uncomfortable clothes).

The term *alexithymia* was originally coined by Sifneos (1973), based on his clinical observations of patients suffering from psychosomatic diseases. However, early measures of alexithymia were poorly designed, unreliable, and largely unvalidated. Thus, any findings with these early scales are highly questionable. More recently, Taylor and his colleagues (Taylor et al., 1985) have developed the Toronto Alexithymia Scale (TAS), using empirical scale construction techniques. Two revised versions of the TAS have also been developed—the TAS-R (Taylor, Bagby, & Parker, 1992) and the TAS-20 (Bagby, Parker, & Taylor, 1994; Bagby, Taylor, & Parker, 1994). The latest version, the TAS-20, shows the best psychometric scale properties, but all versions of the TAS have demonstrated good reliability as well as convergent, discriminant, and criterion validity, and thus provide meaningful results. Sample items from the TAS-20 are "I am often confused about what emotion I am feeling," "I have feelings that I can't quite identify," and "It is difficult for me to find the right words for my feelings."

Because adequate measures of alexithymia are relatively new, most of the longitudinal studies necessary to evaluate the consequences of alexithymia have not been done. However, cross-sectional data provide some intriguing findings. In terms of psychological outcomes, alexithymia is much more common among psychiatric outpatients than in the general population, and it is associated with general dysphoria (Taylor, Parker, Bagby, & Acklin, 1992). Alexithymia is also prevalent among patients with eating disorders and substance use disorders, which are thought to be conditions associated with poor ability to discriminate and modulate affect (Taylor et al., 1991). The original clinical conceptualization of alexithymia was intended to identify patients who responded poorly to insight-oriented psychotherapy. There is indirect evidence of this in that alexithymics score low on psychological mindedness, and lack of psychological mindedness has been found to be related to poorer psychotherapy outcome (Bagby, Taylor, & Parker, 1994; Conte et al., 1990).

One underresearched area is the interpersonal functioning of alexithymics. Clinical lore says that therapists tend to find alexithymics difficult and boring (e.g., Taylor, 1984). (Therapists' lack of enthusiasm for alexithymic clients may be partially responsible for their poor prognosis in psychotherapy.) There is also some suggestion that alexithymics may be impulsive and/or dependent (Taylor et al., 1991), perhaps in an effort to modulate their vague feelings of distress. It seems likely that alexithymics' gross deficits in emotional understanding and communication would cause difficulties in their interpersonal relationships, as well.

In terms of physical outcomes, alexithymics report more somatic symptoms and bodily concerns than nonalexithymics. There is also some evidence of alexithymia being associated with somatization (Acklin & Alexander, 1988) and rheumatoid arthritis (Fernandez, Sriram, Rajkumar, & Chandrasekar, 1989). The traditional psychoanalytic view of somatization is that physical symptoms represent attempts to resolve internal conflict and serve as a defense against painful affect (e.g., Kellner, 1990). This is clearly *not* the case with alexithymics, since they report both dysphoria and physical symptoms. Physiological and longitudinal studies are needed to sort out the relationship between physical and psychological symptoms in alexithymia. Are alexithymics' physical symptoms the cause or the consequence of psychological distress? Are their physical symptoms actual indices of illness or are they simply mislabeled somatic signs of psychological distress? (See Goldman, Kraemer, & Salovey, 1996, and Stretton & Salovey, 1997, for general discussions of the relationship between emotional experience and physical symptom reporting.)

Alexithymia involves both a lack of emotional insight and diminished emotional expression. Conceptually, in terms of the model presented in Chapter 1, these difficulties stem from skill deficits in emotional processing rather than a motivated lack of awareness of emotional experience. (We consider motivated lack of awareness in the next section.) It is not that alexithymics consciously or unconsciously block awareness of painful feelings. Rather, they have difficulty understanding and processing *any* emotions. Larry readily acknowledged that he felt "out of sorts," but he was completely unable to understand or articulate his feelings.

Several types of evidence support a nonmotivational, skill-deficit view of the lack of emotional expression and emotional insight in alexithymia. The simplest form of evidence is that alexithymia has been found to be unrelated to self-report measures of defensiveness (Graham, 1987; L. A. King, Emmons, & Woodley, 1992).

A second form of evidence for a nonmotivational view involves the content of alexithymic deficits. Alexithymia involves the lack of awareness of positive as well as negative emotions. In both clinical observations and empirical findings, alexithymia has been linked to a constricted ability to experience pleasant emotions as well as an increased likelihood of experiencing diffuse, poorly differentiated, unpleasant emotional states (Bagby, Taylor, & Parker, 1994; Krystal, 1988). Defensive processes are unlikely to be necessary as protection against positive feelings. Moreover, alexithymics' limited emotional understanding extends to other people as well as themselves. They show poorer ability to recognize facial expressions of emotions (mentioned in Bagby, Taylor, & Parker, 1994). Again, defensive processes would not be necessary in dealing with others' emotions.

A third form of evidence for a nonmotivational view involves the quality of alexithymic deficits. The limited emotional expression of alexithymics is characterized by struggle rather than denial. Alexithymic individuals do not minimize the importance of disclosing personal information to others, but they report significantly more difficulty in discussing personal feelings and problems than do nonalexithymic individuals (Loiselle & Dawson, 1988). Moreover, although their communication is emotionally constricted (e.g., L. A. King et al., 1992), alexithymics do express their feelings to some extent. Clinically, they may show nonverbal signs of emotion, and they may even use words such as *sad* or *angry*, but they are unable to elaborate on these feelings. They may even demonstrate sudden, apparently random, outbursts of rage or sobbing. However, they are unable to connect these feeling words or behaviors with specific memories or situations or with accompanying physical sensations, and they fail to derive any understanding from them (Nemiah, 1978; Nemiah, Freyberger, & Sifneos, 1976; Nemiah & Sifneos, 1970). In defensive processes, we would expect a complete lack of public acknowledgment of threatening feelings.

Thus, alexithymia refers to a limited ability to process emotion rather than motivated avoidance of painful feelings. We consider motivated lack of emotional insight in the next section.

Lack of Defensiveness

"Quit that howling!" he demands. "Somebody do something about that kid or I'll give him a reason to cry!" Eight-year old Dora moves quickly past her father and picks up her little brother, Tommy. Tommy buries his face in her hair and continues to sob, loudly. Dora carries him out of the room. She sits down in their special spot, behind the door, with Tommy on her lap. Mom and Dad are fighting, again. Dad is yelling and swearing and throwing things. Mom is yelling and crying. They are both drunk. Pretty soon he will start punching her. Then Dad will leave, and Mom will pass out on the couch. That's the way it usually goes.

Tommy is still whimpering. Dora pulls her shirtsleeve down over her hand and uses it to wipe his nose. Softly, so that only the two of them can hear, she starts to sing the song she made up for Tommy, "Don't cry. Everything's all right. Don't cry. Everything's all right." She can feel Tommy's body relax against her as he sucks noisily on his thumb. They just have to wait until Dad leaves. Then it will be safe to come out. "Don't cry. Everything's all right."

A third prerequisite of emotional insight is that the perception and interpretation of emotional experience not be blocked or distorted by motivational factors. We will refer broadly to the motivated lack of awareness of emotional experience as defensiveness. In the anecdote above, Dora's song is as much an effort to convince herself that she feels no fear or vulnerability as it is an attempt to soothe her little brother. No one would suggest that it would be a good idea for Dora to "get in touch with her feelings" at this time. She is a child, dependent on grossly inadequate parents, and responsible for a younger sibling. The issue for her is survival, not self-understanding. Under these harrowing circumstances, pushing her feelings out of awareness is probably the most adaptive thing she can do. We suspect, however, that many years of practice denying her feelings will make it difficult for her to respond adaptively to her feelings in later life, under more benign circumstances. Negative feelings, if she acknowledges them at all, will feel threatening and dangerous to her. She will have difficulty opening up to others and cultivating intimacy. In other words, the extreme coping strategy that is necessary to her survival as a child is likely to interfere with her functioning as an adult.

Emotional defensiveness is a self-protective response to feelings that are perceived as not just unpleasant but unbearable and highly threatening to one's sense of self (Weinberger, 1990). It can take many forms. We will discuss three of them, which entail excluding feelings from awareness with varying degrees of completeness. One form of emotional defensiveness involves a deconstructed state, in which emotions are processed at only the most primitive level. A more subtle form of emotional defensiveness involves emotional substitution, in which painful emotions are transformed into less threatening feelings. Finally, an enduring form of emotional defensiveness involves a repressive coping style, in which awareness of all negative feelings and unacceptable impulses is avoided. We describe these three forms of defensiveness in order to help therapists recognize some of the processes that can interfere with the acquisition of emotional insight, to perceive the role of emotional expression in these processes, and to understand their consequences for well-being.

Cognitive Deconstruction

Baumeister has articulated a theory of cognitive deconstruction as a means of escaping self-awareness (Baumeister, 1990a, 1990b; Heatherton & Baumeister, 1991). Cognitive deconstruction involves limiting self-awareness by processing information only in a very restricted, concrete way. When life circumstances lead individuals to view themselves as fundamentally flawed, inadequate, or incompetent, self-awareness generates excruciatingly painful affect. Individuals are then motivated to escape from self-focus and the accompanying painful feelings. Deliberately *not* thinking about oneself, through brute cognitive force, is difficult. Trying to do so may make the self more salient (cf. Wegner et al., 1987), and paradoxically, monitoring one's efforts to avoid self-awareness implies self-awareness. Thus, rather than attempting to redirect attention in order to escape self-awareness, individuals may do so by limiting the cognitive level at which they process information. They avoid meaningful, integrative, interpretive thought and instead process information only in terms of unelaborated stimuli, immediate sensations, and simple associations. It is as if individuals in a deconstructed state are telling themselves, "Don't think; don't feel; just exist." They attempt to immerse themselves in the concrete, trivial details of the present in order to block out self-awareness.

There are a number of consequences of cognitive deconstruction. From the individual's perspective, the goal and the most important consequence of deconstruction is a deadening of emotional responses. Neither positive nor negative affect occurs spontaneously. Trained clinicians may be able to detect some signs of negative affect, but on the surface individuals in a deconstructed state appear completely nonexpressive. Their emotions are available, but they struggle to keep them out of awareness by refusing to engage in meaningful thought that might foster emotional insight. Sometimes, cognitive efforts at deconstruction are insufficient to reduce negative feelings to a tolerable level, and individuals may resort to physical strategies such as consuming excessive alcohol or binge eating in order to bolster their efforts to avoid emotional awareness.

A second consequence of deconstruction is passivity. Because they reject meaningful thought, individuals in a deconstructed state cannot engage in active efforts to solve their problems. Such efforts would require facing the problems, through examination of the implications of existing circumstance, planning, goal setting, and self-evaluation. All of these are incompatible with the desire to stay narrowly and concretely focused on the present in order to avoid painful feelings. Thus, deconstruction is likely to be associated with diminished coping abilities.

A third consequence of cognitive deconstruction is behavioral disinhibition. Lack of self-awareness removes certain inner restraints that depend on perception of emotional experience. Normally, behaviors that seem irrational or contrary to one's values evoke feelings of discomfort or distress. People in a deconstructed state do not recognize or process these internal emotional warning signals, so these behaviors do not seem objectionable. Examples of such behaviors, which are associated with lack of self-awareness and disinhibition, include risk taking, sexual masochism, and suicide. These behaviors may occur simply as a result of the lack of awareness of normal inhibitions, or they may entail extreme efforts to avoid emotional self-awareness, which seem acceptable because of disinhibition. Thus, in addition to impairing coping efforts, a state of cognitive deconstruction may lead to self-destructive behaviors.

Baumeister (1990b) emphasizes several important aspects of cognitive deconstruction:

1. It is a transient state, rather than a chronic disposition. Usually people emerge from this state when they construct new, more benign, interpretations for events. However, it is not clear how this transition occurs.
2. It seems to be a fairly deliberate strategy. Baumeister states that deconstruction may even be a normative response to personal crises and the accompanying intense negative feelings.
3. It is unlikely to be entirely successful: Awareness of meaning and affect are extremely impoverished during deconstruction, but not altogether eliminated.

Emotional Substitution

A second means of avoiding awareness of painful emotions is to focus on other feelings. Emotional substitution involves replacing one emotional reaction with another less threatening one. Like cognitive deconstruction, it tends to be a state rather than a trait. That is, this strategy is evoked in response to a particularly painful emotional experience rather than being an enduring, pervasive personality characteristic. However, substitution entails less conscious employment and less broad application than deconstruction. Deconstruction involves an attempt to block awareness of all feelings, whereas substitution is directed at blocking awareness of a particular emotion or emotions. In this sense, emotional substitution is more like an emotional blind spot rather than a wholesale lack of emotional insight. Behaviorally, whereas lack of emotional insight in deconstruction is associated with lack of emotional expression, in substitution it is associated with a great deal of emotional expression.

Based on clinical observation, Lewis (1992) describes a specific form of emotional substitution, in which the painful emotion of shame is bypassed by converting it to sadness or anger. Shame implies a focus on the self and a global evaluation of the self as profoundly inadequate. Phenomenologically, it is associated with a desire to hide or disappear, intense discomfort, confusion, and disruption of ongoing activity. The shamed person can't think, can't talk, can't act. The experience of shame is so aversive that individuals are highly motivated to avoid acknowledging it. One way to do so is to focus on other feelings to block out awareness of shame. The occurrence of shame is marked by a nonverbal wince or "wordless shock," but then is quickly transformed into another emotion. Because they share some features with shame, sadness and anger are the most likely candidates for this substitution. Although sadness and anger are also unpleasant emotions, they are not paralyzing like shame, and they carry less devastating implications for the self.

L. S. Greenberg and Safran (1987) discuss emotional substitution more broadly, also drawing from clinical observation. They identify three classes of emotional expression: *Primary emotional reactions* convey biologically based, basic emotions, which provide adaptive information for functioning. Often, clients entering therapy are unaware of these underlying feelings. *Secondary emotional reactions,* which include emotional substitution, are defensive coping efforts aimed at self-protection. These feelings are readily available to consciousness. Expression of such feelings may have the quality of a well-rehearsed, often-repeated litany. Even though these feelings may be negative, and may motivate clients to seek therapy, there is a sense of comfort and familiarity with these feelings. The third class of emotional expression, *instrumental emotional reactions,* involves efforts to influence others, such as expressing sadness to gain sympathy or anger to avoid responsibility. This last type of emotional reaction entails a lack of correspondence between overt emotional expression and covert emotional experience. It is easily noticed and controlled by clients.

In therapy, evocation or intensification of secondary emotional reactions is not helpful and is often harmful. In contrast, evocation of primary emotional reactions elicits responses similar to those described in moments of affective insight (Kuiken et al., 1987) and results in therapeutic change. The primary emotions are felt with a profound sense of authenticity. Recognition and expression of these emotions leads to increased motivation, improved interpersonal communication, and greater understanding, all of which translate into improved problem solving and better general functioning. Thus, the therapist's goal is to use nonverbal cues and clinical judgment to distinguish between primary and secondary emotional reactions in order to explore authentic emotional responses, and promote adaptive awareness and use of the information entailed in these reactions (L. S. Greenberg & Johnson, 1990).

Emotional substitution is intriguing because it involves using emotional expression to avoid emotional awareness. In all the other instances we have mentioned in this chapter, expression and insight have positively covaried. In this case, they are inversely related. Expression of the substituted emotion is used to drown out awareness of the primary emotion. Essentially, emotional substitution involves creating too much emotional noise to hear how one really feels. The cost of emotional substitution, however, is that it entails misdirection of attention and coping efforts. As long as attention is focused on the substitute emotion, the underlying issues or difficulties can't be addressed.

Repressive Coping Style

The last form of emotional defensiveness that we describe is repressive coping style. Repressors have a strong desire to maintain a self-perception that they experience little negative emotion, despite physiological and behavioral indications that they feel very distressed (see Weinberger, 1990, for a review). This form of defensiveness seems to be a stable personality trait rather than a transitory strategy. Like emotional substitution, it tends to be employed without conscious intent. However, its application is more pervasive than emotional substitution, since it is aimed at blocking not just a specific painful emotion but all negative emotions and unacceptable impulses.

Repressors are characterized by oversocialization and overcontrol of impulses and affect. In the original study identifying repressive copers (Weinberger, Schwartz, & Davidson, 1979), college student volunteers completed a trait measure of anxiety as well as the Marlowe–Crowne (MC) scale (Crowne & Marlowe, 1964), which is a self-report measure of defensiveness.[1] The MC scale contains items reflecting behaviors and responses that are culturally sanctioned but improbable, such as "I never hesitate to go out of my way to help someone," "I am always courteous, even to people who are disagreeable," and "I have never intensely disliked anyone." MC scores were used to classify volunteers who reported little anxiety into two groups: truly Low-Anxious individuals (low anxiety plus low MC scores) versus defensive Repressors (low anxiety plus high MC scores).[2] In response to laboratory stressors, Repressors showed greater behavioral and physiological signs of anxiety compared to truly Low-Anxious individuals.[3] In fact, Repressors showed even greater signs of anxiety than a third group of moderately High-Anxious individuals (high anxiety plus low MC scores). Numerous other studies have documented similar findings among Repressors of greater than average physiological or behavioral responses to stress coupled with less than average self-report of discomfort.

In terms of emotional behavior, Repressive coping style is unrelated to global measure of self-reported expressiveness (L. A. King et al., 1992). Instead, Repressive coping entails a more targeted form of nonexpression, involving an unwillingness to acknowledge the experience of negative emotions (Weinberger & Davidson, 1994). In a study of facial expression while watching a stressful videotape, Levenson and Mades (1980) noted that Repressors maintained greater overt composure compared to Low-Anxious individuals, who were more facially expressive. T. L. Newton, Haviland, and Contrada (1996) observed that, compared to Nonrepressors, Repressors show more social smiles (i.e., smiling with the mouth but not the eyes) when asked to disclose their most undesirable characteristic while supposedly being watched by an audience. However, under some circumstances, Repressors may show signs of expressive leakage, indicating high levels of (unacknowledged) anxiety (see earlier discussion on identifying lack of emotional insight). Asendorpf and Scherer (1983) observed that when competing task demands make it difficult for Repressors to focus attention on their facial expressions, they actually show greater facial expressions of anxiety than Low-Anxious individuals. Other investigators have found that Repressors tend to show paralinguistic signs of anxiety such as stuttering (Kiecolt & McGrath, 1979; Weinberger et al., 1979).

In general, Repressors act as if they do not know and do not want to know that their negative emotional reactions are often stronger than their self-reports indicate. It is as if they have erased the boundary between what they believe they should feel and what they actually feel (Horney, 1950). Experiencing especially low levels of negative affect is central to their identity. Instructions or experimental conditions designed to encourage honest self-report and discourage lying do not change Repressors' answers. In fact, being stressed tends to increase Repressors' defensiveness. Participating in a stressful laboratory task leads Repressors, but not other volunteers, to claim even lower levels of trait anxiety compared to pretask assessments

(Weinberger et al., 1979). In one study (Mosher, 1965), participants with high MC scores (who are primarily Repressors) were more likely than low scorers to risk offending a high-status therapist by denying unflattering test assessments. Weinberger and Davidson (1994) quote one Repressor who responded to feedback about his elevated heart rate during a stressful task by saying, "I'm hard pressed to say there is any logical reason for your finding that my heart rate was elevated. Maybe it was random variation" (p. 605).

In terms of physical consequences, repressive coping style has been linked to greater risk of physical illness and exacerbation of health problems such as cancer, asthma, and hypertension (see G. E. Schwartz, 1990, for a review). This could be the result of physiological processes involving excessive release of stress hormones and/or immunosuppression. Or, it could stem from behavioral mechanisms. In keeping with their desire to avoid threat, Repressors are likely to delay seeking medical diagnosis or treatment.

The psychological consequences of repressive coping are more subtle. In some ways, Repressors seem to be functioning extraordinarily well. They report few psychological symptoms, and they show a lower lifetime prevalence of psychiatric disorder compared to Nonrepressors (R. D. Lane, Merikangas, Schwartz, Huang, & Prusoff, 1990). However, some studies suggest that Repressors may experience interpersonal difficulties related to lack of assertiveness, poor empathy, and diminished ability to accurately recognize and predict their own and others' behavior (e.g., Kiecolt-Glaser & Murray, 1980; Nielsen & Fleck, 1981).

In our opinion, the greatest psychological cost of repressive coping has to do with the grim self-control it entails. Repressors' rigid preoccupation with denying distress seems to interfere with their ability to fully experience and enjoy life. Weinberger et al. (1979) asked Repressors and Nonrepressors to provide open-ended self-descriptions. Statements by Repressors reflected concern with self-control and appropriate, even dutiful behavior: "I do not get upset easily"; "I like to deal with people and objects on a nontrivial level"; "not overly worried; I reason rationally"; "I can make an important contribution to humanity." These self-descriptions contrast starkly with the open, happy, vital self-descriptions of the truly Low-Anxious individuals, which included "enjoying life," "interact with people easily and naturally," "a diverse person who enjoys doing active things." In another study (Tublin, Bartholomew, & Weinberger, 1987) peer ratings of Repressors were found to echo these self-reports of being low in expression of negative affect without being particularly high in positive affect. Although this type of stern joylessness and effortful self-control may not interfere with day-to-day functioning or prompt Repressors to seek therapy, we believe that there is more to mental health than simply not being upset (cf. Langston, 1994).

CONCLUSION

In summary, although lack of awareness of one's feelings may be adaptive in some instances, such as in a short-term crisis or unusually traumatic circumstances (G. E. Schwartz, 1990), in general, greater emotional insight is associated with better intrapersonal and interpersonal functioning. Recognizing and understanding one's feelings facilitates coping efforts and contributes to better interpersonal relationships.

The relationship between emotional expression and emotional insight is complex. In some cases, expression is simply a consequence, a direct sign of the presence of emotional insight. In other cases expression is a cause of emotional insight, fostering emotional understanding through self-observation, verbalization, or social feedback. In still other cases, certain forms of emotional expression may be a sign of lack of insight. For instance, when expression involves perseverative attention to poorly understood emotional distress, such as repeated expressions of "I feel bad," it indicates a lack of emotional understanding. Expression can also be used as a means of defensively avoiding emotional awareness through emotional substitution, such as when anger is expressed to avoid acknowledging feelings of sadness.

The implication of all of this is that when clients show deficits in emotional insight, it is important for therapists to determine whether these deficits are related to a lack of attention to inner experience, to skill deficits in emotional processing, or to a motivated lack of awareness of emotional experience. Therapists need to assess the role of emotional expression or nonexpression in contributing to or correcting a lack of emotional insight. When emotional expression enables individuals to label and understand their emotions, and to extract information from them, it fosters emotional insight, directs coping efforts, and should lead to enhanced well-being. When expression persists at the lowest levels of emotional awareness, or when it disguises genuine feelings, it is not related to emotional insight. In these cases, emotional expression may be harmful because it merely intensifies negative feelings and interferes with functioning.

NOTES

1. The MC scale was originally developed as a measure of socially desirable response bias. The developers wanted to identify people who answered questionnaires by saying what they thought was the "right" or socially desirable answer rather than answering truthfully. However, subsequent investigations showed that, rather than measuring a response bias, the MC scale actually taps a substantive individual difference in defensiveness and protection of self-esteem involving rigid standards of self-control (Crowne & Marlowe, 1964; Weinberger, 1990; Weinberger & Davidson, 1994).

2. This method of identifying Repressors can be questioned on psychometric grounds because the two component measures, the MC scale and the Taylor Manifest Anxiety scale measure are not orthogonal ($r = .19$, $p < .05$; Turvey & Salovey, 1993). This overlap may stem from limitations of the measures, or it may indicate that many people who are especially low in anxiety also tend to be Repressors. We believe that the mountain of evidence supporting the validity of the MC scale as a measure of Defensiveness, either alone or in combination with the Taylor Manifest Anxiety scale, warrants our attention (see Weinberger, 1990, for a review). Weinberger also has a newer measure of defensiveness—the Defensiveness scale of the Weinberger Adjustment Inventory (Weinberger, 1991; Weinberger & Schwartz, 1990)—which looks promising in terms of scale properties, such as having a normal distribution and internally consistent items (Turvey & Salovey, 1993), but as yet there is little research with it.

3. The heightened autonomic reactivity to negative emotional stimuli that occurs in Repressors is *not* characteristic of alexithymic individuals (Wehmer, Brejnak, Lumley, & Stettner, 1995).

4

The "Shoulds," "Oughts," and "Musts" of Emotional Behavior: Expressive Goals and Values

INTRODUCTION

With the possible exception of sexual activity, no other behavior is more subject to proscriptive beliefs and evaluative judgments than emotional expression. We see this in *broad cultural dicta* such as "Keep a stiff upper lip" or "Let it all hang out." We see it in *situational norms* or "display rules" (e.g., Ekman, 1972; Hochschild, 1983; H. S. Friedman & Miller-Herringer, 1991) such as "It's important to cry at a funeral, but never cry at work" and in the negative evaluations by others when such situational norms are violated (Heise, 1989). Moreover, we see it in our *personal goals and values* concerning how we behave emotionally. Do we generally prefer to be emotionally discreet or more open? How comfortable are we being the center of attention? Which is more salient to us when developing personal relationships: the potential risks of vulnerability from self-disclosure or the potential rewards of intimacy from sharing our feelings? The answers to these and other questions indicate what sort of emotional behavior we consider to be desirable. They represent our subjective "shoulds," "oughts," and "musts" concerning expression and nonexpression.

Our focus in this chapter is on describing the sorts of expression-related goals people can have and the consequences of having these goals. We use the term *goals* to mean cognitive representations of desired states that reflect an individual's values or ideals (cf. Pervin, 1989). Expressive goals and values pertain to the reflection component of emotion (see Chapter 2), which entails thoughts about emotional responses. In terms of the process model of emotional expression presented in Chapter 1, this chapter

91

concerns the steps involving evaluation of emotional responses and perception of the social context.

In the next section, we provide some background concerning theoretical links between emotional behavior and goals. We then describe various goals associated with expression or nonexpression. We discuss emotional behavior in the context of goal-based models of personality, and we identify a number of personality traits associated with particular goals and particular patterns of emotional behavior. Finally, we look at goal-related problems involving emotional behavior. We consider the consequences of extreme goals, failed goals, and conflicting goals, and we describe the clinical implications of these difficulties.

THEORETICAL LINKS BETWEEN EMOTIONAL EXPRESSION AND GOALS

Recent work in social psychology and emotion theory has focused on the links between affect and goals (see L. L. Martin & Tesser, 1996). Most of this work looks at the informational and motivational functions of emotional *experience*. The quality and intensity of emotional experience can provide information about the salience of a particular goal (e.g., Frijda, 1986; R. S. Lazarus, 1991; Roseman, Wiest, & Swartz, 1994; Singer & Salovey, 1993) or the status of goal-directed efforts (e.g., Carver, Lawrence, & Scheier, 1996). For example, according to R. S. Lazarus (1991), the feeling of compassion informs individuals that they are moved by another's suffering and want to help; the feeling of jealousy says that they resent a third party for the loss or threat to another's affection; the feeling of happiness means that they perceive that they are making reasonable progress toward a goal. Emotional experience can also energize goal-directed behavior or determine one's commitment to achieving a particular goal (e.g., Higgins, 1997; Singer & Salovey, 1996). A student who feels moderately anxious before a test is more strongly motivated to study than other students who feel either confident of their knowledge or unconcerned about their performance.

By extension, emotional *expression* can also provide information about goals and motivate goal-directed behavior by helping people to recognize and process their emotional experience. For example, a woman in a troubled marriage may find that talking about her feelings with a friend helps her to clarify what sort of relationship she really wants and to bolster her resolve to act in ways that can create this type of relationship.

However, in addition to these informational and motivational functions, expression is also linked to goals in a more direct way: Emotional behavior can be a means of achieving or failing to achieve certain goals. When we cry, or yell, or gaze adoringly at another person, we not only communicate how we are feeling, we also communicate how we would like the other person to react, and we often evoke some sort of corresponding emotional response in that person (cf. Benjamin, 1996; Kiesler, 1991). Through our emotional behavior, we can elicit support or push people away. Expression and nonexpression are means of creating, destroying, or changing relationships (see Chapters 6 and 7).

We believe that understanding people's goals and values pertaining to emotional behavior is critically important for several reasons. First, expressive goals and values influence whether and how people express their feelings. For instance, people with negative attitudes toward expression, who endorse statements such as "I think you should always keep your feelings under control," "I think you ought not to burden other people with your problems," and "I think getting emotional is a sign of weakness" are less likely than other people to seek social support (Joseph et al., 1994). Expression-related beliefs can also determine qualitative aspects of expression, such as whether a husband shows his love for his wife by holding her hand during a romantic moonlit walk or by building shelves for her.

Second, expressive goals and values are important because they determine the meaning that expression or nonexpression carries for particular individuals. For example, after bursting into tears, expression-related beliefs might lead one person to feel ashamed of crying while another person accepts this as a natural and desirable response to distress. Expressive goals and values influence not only our interpretation of our own emotional behavior, but also how we react to other people's emotional behavior. Suppose that while on a first date with a woman, a man makes an intimate self-disclosure about his feelings of loss following the recent death of his mother. Depending on her own expressive values, the woman might interpret his self-disclosure as a positive sign of openness, sensitivity, and trust, or she might perceive it as a negative sign of poor emotional control or a premature bid for intimacy.

Finally, expressive goals and values are important for clinical understanding and therapeutic intervention. Understanding clients' emotional behavior requires that we see it in the context of their expression-related beliefs. Knowing about these beliefs may help guide clinical interventions. As we have pointed out in previous chapters, therapists should *not* assume that "more" expression is always good for all clients. R. S. Lazarus and Folkman (1984) note that coping strategies, such as expression or non-expression, that are inconsistent with one's values "are likely to be used reluctantly or without conviction and are likely to fail" (p. 189). Sometimes this means that therapists need to devise and implement treatment plans in a way that is consistent with a particular client's expressive goals and values (see discussions by Safran & Muran, 1995, and J. C. Watson & Greenberg, 1995, on agreement between therapists and clients on therapeutic goals and tasks). Other times, a client's expressive goals and beliefs

themselves are a focus for clinical intervention. As we describe later, helping clients to articulate their expression-related beliefs can enable clients to
understand the influence of these beliefs on their own emotional behavior
and their responses to others. It can also help them to revise these beliefs, if
necessary.

So far, we have talked about expression-related goals in broad terms,
focusing on their theoretical importance. In the next section, we look more
specifically at the types of goals that people might hope to achieve through
their emotional behavior.

GOALS ASSOCIATED WITH EXPRESSIVE
AND NONEXPRESSIVE STRATEGIES

Goal-Based Models of Personality

Goal-based models of personality (e.g., Miller & Read, 1987; Emmons,
1986, 1992; Emmons, King, & Sheldon, 1993; Pervin, 1989; see also
Baxter, 1987, for a related communications perspective) see behavior as
strategic, aimed at particular goals, and reflecting particular values. Stable
personality traits involve specific, enduring patterns of strategies, goals,
and values, whereas within-person variability in behavior can stem from
situational differences in the salience of particular goals (e.g., wanting to
appear confident at work but wanting to confide worries at home) or in the
availability of coping resources required to achieve certain goals (e.g., being
too tired or too emotionally distraught to focus on one's usual concerns
about making a good impression on others). Most (if not all) personality
traits can be understood within a goal-based framework. However, our
concern is with personality traits and goals associated with expression or
nonexpression.

Table 4.1 lists examples of a number of personality traits corresponding to particular patterns of expressive strategies, goals, and values. This
list is not exhaustive. Undoubtedly, other goals as well as other traits are
relevant to emotional behavior. Our point is to indicate that emotional behavior can serve a variety of goals and to illustrate how various personality
traits can be understood as involving a particular combination of expressive strategies, goals, and values.

Before we consider the contents of Table 4.1 in detail, we want to
make several general observations. First, the expression-related goals in this
table are relational—they refer to either how people want to interact with
others or what they want to gain from their relationships. This focus on relational goals is consistent with our emphasis throughout this book on the
interpersonal consequences of expression, as well as evidence that personality traits are best illustrated in an interpersonal context (Brokaw &
McLemore, 1991). Second, the goals listed in Table 4.1 are universal (to

TABLE 4.1. Patterns of Expressive Strategies, Goals, and Values

Expressive strategy	Goal	Value	Trait
Expression	Attention	I like to be the center of attention. Passion and drama make life richer.	Charismatic; Histrionic
Expression	Intimacy	Getting close to others and sharing at a deep level makes life meaningful.	Opener
Nonexpression	Self-Protection	It's dangerous to be too open with others. It's best to proceed slowly and cautiously when getting to know someone.	Socially Anxious; Fearful of Intimacy
Nonexpression	Emotional Self-Control	It's important to approach life rationally and to keep one's emotions under control.	Rational/ Antiemotional; Masculine Role
Expression of desirable emotions; nonexpression of undesirable emotions	Social Approval	Creating a good impression and having others like me is very important to me.	Self-Monitoring; Oversocialized; Type C
Expression of dominant emotions; nonexpression of vulnerable emotions	Power	I like to be in charge in social situations.	Type A; High Need for Control/ Dominance

some extent, we all want attention, intimacy, approval, etc.), but for people with the corresponding traits, these goals are extremely salient. These individuals have a subjective sense of the relevant goal as vitally important and central to their identity (cf. Singer & Salovey, 1993). The values listed in this table are strong but not necessarily dysfunctional statements of beliefs underscoring the importance of a particular goal for a particular individual. Third, it is not clear how conscious people are of either their expression-related goals or their corresponding values. However, we suspect that individuals for whom a particular expression-related goal or value is especially central would generally be able to recognize or resonate with statements of that goal or value, and they could probably articulate such beliefs, to some extent, given appropriate questioning.

We now turn to a closer look at some examples of goals associated with expressive, nonexpressive, or mixed behavioral strategies. In each case, we briefly mention some personality traits that are conceptually and sometimes empirically linked to the relevant expressive strategy and goal. We will talk about some of these traits in more detail later in this chapter. For now, the specific traits we mention are less important than the general idea that emotional behavior can serve a variety of relational functions and can carry very different meanings for different people.

Goals and Traits Associated with Expression

Expression can be a means of achieving a number of different goals (see Table 4.1). One such goal is *Attention*. Emotional expression is highly salient: Other people notice and remember it. Politicians and actors cultivate their expressive abilities. People for whom the goal of Attention is especially important tend to value drama and having others notice them. This goal may be particularly important for individuals with Charismatic (H. S. Friedman, Prince, Riggio, & DiMatteo, 1980) or Histrionic traits, who are very expressive of both positive and negative emotions.

Expression can also be a means of cultivating *Intimacy*. Communicating our feelings to others is a way of letting them get to know us. Expressive behavior also tends to elicit expression from others, allowing us to get to know them (Derlega, Metts, Petronio, & Margulis, 1993). More expressive people tend to create a more positive first impression (Buck, 1989), and, in general, increasing intimacy in personal relationships is associated with greater expression (Altman & Taylor, 1973). One trait associated with the goal of Intimacy is being an Opener (Miller, Berg, & Archer, 1983). These individuals value and tend to elicit intimate disclosures from others. Openers are exceptionally expressive in the sense of communicating empathy and responsiveness while listening to others. We know of no direct evidence concerning whether Openers are also expressive when it comes to their own emotional disclosures. However, Openers tend to be well-liked and have many close friends, which (because of reciprocity norms) presumably would not be the case if their emotional communication involved only listening to others and never talking about their own feelings.

Goals and Traits Associated with Nonexpression

Nonexpression can also be an effective strategy for achieving certain goals. For example, active avoidance of emotional expression may stem from the goal of *Self-Protection*. Some people have a particularly strong sense of themselves as vulnerable and other people as dangerous. These individuals value caution in interpersonal interactions. They approach others guardedly, trying to reveal as little as possible about themselves, in order to ward off potential threats such as criticism or rejection. Emotional topics seem particularly dangerous to them. The goal of Self-Protection may be especially important to individuals who are Socially Anxious (Meleshko &

Alden, 1993) and those who Fear Intimacy (Descutner & Thelen, 1991; Doi & Thelen, 1993; Pilkington & Richardson, 1988).

Nonexpression can also be a means of achieving the goal of *Emotional Self-Control.* This goal is held by people who value appearing calm and unemotional at all times and especially in their interactions with others. They may see emotional expression as a sign of being weak or a "sissy." The goal of Emotional Self-Control is especially important for individuals who prefer a Rational/Antiemotional coping style (e.g., Grossarth-Maticek, Kanazir, Vetter, & Schmidt, 1983). It may also be important for men whose sense of masculinity is tied to appearing unemotional, such as those who endorse the restrictive emotionality and inhibited affection components of the Masculine Role Inventory (Snell, 1986; see also Eisler & Blalock, 1991).

Goals and Traits Associated with a Mixed Pattern of Emotional Behavior

A mixed pattern of expression and nonexpression is relevant for still other goals. One such goal is *Social Approval.* People for whom this goal is central are acutely aware of how others are reacting to them, and they consider it extremely important to create a positive impression. The goal of Social Approval is likely to be associated with nonexpression of socially undesirable (usually negative) emotions coupled with expression of socially desirable (usually positive) emotions. Traits relevant to this goal are Self-Monitoring (Snyder, 1974), Oversocialization (Weinberger & Schwartz, 1990), or Type C (e.g., Eysenck, 1985, Temoshok, 1987). Self-Monitors seek approval by actively trying to create a positive impression in others, whereas Oversocialized or Type C individuals seek approval more passively, by being extremely cooperative, submissive, and unassertive, and by focusing on the needs of others rather than themselves.

Another relationship goal associated with both expression and nonexpression is *Power.* This goal refers to a desire to influence others and to be in a position of authority in social interactions. We expect this goal to be associated with expression of dominant emotions such as anger and the avoidance of expression of vulnerable emotions such as sadness. Power is an important goal for individuals with a High Need for Interpersonal Control or Dominance (H. A. Murray, 1938; see also Weary, Gleicher, & Marsh, 1993) and perhaps also for Type A individuals (M. Friedman & Rosenman, 1974; Thoresen & Powell, 1992).

Summary

To summarize, our discussion of goals related to expression and nonexpression suggests that the same form of emotional behavior can stem from different goals. Moreover, depending on their expression-related goals and beliefs, different people may have very different views of emotional behavior and adopt very different expressive strategies. Some people see expression as a highly desirable behavior and an effective means of getting what they want or need from their social environment. Other people view emotional expression as "wimpy" or dangerous and strenuously avoid it. Our key point in this section is that to understand a person's emotional behavior, we need to view it in the context of his or her expression-related goals and values.

We have described individual personality traits related to particular constellations of expressive strategies, goals, and values. Some cultural differences can also be understood in this manner. For instance, members of individualistic cultures may use the strategy of emotional expression to achieve their goal of self-assertion. Members of communal cultures may use nonexpression to achieve social harmony.

GOAL-RELATED PROBLEMS WITH EMOTIONAL BEHAVIOR

So far, our discussion of expression-related goals and values has been descriptive. Our aim has been to illustrate some of the variety of expressive beliefs underlying emotional behavior, without focusing particularly on the consequences of either these beliefs or their associated emotional behavior.

However, research suggests that there are instances of goal-related problems with emotional behavior. As we explain below, we believe that goal-related problems with emotional behavior are *not* so much a function of the specific content of expressive goals, such as the particular value or concern they involve, or whether these goals are aimed at expression or nonexpression. Rather, these problems stem from the psychological costs and consequences of achieving or failing to achieve expression-related goals. Specifically, we suggest that expression or nonexpression may be maladaptive when associated with (1) extreme goals, (2) failed goals, or (3) conflicting goals.

Extreme Goals

Elliot's wife, Evelyn, died 2 weeks ago of a heart attack. They had been happily married for 25 years. Friends and family members are constantly urging Elliot to let his feelings out, but he insists he is fine. Elliot prides himself on coping well with adversity. Over the course of his lifetime, he has dealt calmly and effectively with many stressful circumstances, including being laid off from his job, moving his family across the country, and having an alcoholic brother. The last thing he wants to do now is fall apart.

An expressive goal can be maladaptive if it is so extreme that achieving the goal is associated with great psychological cost or strain. When we talk about extreme expressive goals, we are *not* necessarily referring to goals that are statistically rare or subjectively vehement. Instead, we are referring to goals that are inordinately difficult for a particular individual, demanding all-consuming effort.

Elliot may or may not be an example of someone with this type of extreme expressive goal. Clearly, the goal of Emotional Self-Control is important to him. He prefers to use a stoic coping style in dealing with major difficulties, and he has found this strategy useful in the past. It may be that this strategy is the best possible response for this particular individual at this particular time. If Elliot's goal of Emotional Self-Control represents a preference rather than a severe, unyielding self-prohibition, if he feels comfortable with this goal, and if he is functioning well in other areas of his life, we would conclude that he is coping well and that his nonexpressive strategy is adaptive.

Some empirical evidence backs up this conclusion concerning the adaptiveness of Elliot's nonexpression. Longitudinal studies of bereavement show that a substantial minority of people report low levels of distress shortly after the loss and *continue* to show minimal distress at follow-up (Bonanno et al., 1995; Wortman & Silver, 1989). Moreover, laboratory data suggest that people's preferred emotional coping style is their most adaptive. In one study (Engebretson et al., 1989), volunteers completed a questionnaire indicating their preference for an anger-outward versus an anger-inward expressive style. They then completed a task with either a pleasant or a harassing research assistant and subsequently were asked to write either a positive or a negative evaluation of the assistant. Volunteers who interacted with the harassing assistant showed the least systolic blood pressure reactivity when the evaluation-writing instructions they received matched their preferred expressive style.

On the other hand, in talking to Elliot, we might find out that his preference for emotional control is extremely rigid and achieved only at the cost of great effort. Perhaps he allows himself no room whatsoever for emotional expression of any sort, under any circumstances. Maybe he considers any lapses in his emotional control catastrophic. We might see signs of strain associated with this goal. Maybe he thinks constantly about the need to control his feelings or worries desperately about falling apart emotionally. Perhaps he tells us that it takes constant, strenuous vigilance to keep his feelings under wraps, to the extent that he can't concentrate in his day-to-day life. Maybe he reports vague physical complaints that weren't there before his wife died. Under these circumstances, we would suspect that Elliot's goal of Emotional Self-Control is extreme and that the strain of meeting such a goal is detrimental to him psychologically and perhaps also physically.

One trait that may involve an extreme form of the goal of Emotional Self-Control is Rationality/Antiemotionality (R/A) (e.g., Grossarth-Maticek,

Bastiaans, & Kanazir, 1985; see discussions by Eysenck, 1991a, 1991b). Individuals with this trait try to use reason rather than emotion to guide their behavior at all times. In a prospective study, R/A was found to be associated with cancer and/or cardiac mortality at levels comparable to or exceeding organic predictors such as smoking or blood cholesterol level (Grossarth-Maticek, Bastiaans, & Kanazir, 1985; Grossarth-Maticek, Kanazir, Schmidt, & Vetter, 1985).

R/A has been assessed using a variety of methods by the original investigators. This makes it difficult for other investigators trying to replicate or extend work in this area. However, the fact that generally similar results have been obtained using different questionnaires as well different methods of administration and scoring is indicative of the robustness of the construct. One version of the questionnaire uses a format consistent with a goal-based approach (e.g., Grossarth-Maticek, Bastiaans, & Kanazir, 1985). Example items are "Do you always try to do what is reasonable and logical?" and "Do you try to act rationally in all interpersonal situations?" Most of the items refer to effort toward rationality (i.e., "try") rather than actual behavioral success or failure at emotional control, which suggests to us that R/A is a measure of an expression-related goal rather than a measure of actual emotional behavior.

Unfortunately, there is no information about the mechanism by which R/A influences mortality. One possibility is that health problems stem from chronic arousal associated with the strain of trying to achieve such an extreme version of the goal of Emotional Self-Control. Another possibility is that the effort required to live up to the R/A goal may not be difficult or detrimental in day-to-day life, but it may be substantial enough following major stressful life events to compound distress and interfere with coping abilities.

How might someone with problems in emotional behavior due to an extreme expressive goal be approached clinically? Simply "forcing" Elliot, the nonexpressive widower, to vent his feelings is unlikely to be an effective intervention. His goal of Emotional Self-Control is so central to his identity that he is likely to feel frightened or ashamed if a therapist suddenly induces him to express. A more sensitive therapeutic approach involves first laying some groundwork, creating an opportunity for Elliot to reconsider his expressive goals and values, before explicitly addressing his emotional behavior.

The therapeutic relationship is critically important to this process. Elliot will only be able to reconsider his extreme goal of Emotional Self-Control in a context of interpersonal safety, trust, and respect. Having a therapist blunder in, stating or implying, "No, your deeply held conviction is completely wrong and irrational" is not helpful. To connect with Elliot, his therapist needs to be able to see this issue through Elliot's eyes. This is especially important if the therapist's own expressive goals and values are very different from Elliot's. How does Elliot describe his expressive goals?

What are the values underlying his expressive goals? What are the origins of these goals and values? What is likely to emerge from this discussion is that Elliot's extreme goal of Emotional Self-Control *makes sense* given certain past assumptions or experiences, even though it may not be adaptive in the current context. The therapist needs to communicate this understanding.

After Elliot has articulated his expressive goals and values, his therapist can help him consider the consequences of complying or not complying with his extreme goal. On the side of compliance, in this case, it is important to acknowledge that Elliot's goal of Emotional Self-Control has served him well through most of his life. However, the therapist might also help Elliot to become aware of the strain he is currently experiencing because of his extreme goal. On the side of noncompliance, the therapist should encourage Elliot to spell out what consequences he fears or dreads and what it would mean to him if he did not act in accordance with his goal of Emotional Self-Control. Maybe Elliot fears that if he starts expressing his feelings he won't be able to stop. Maybe Elliot's extreme goal stems from his deep respect for his father, who was always very stoic, and so expressing his feelings would seem like a rejection of his father and of everything his father ever taught him about being a man. The therapist can help Elliot to consider how likely it is that these feared consequences will actually occur as well as whether these consequences are truly unbearable.

Finally, after laying all of this groundwork pertaining to expressive goals and values, the therapist can encourage Elliot to express his feelings, preferably starting with small, manageable doses, so that Elliot can test and disprove his catastrophic beliefs about the consequences of expression, and thereby gradually modify or temper his extreme expressive goal. The issue here is not necessarily trying to turn Elliot into a "Let it all hang out" sort of person, but rather helping him to discover a pattern of expressive strategies, goals, and values that work for *him* in his particular circumstances.

Failed Goals

Fiona is dreading going to work today. Yesterday, she got into a heated argument with Frank, one of her coworkers. The two of them were supposed to be working together on a proposal, but Frank had claimed to be tied up with other commitments, so Fiona had put in a lot of overtime and done 90% of the work. Yesterday, she heard their boss raving enthusiastically about what a thoughtful, thorough, and timely job Frank had done with this proposal. She found out that Frank had gone behind her back and presented the proposal to their boss, claiming credit for her work, and mentioning her contribution only as an aside. When Fiona confronted Frank about this, he dismissed her concerns by saying that it wasn't a big deal and that she was getting worked up over nothing. Finally, out of sheer anger and frustration, Fiona burst into tears. Frank made a derisive remark about her getting "hysterical." They work in a small office, so Fiona is sure that everyone in the company will have heard about this interaction by now. When she thinks about the fact that she cried at work, she feels mortified. What gets to her most is that she gave Frank the satisfaction of seeing how much he had upset her.

Failed expressive goals can also be detrimental. Fiona is an example of this. She is feeling distressed not only because Frank took credit for her work and dismissed her concerns, but also because her own emotional behavior violated her expression-related goals. Fiona failed her goal of achieving Power in her relationship with Frank because she was not able to effectively influence him. She failed her goal of Emotional Self-Control because she was not able to control or modify her display of frustration and rage. Failing at her expression-related goals makes Fiona feel ashamed and humiliated.

One empirical example of a failed goal relevant to emotional behavior is a study involving distress disclosure and Self-Monitoring. High Self-Monitors are extremely concerned with the goal of Social Approval. They endorse items such as "In order to be liked, I tend to be what people expect me to be rather than anything else" (Snyder, 1974). In a questionnaire study involving college students, Coates and Winston (1987) found an interesting interaction involving expression and Self-Monitoring: Among individuals who expressed little distress, high and low Self-Monitors had equivalent low levels of depression. However, among individuals who expressed moderate or high levels of distress, high Self-Monitors were significantly more depressed than low Self-Monitors. One possible explanation for these findings is that the distress of high Self-Monitors is compounded when they express negative feelings because, for them, distress expression entails a failed expressive goal. Expressing distress works against their central goal of obtaining Approval from others. As Coates and Winston note (1987), "When we disclose our distress, we let others know that we are hurt and suffering, which is apparently not a very good way to win friends" (p. 235).

Another example that may involve failed expressive goals is a group of men identified by Friedman and his colleagues (H. S. Friedman & Booth-Kewley, 1987b; H. S. Friedman, Hall, & Harris, 1985), whom we will call discrepant Type Bs. Type B individuals are the opposite of Type As. They do *not* see themselves as impatient, work-oriented, or competitive. Discrepant Type Bs qualify as having a Type B personality (based on a self-report questionnaire called the Jenkins Activity Survey; Jenkins, Zyzanski, & Rosenman, 1979) but they show a discrepancy between how they and others perceive their emotional behavior. Discrepant Type Bs claim to be very expressive in a charismatic way, whereas other people see their expressive behavior as nervous, tense, and inhibited. Although their words are friendly, their tone of voice comes across as unfriendly. Discrepant Type Bs report feeling more depressed, anxious, powerless, and alienated than other individuals. It may be that this distress stems, at least in part, from their failure to live up to their expressive goals. These men want to express their feelings openly and to be the center of attention, but they lack the social competence and confidence to do so.

Still another example of failed goals relevant to expression can be inferred from work by Pennebaker and his colleagues (e.g., Pennebaker & Beall, 1986; Pennebaker et al., 1988). As we described in Chapter 2, these investigators have conducted a series of studies pointing to the benefits of talking or writing about trauma-related feelings.

A close look at Pennebaker's methodology and results suggests that in understanding these results it may be important to consider goals related to emotional expression. For ethical reasons, potential participants in these experiments are informed that they might have to talk or write about their traumatic experiences. For example, in Pennebaker et al. (1988), volunteers are warned about possibly having to express their traumatic feelings in the initial description when they sign up for the experiment, again when they later come in to provide baseline physiological data, and again, the following day, when they begin the writing portion of the experiment. In Pennebaker et al. (1987) volunteers are asked four different times whether they would be willing to talk about their traumatic feelings. We suspect that individuals for whom *nonexpressive* goals are central would not sign up for these experiments. Even individuals who are ambivalent about expressing seem unlikely to say on multiple, separate occasions, "Yes, I'm willing to express my traumatic feelings." Thus, it seems likely that the participants in Pennebaker's experiments are people who very strongly *want* to express their feelings. Moreover, looking closely at the results of Pennebaker's studies, it appears that many of the health effects represent a deterioration in health among nonexpressive participants relative to initial baseline compared to relatively stable health among expressive participants.

One possible interpretation of the above is that participants in Pennebaker's studies have certain goals (perhaps *Attention* or *Acceptance* from the experimenter or else *Self-Understanding*) that can be met through a strategy of emotional expression. Expressive participants have the opportunity to implement this strategy and achieve their goal. On the other hand, nonexpressive participants are unable to express, *even though they want to,* and suffer the consequences of failing to achieve a goal that is important to them.[1] This interpretation does not in any way diminish the importance of Pennebaker's work, but it does suggest that we need to consider expressive goals when predicting the effects of emotional behavior. Expression is most likely to be helpful when it is consistent with people's goals. Nonexpression is likely to be detrimental when it involves a failed goal.

Along these lines, Pennebaker himself (1985) has commented that nonexpression is *not* pathogenic in and of itself. Rather, it is the combination of nonexpression plus a desire to express that causes health difficulties. This interpretation is consistent with a study by Ogden and Von Sturmer (1984) which found that (1) individuals who report regularly expressing their negative feelings and (2) individuals who say that they do not express their feelings but are not troubled by them are equally healthy both physically and psychologically. In both of these groups, behavior is consistent with expressive goals, albeit different goals. In contrast, a third group of individuals who say that they don't express their negative feelings but continue to experience them report greater dissatisfaction and more physical symptoms than the other two groups. This may be due to distress associated with a failed expression-related goal.

Clinically, there are several options for addressing distress related to failed expressive goals. One option is to bolster clients' abilities to meet their existing expressive goals, either by modifying their circumstances or increasing their skills. In Fiona's case, this might involve helping her to come up with strategies to avoid or outmaneuver Frank, so she doesn't get upset by him in the first place. Other clients who want to express their feelings but can't may benefit from a therapist's help and encouragement in putting their feelings into words. Another option for addressing failed goals is to help clients to modify their expressive goals so that they are more achievable. For instance, Fiona might decide that rather than trying never to express distress at work, she will only try to avoid expressing distress in front of Frank, and she will seek emotional support from some of her women colleagues. A third option in dealing with failed goals is to help clients to perceive the consequences of failing to achieve their expressive goals in less drastic ways. Fiona fears that everyone in the office will think less of her because she cried at work, but if she talks to sympathetic friends and colleagues she may find that this is not the case. Imagine how much better Fiona would feel if one friend told her, "I would have reacted the exact same way!" and another friend told her, "I remember a time when I started crying at work . . ." and still another friend told her, "*You* are not the problem. Frank was being a complete jerk!"

Conflicting Goals

Akeisha has been dating Alex for almost a month now, and things are starting to get serious. Akeisha thinks they are falling in love. This is wonderful but also frightening because it brings up the issue of what she should do about her secret: Two years ago, she was raped by a neighbor in her previous apartment building. Akeisha believes that openness and honesty are important in a relationship, but she can't bring herself to tell Alex about the rape. How can she tell him that when he hugs her close she relives the terror of being trapped and help-less? How could Alex possibly understand the humiliation she went through or the shame she still feels? How could he possibly accept that the idea of having sex, even with someone as wonderful as Alex, fills her with dread and revulsion? Alex is a fairly traditional man. Maybe he would blame her and think she led on her neighbor. Or, Akeisha sighs, maybe he just wouldn't want to be involved with someone as emotionally "messed up" as she is. Akeisha thinks she is being dishon-est and cowardly in not telling Alex about the rape, but she still avoids bringing it up. She wonders if it would be better just to break up with him.

Probably the most common type of goal-related problem with emo-tional behavior involves ambivalence. This ambivalence may stem from conflicting reactions to a particular goal or conflicting goals. Akeisha, who is torn between telling and not telling her boyfriend about having been raped, is an example of someone with conflicting goals. She wants Inti-macy, but she is also concerned about Self-Protection. These goals conflict because the strategies associated with them (i.e., expression vs. non-expression) are incompatible. Akeisha is struggling not only with her feel-ings stemming from the rape, but also with her distress stemming from her conflicting expressive goals.

Conflict between the goals of Intimacy and Self-Protection is particu-larly relevant for lonely and socially anxious individuals. These individuals have a strong desire to be close to others but doubt that they will be ac-cepted or liked. They therefore adopt a nonexpressive strategy in the inter-est of self-protection, while feeling torn apart inside by their conflicting fear and desire for intimacy (e.g., Meleshko & Alden, 1993; Stokes, 1987).

Emmons (Emmons & King, 1988; Emmons et al., 1993; L. A. King & Emmons, 1990) has written extensively about goal conflict and ambiva-lence. In particular, he has found that emotional expression is often the fo-cus of conflicting goals. L. A. King and Emmons (1990) developed a questionnaire measure of ambivalence over expression. Sample items are "I want to tell someone when I love them, but it is difficult to find the right words" and "I'd like to talk about my problems with others, but at times I just can't." Interestingly, self-report of expressive behavior was *not* related to well-being, but ambivalence over expression was associated with psy-chological distress as well as questionnaire measures of physical symptoms. These findings underscore our point that emotional behavior needs to be understood in the context of expressive goals and values.

Clinically, the issue in dealing with problems stemming from conflict-ing expressive goals is to help clients resolve their ambivalence in some way (cf. Emmons, 1989, 1992). This may involve (1) choosing one goal over an-other, (2) compartmentalizing goals, so that one goal applies under certain circumstances, whereas another goal applies under other circumstances, or (3) creating new goals that represent some sort of compromise between the values underlying the original goals. Before clients can effectively choose one or several of these solutions, they need to fully articulate their expressive goals and values, and to carefully consider the consequences of complying or not complying with these goals. In Akeisha's case, her therapist might help her to explore the possible risks and costs of confiding in Alex. In some cases, dealing directly with emotional behavior can help resolve ambivalence surrounding conflicting goals. For instance, Akeisha may want to practice how she might confide in Alex by role playing with her therapist. Socially anxious clients might benefit from social skills training to bolster their confidence and make positive responses from others more likely.

CONCLUSION

In this chapter we have argued that emotional behavior must be understood in the context of goals and beliefs about that behavior. We described a number of expression-related traits in terms of patterns of expressive strategies, goals, and values. We also noted that problems involving emotional behavior can occur when expression-related goals are extreme, failed, or conflicting.

Clinically, knowing about clients' goals and values related to emotional behavior is essential for understanding the subjective meaning of their emotional responses and for designing effective treatment strategies. In general, people feel most comfortable with emotional behavior that is consistent with their expressive goals and values. Encouraging clients to articulate these expression-related beliefs is a means of helping them to understand the influence of these beliefs on what they express, how they express, and how they respond to other people's expression. In some cases, clients may want help in bolstering their ability to achieve their existing expressive goals. In other cases, therapists may need to gently and respectfully help clients to modify their expressive goals.

NOTE

1. In Pennebaker and Beall (1986) and Pennebaker et al. (1988), experimental instructions prevent the nonexpressive participants from expressing. In Pennebaker et al. (1987), the failure of nonexpressive subjects to express is due to some individual difference characteristic—perhaps a skill deficit in recognizing or verbalizing feelings. Nevertheless, we maintain that all of Pennebaker's participants indicate a strong desire to express their feelings.

PART III

Interpersonal Processes

5

Family Socialization
of Emotional Behavior

INTRODUCTION

Families provide the context for earliest learning about emotional behavior. They can be the source and subject of very intense feelings. They provide the setting for our first attempts to communicate our emotional experience. They embody our first models of the way in which emotions can be expressed, should be expressed, and typically are expressed.

Family socialization of emotional behavior consists of what and how families teach children about expression and nonexpression. From infancy onward, children learn a great deal about emotional expression. Typically, according to Dunn (1994), children learn "to argue rather than assault, to wait rather than wail, . . . to control their impatience or frustration, . . . to explain their own state and enlist aid or comfort when distressed, . . . to express their affection and ask for love" (p. 354). The family environment can influence the extent to which children achieve these milestones of emotional development (e.g., Gaensbauer, 1982; R. A. Thompson, 1991).

Clinically, understanding family socialization of emotional expression is important for several reasons. First, a family socialization perspective can provide important clues to understanding the style and content of clients' current emotional behavior. Second, by outlining the processes by which expressive norms and values are established, a family socialization perspective provides therapists with a context for respecting clients' current beliefs concerning expression and helping clients to articulate these beliefs explicitly (see Chapter 4). Third, a socialization perspective suggests possible avenues of clinical intervention for modifying problematic emotional behavior. These possibilities include helping clients to reconsider early expression socialization experiences in light of current circumstances, supplying new, therapeutic experiences concerning the social consequences of emotional expression, and intervening directly to alter current maladaptive patterns of family interactions surrounding emotional expression.

The Content of Expressive Socialization

The content of expressive socialization (i.e., *what* is taught) entails norms, values, and beliefs concerning expression. These can often be stated in terms of *display rules*, which are standards or guidelines concerning what constitutes socially acceptable emotional behavior in a particular context (e.g., Ekman, 1972; H. S. Friedman & Miller-Herringer, 1991; Matsumoto, 1993; see also Hochschild, 1983). Display rules pertain both to the quality and the intensity of emotional expression. They vary across different social situations, different cultural groups, and even different families. They reflect the values and expectations of a particular social group. Some examples of display rules are "One should express only sadness, not humor, at a funeral," "Parents should not argue in front of their children," or "Kissing in public is romantic."

In early infancy, emotional expression and emotional experience are isomorphic. Young babies express what they feel. However, as they get older, children develop the capacity to disconnect expression and experience in order to comply with either display rules or personal goals (see Saarni, 1993). They may modify their spontaneous expressions of emotion by intensifying or deintensifying overt signs of an emotion they feel. They may also feign an emotion they do not feel. Older children are capable of inhibiting expression of an emotion they feel or masking it by expressing a different emotion.

Children acquire increasing knowledge of relevant display rules as they grow up (e.g., Saarni, 1993). They are able to act in accordance with display rules even when they are too young to articulate such rules. For example, Cole (1986) observed that even 3- and 4-year old children attempt to hide their feelings of disappointment when presented with a disappointing gift. Halberstadt (1991) argues that the fact that the similarity in expressive behavior between mothers and their children is evident even when children are assessed while not in their mother's presence (e.g., Brody & Landau, 1984; Camras et al., 1990) and the fact that this similarity increases over time (e.g., Malatesta & Haviland, 1982) suggest that children gradually internalize the expressive style and values of family members.

The precise direction of socialization of emotional expression varies across families from different cultures, ethnic backgrounds, and social classes. Cross-cultural studies of facial expressions find evidence for both universality and cultural specificity in how people express emotions (see reviews by Ekman, 1993; Kitayama & Markus, 1996; Mesquita & Frijda, 1992; R. E. Porter & Samovar, 1998), which suggests that facial expression is both biologically driven and socially taught. Studies looking more broadly at values and beliefs concerning expression find considerable variability across different cultural and ethnic groups. For instance, Italian and English parents report being more accepting of their children's expressions of anger than do French-Belgian or English-Canadian parents. Black Americans value emotional expression more than white Americans (e.g., Hanna, 1984), and they are more likely to express themselves through touch (Halberstadt, 1985). Halberstadt (1991) points out that when comparing parents from diverse cultural backgrounds, the same infant behavior can elicit different parental responses. For instance, a baby's expression of alertness tends to elicit chatting from American mothers but lulling from Japanese mothers. Moreover, different infant behaviors can elicit the same parental response: Happy infant vocalizations tend to elicit chatting from American mothers, but unhappy infant vocalizations are more likely to evoke chatting responses from Japanese mothers (see Porter & Samovar, 1998, for a more detailed discussion of emotional expression and culture).

Display rules also vary depending on characteristics of the individual, such as sex and age. What is considered appropriate emotional behavior in a young girl may not be appropriate for a middle-aged man. In general, parents and other adults are less tolerant of temper tantrums as children get older (Lemerise & Dodge, 1993; see also Caspi, Elder, & Bem, 1987). Malatesta and Haviland (1982) note differences in the way mothers respond to the facial expressions of their boy or girl infant. Although there are no sex differences in the type or rate of babies' facial expressions, mothers of boys tend to match their baby's facial expressions, whereas mothers of girls tend to respond with different facial expressions. American parents tend to be less tolerant of anger expression in girls compared to boys, whereas they are less tolerant of sadness expression in boys compared to girls (Fuchs & Thelen, 1988). Noller (1978) observed parents leaving their children at preschool and noticed differences in the way mothers and fathers interact with their child. Fathers are less likely than mothers to express affection, and the least affection is shown between fathers and sons. Noller interprets this to mean that little boys learn through both observation and experience that males express less affection than females. The fact that gender differences in emotional expression are generally not evident until after preschool suggests that these differences reflect socialization processes rather than innate tendencies.

The Process of Expressive Socialization

The process of expressive socialization involves both implicit modeling and explicit teaching (Saarni, 1993; Saarni & Crowley, 1990). Parents influence their children's expressive behavior in numerous ways, including "channeling children into appropriate settings and experiences, encouraging or punishing certain behaviors, actively coaching their children with nonverbal examples or verbal descriptions of appropriate behavior, and labeling children's behavior as appropriate, inappropriate, and/or typical for that child" (Halberstadt, 1991, pp. 110–111).

Socialization of emotional expression begins immediately. Even newborn babies imitate facial expressions. Malatesta and Haviland (1982) documented socialization influences on expressive behavior within the first 6 months of life. Three- and 6-month old babies show similar facial expressions to their mothers during play and reunion interactions. Older babies are more expressively similar to their mothers than younger babies. In an observational study of mother–infant interactions, Malatesta and Haviland (1982) found that mothers send about eight signals per minute teaching their babies when and how to express their feelings. In a longitudinal study (Malatesta, Grigoryev, Lamb, Albin, & Culver, 1986), Malatesta and her colleagues found that mothers' modeling of expressions of joy and interest with their 5-month-old babies leads to increases in the babies' expressions of joy and interest 2½ months later.

Interaction of Temperament and Socialization

Socialization is not the whole picture when it comes to expressive behavior. The style with which individuals typically express their emotions is also influenced by innate temperamental characteristics. By temperament, we mean biologically based patterns of behavior that appear early in life, are relatively enduring, but are influenced over time by maturation and experience (Rothbart & Derryberry, 1981).

Individual differences in emotional expression are evident shortly after birth (e.g., Field, 1982). This means that babies are born with innate tendencies to be more or less expressive. Most attempts to classify infant temperament incorporate dimensions referring to the quality and intensity of babies' emotional responses. For instance, babies rated high on *Emotionality* are easily distressed by ordinary experiences (e.g., Buss & Plomin, 1984). Infants rated high on *Sociability* (e.g., Buss & Plomin, 1984) or low on *Inhibition* (Kagan, 1992) tend to be outgoing and enjoy novelty. Babies with high *Intensity of Emotional Response* (A. Thomas & Chess, 1977; Eisenberg & Fabes, 1992) evidence particularly strong or energetic emotional reactions, both positive and negative.

For our purposes, temperamental expressive tendencies are important because they can influence socialization processes and outcomes. Child temperament can influence family socialization, and family socialization can influence child temperament. As we explain below, children's expressive behavior can influence how parents react to them. Furthermore, temperamental expressive tendencies continue to be reflected in emotional behavior as children grow and develop, although they can be influenced by environment and experience. Emotional temperament can be thought of as a starting point in terms of expressive behavior, which socialization influences can either reinforce or modify.

Although most research on family socialization of expression emphasizes parental influence on children's expressiveness, this influence is reciprocal: Children can and do influence emotional communication within a family (e.g., Cappella, 1981; Halberstadt, 1991; McCoy & Masters, 1985). Various theorists (e.g., Buck, 1991; D. G. Gilbert, 1991; Scarr & McCartney, 1983) have suggested that from the first months of life, infants with different temperamental characteristics help create different social-emotional environments. For instance, Buck (1991) argues that more expressive children evoke more responses from caretakers than less expressive children. Smiling, active babies tend to elicit positive reactions from caretakers; irritable babies tend to elicit more negative reactions and perhaps even rejection; emotionally intense babies, who experience and express all of their emotions in an extreme way, are likely to elicit a more emotionally charged interpersonal environment than their more mild-mannered counterparts (cf. D. G. Gilbert, 1991). Corresponding feedback from the environment tends to reinforce these temperamental traits.

However, temperamental traits are by no means immutable. Socialization experiences, through interactions with family members and others, serve to intensify or restrict, expand or redirect innate expressive tendencies.

Clear evidence of both stability and modifiability of expression-related temperamental traits comes from Kagan's (1992) work with inhibited and uninhibited children. Inhibited children are timid when confronted with novel stimuli, whereas uninhibited children tend to be outgoing, eager to meet new people and explore new situations. Based on LeDoux's research with rats (summarized in LeDoux, 1996), Kagan believes these temperamental differences stem from differences in the excitability of the amygdala. Inhibited children have a low threshold for arousal and therefore try to avoid overstimulation, whereas uninhibited children have a much higher threshold for arousal and are therefore less easily overwhelmed. This type of biological explanation for temperament may seem to suggest that temperament is unalterable, but Kagan presents evidence that inhibition can change over time, given particular types of experience. In one study, Kagan, Reznick, and Snidman (1987) observed children in a social, free-play situation when the children were 21 months old and again, 4 years later, when these same children were in kindergarten. None of the uninhibited children later became inhibited. Among the inhibited toddlers, two-thirds were still inhibited in kindergarten, but one-third were no longer inhibited. According to Kagan's research (Kagan, 1992; Kagan et al., 1987), children who "outgrow" their inhibition are especially likely to have mothers who do not focus on protecting their children from distress, but rather gently and gradually encourage their children to learn to overcome their timidity, and who provide clear, firm limits for their children.

Summary

So far in this chapter, we have suggested that the content of expressive socialization is display rules and the process of expressive socialization involves direct and indirect learning. We have also noted that expressive styles reflect a combination of innate temperamental characteristics and socialization experiences, and that the influence between parents and children is often reciprocal.

In the rest of this chapter we describe research and theory concerning how children's emotional behavior is shaped by socialization processes within the family. We highlight several different approaches, emphasizing both indirect and direct influences on expression. First, we examine *expressive matching*, reviewing research addressing how quantitative and qualitative aspects of the overall climate of emotional expression within families influences children's expressive behavior. Second, we consider *expressive coaching*, which pertains to parents' responses to children's expressions of distress and how this shapes children's self-regulation. Finally, we discuss *attachment and expression*, concerning the effects of different types of parent–child relationships on expression. As we describe below, family socialization of expressions influences not just children's expressive behavior but also the meaning that emotional expression carries for them.

EXPRESSIVE MATCHING

Hatfield, Cacioppo, and Rapson (1994) describe emotions as social viruses that are easily spread from one person to other people in the social environment. Such spreading or contagion of emotional responses is one way that family context can influence children's emotional expression. More specifically, *expressive matching* refers to the tendency of individuals within a particular social environment to display similar emotional behavior. This matching involves both quantitative and qualitative aspects of emotional behavior: how much people express as well as what and how they express.

Expressive matching is well-documented in research and readily apparent in daily life. It's hard to be around someone who expresses hostility without reciprocating that expression. When we see other people whooping with laughter, we often find ourselves grinning, even if we don't know the cause of their hilarity. Expressions of joy, sadness, fear, and anxiety seem to be especially "contagious" (Klinnert, Campos, Sorce, Emde, & Svejda, 1983).

Sometimes expressive matching comes in the form of reciprocity, when one person responds to another person's expression by displaying comparable emotional behavior (Burgoon, Stern, & Dillman, 1995). Other times expressive matching is more of a two-way street, involving convergence, as both participants in an interaction adapt their expressive behavior to become increasingly similar over time (Giles, 1980). Expressive matching can occur on a large scale, as evidenced by mob panic or mass euphoria, but it is most likely to occur between people in close relationships, which suggests that it can play an important role in family socialization of expression.

While the phenomenon of expressive matching has been widely noted, the mechanisms underlying it are not well understood. P. A. Andersen and Guerrero (1998) outline a number of possible mechanisms, some of which seem particularly relevant to family socialization of expression.

One such mechanism involves *social referencing*. This occurs when children look to their parents' expressive behavior as a cue to help them figure out how to respond in a given situation. For instance, a child might interpret her mother's expression of nervousness near a large dog as a sign that she should also feel and express fear.

Another possible mechanism underlying expressive matching is conscious or unconscious *imitation* of nonverbal expressive cues (e.g., Capella, 1981). Even newborn babies tend to match the facial expressions of interaction partners. Vocal expressions also tend to elicit imitation in infants and others (Magai & McFadden, 1995). Interaction partners tend to match each others' speech rate and volume (Feldstein & Welkowitz, 1987). Cappella (1993) posits an interpersonal facial feedback hypothesis, which suggests that this matching of nonverbal emotional expression influences moods through facial feedback, ultimately resulting in interaction partners having shared emotional experience as well as shared emotional expression. The effects of this type of feedback are likely to be subtle. Burgoon, Buller, and Woodall (1996) conclude, based on their review of facial feedback experiments, that "facial expressions may affect the intensity of the felt emotion or create general emotional feelings such as pleasantness or unpleasantness, but facial expressions may not produce specific emotional experiences such as disgust, anger, and contempt" (p. 275).

Emotional matching not only implicitly teaches children about expression, it can also play a key role in cementing relationships. Oatley and Johnson-Laird (1987) describe how shared expressions of happiness make partners aware of each other's feelings, leading to a shared sense of euphoria. Bavelas and her colleagues (Bavelas, Black, Chovil, Lemery, & Mullett, 1988; Bavelas, Black, Lemery, & Mullet, 1986) argue that motor mimicry, which occurs when an observer simultaneously and symmetrically mirrors another person's affect (e.g., wincing at another person's pain, smiling at another person's delight), communicates not just empathy, but also a shared emotional state. P. A. Andersen (1985) notes that synchronous and congruent positive expressive behaviors contribute to a sense of intimacy (see Chapter 6).

We turn now to a closer look at expressive matching within a family context, looking at how children are influenced by quantitative and qualitative aspects of family expressiveness.

Quantitative Aspects of Family Expressiveness

"How often did this situation occur in your family, relative to other families?"
    "Showing contempt for another's actions."
    "Expressing sympathy for someone's troubles."
    "Expressing deep affection or love for someone."
    "Telling a family member how hurt you are."

The question and items above are part of the Family Expressiveness Questionnaire (FEQ) developed by Halberstadt (1983, 1986). This questionnaire asks respondents to provide retrospective reports of the overall frequency of emotional expression within their families.

One caveat to bear in mind regarding the FEQ is that it does not separate the frequency of emotional expression from the frequency of emotional experience or the eliciting context. Consider the item "Expressing sorrow when a pet dies." Someone who says that this occurred "not at all frequently in my family" may have grown up in a family where expression of sorrow was inhibited, or they may have had few or long-lived pets. Similarly, someone who reports that "Crying for being punished" occurred "very frequently in my family" may have grown up in a context where such crying was accepted or even expected, or they may have been punished particularly frequently. Nevertheless, the FEQ does provide a measure of a quantitative aspect of the overall expressive climate of a family. It shows excellent reliability, reasonable patterns of relationships with other measures, and moderate agreement when completed by different family members.

What are the effects of growing up in a family that is high versus low in emotional expressiveness? Consistent with the idea of expressive matching, research by Halberstadt and others suggests that individuals tend to adopt the expressive style of their families. For instance, Halberstadt (1986) selected college students with high or low scores on the FEQ, then unobtrusively videotaped them while they conversed with confederates about emotionally significant topics of their own choosing. Based on observer ratings, individuals from high-expressive families were more facially and vocally expressive than individuals from low-expressive families.

Moreover, family expressiveness is related to individuals' skill at receiving and sending nonverbal communications of emotion. In terms of receiving skills, it seems that the pattern of relationship between family expressiveness and the ability to interpret other people's emotional expression accurately changes over time. Research with young children between 3 and 7 years old consistently shows that children of more expressive mothers are more accurate at decoding emotional expressions (e.g., Daly, Abramovitch, & Pliner, 1980; Camras et al., 1990). In contrast, research using the FEQ with college students consistently shows that individuals from *low*-expressive families are *more* accurate than individuals from high-expressive families at judging other people's spontaneous emotional expression (Halberstadt, 1983, 1986). The relatively stronger receiving skills of college-age individuals from low-expressive families are especially apparent with difficult or negative emotional communications. In other words, among children, there is a positive relationship between family expressiveness and receiving skill in emotional communication, but among adults there is a negative relationship between family expressiveness and receiving skill.

Halberstadt (1991) speculates that this pattern of results reflects a crossover effect in which children whose social context involves low family expressiveness (low FE) initially lag behind their high-FE peers in receiving skills but eventually outpace them. Initially, people growing up in low-expressive families may be slower to learn to interpret emotional communication simply because they are exposed to less of it, but over time they may become especially adept at discerning subtle signs of emotion in order to deduce family members' reactions. In contrast, people growing up in high-expressive families, where emotions are readily apparent, would have had plenty of exposure to emotional communication, and they probably didn't have to work as hard to understand family members' emotional reactions. However, high-FE individuals may have had less practice interpreting more subtle, masked, blended, or partial expressive signs.

In terms of expressive sending skills, the influence of family expressiveness is also complex. As we mentioned above, observers rate high-FE individuals as more spontaneously expressive than low-FE individuals. However, just as high volume on a radio doesn't necessarily mean greater message clarity, expressing a lot doesn't necessarily mean that one is skilled at getting across the desired emotional message (Halberstadt, 1991). When volunteers are asked to express deliberately by acting out particular emotional situations, individuals from low-expressive families do a better job of accurately sending the easier items, whereas individuals from high-expressive families are relatively more adept at posing the more difficult emotional communications (Halberstadt, 1986). It may be that low-FE individuals haven't had sufficient practice to communicate complex emotional messages effectively. High-FE individuals may have had lots of practice communicating complex emotional messages, but the clarity of their emotional communication may be compromised with simple messages if they are not concentrating and fail to inhibit their expression of irrelevant messages (see Halberstadt, 1991).

Family expressiveness also appears to influence social relationships. High family expressiveness yields some social advantages among young children. Cassidy and Parke (1989) found that, according to peer and teacher ratings, kindergarten and first-grade children with high-expressive parents were more popular, less aggressive, and more prosocial than children with low-expressive parents. On the other hand, a study by Halberstadt, Fox, and Jones (1993) suggests that there may be some socioemotional advantages to growing up in a low-expressive environment: They found that children of high-expressive mothers were more expressive of negative emotions, whereas children of low-expressive mothers were more expressive of positive emotions. By college age, however, similarity of expressive style is more important in social relationships than quantity. Most people prefer to interact with others whose expressive style or background of family expressiveness matches what they are used to in their own family (see discussion in Halberstadt, 1991). Perhaps people find more familiar expressive styles to be more comfortable or more understandable.

To summarize, how much people express tends to match the overall frequency of expression in their families of origin. People who grow up in more expressive families tend to be more expressive themselves. However, our reading of this literature suggests that, at least in the ranges occurring within the normal populations studied by Halberstadt, neither high- nor low-frequency expression is clearly optimal. High-FE individuals are somewhat better under some circumstances at sending emotional messages, but low-FE individuals are somewhat better under some circumstances at receiving emotional messages. Generally, people feel more comfortable with others who have the same level of expressiveness as they do. Clinically, we believe that these findings suggest that it doesn't make sense to try to get all clients to be more (or less) expressive. Rather, variations in the overall frequency of expressiveness should be regarded as emotional dialects, comparable to the differences between fast-talking New Yorkers and slow-talking southerners. Neither style is intrinsically better, but knowing about the frequency of expression within clients' current or past family context can be one part of understanding their emotional behavior.

Qualitative Aspect of Family Expressiveness

Expressive matching within families is evident not only in terms of how much family members express but also in terms of what and how they express. Two key areas of research examining qualitative aspects of family expressiveness concern parental depression and parental conflict.

Parental Depression

Parental depression is reliably related to impaired emotional communication by parents and negative outcomes in children's emotional behavior.

Although most research focuses on the detrimental effects of maternal depression, paternal depression is also harmful to children (Forehand & Smith, 1986; A. M. Thomas & Forehand, 1991). Children of depressives are at risk for a variety of cognitive, behavioral, and emotional difficulties, including depression (Downey & Coyne, 1990; Gelfand & Teti, 1990; Hammen et al., 1987).

In general, studies of the social and communicative behavior of depressed people show a pattern of negativity, low interpersonal involvement, and unresponsiveness. Not surprisingly, this expressive pattern carries over to their interactions with their children. Depressed parents' emotional behavior toward their children is characterized by negativity, hostility, and complaining (see review by Segrin, 1998). Perhaps because they are preoccupied with their own distress, depressed mothers are less able than nondepressed mothers to interact with their babies in an active and responsive way (e.g., Cohn, Campbell, Matias, & Hopkins, 1990; Field, Healy, Goldstein, & Guthertz, 1990; Wilfong, Saylor, & Elksnin, 1991). Some investigators find that even subclinical levels of maternal depression impair mother–infant communication (Bettes, 1988), but a recent study by Carter and her colleagues (Carter, Little, & Garrity-Rokous, 1998) suggests that only depressed mothers who also suffer from other clinical problems, such as anxiety disorders or substance abuse, are significantly worse than nondepressed mothers at responding sensitively to their babies.

Depressed parents' expressive style tends to be matched by their children. While interacting with their parents, children of depressives spend less time looking at their parents, appear tense and irritable, and express more negative affect than do children of nondepressives (e.g., Cohn et al., 1990; Field, 1984). Field et al. (1985) observed a persistent depressed interaction style in infants of depressed mothers, even when the children were as young as 3 to 6 months.

It is plausible that the expressive behavior of depressed parents while interacting with their children is the mechanism underlying the detrimental effects of parental depression on children (cf. L. Murray, 1992). Some theorists have suggested that the emotional behavior of children of depressives may represent children's "giving up" any attempts to have their nonresponsive parents meet their needs (Tronick & Gianino, 1986). However, it is not clear whether expressive matching between depressed parents and their children occurs because of socialization processes or whether it reflects shared temperamental traits. Most likely, both influences are relevant.

Parental Conflict

Another approach to qualitative aspects of the expressive context within a family looks at the effects of parental conflict. There is a great deal of evidence that children tend to be upset by conflict and anger expression in general. Even 10-week-old infants notice and are distressed by their mother's expressions of anger (Haviland & Lelwica, 1987). Toddlers and preschoolers are also distressed when they witness anger expression, even when the anger is not directed at them (Cummings, Iannotti, & Zahn-Waxler, 1985). Moreover, with repeated exposure to adults engaged in verbal arguments, young children become increasingly distressed (Cummings, Zahn-Waxler, & Radke-Yarrow, 1981). Accumulating evidence suggests that when parents divorce, it is not the breakup of the family per se that produces adjustment problems for children, but rather a high level of parental conflict accompanying divorce (e.g., Amato, 1993; Cherlin et al., 1991). Parental conflict has been linked to a wide range of negative child outcome, such as impaired social competence, aggression, conduct disorder, and anxiety or social withdrawal (see review by Gano-Phillips & Fincham, 1995).

Is parental conflict always detrimental to children? Since at least some conflict in marital relationships seems inevitable, and since most children do not have adjustment problems, it is likely that this not the case. In theory, it is possible that children might even benefit from observing their parents resolve conflict in a constructive way (cf. Grych & Fincham, 1990). This might give them the opportunity to learn adaptive communication and problem-solving skills. However, to our knowledge, there are no studies showing positive effects on children of particular types of parental conflict. Perhaps children's dependence on their parents means that they always experience parental conflict as at least somewhat threatening. Interestingly, Hetherington, Cox, and Cox (1982) found that "encapsulated" conflict, in which parents argue but refrain from doing so in front of their children, does not seem to have detrimental effects on children. Similarly, B. Porter and O'Leary (1980) conclude that the links between parental conflict and negative child outcomes are strongest when children are actually exposed to conflict. Thus parents' ability to limit or contain their conflict may limit the negative impact of conflict on children. Grych and Fincham (1990, 1993) suggest that how children respond to parental conflict depends on children's appraisals or understanding of that conflict. When parents are better able to control their conflict, children may see it as more benign.

Some recent research has attempted to go beyond aggregate relationships between parental conflict and child difficulties to describe which aspects of parental conflict are most pathogenic and in what ways. This research implicates certain qualitative aspects of parents' expressive behavior. Specifically, parental conflict is more closely linked to children's distress when the conflict is frequent, intense, involves physical aggression, and is unresolved (Gano-Phillips & Fincham, 1995).

An impressive study by Katz and Gottman (1993) documents long-term effects of qualitative aspects of parents' anger expression styles on children's social-emotional functioning. These investigators found that parents' interaction style during a laboratory task involving conflict resolution when the children were 5 years old predicted teachers' ratings of children's internalizing and externalizing behaviors *3 years later*. Parents whose conflict discussion involved a *Mutually Hostile* pattern, characterized by both partners' expressions of contempt and belligerence, tended to have children with externalizing difficulties, such as hyperactivity, antisocial behavior, and negative engagement with peers. Parents whose conflict discussions involved a *Demand–Withdraw* pattern, in which the wife expressed anger in a defensive and domineering way while the husband expressed anger indirectly, through a deliberate show of lack of attention or interest in his wife's remarks (i.e., "stonewalling"), tended to have children with internalizing difficulties, such as depression, tension, or having the role of a victim or rejected child. Child temperament assessed at Time 1 did not predict either marital satisfaction or child outcomes at Time 2. General marital satisfaction was also not predictive of child outcomes. The study by Katz and Gottman (1993) is important because it documents specific, predictive links between parents' emotional communication styles and children's emotional well-being and expressive style

Precisely why these links occur between particular types of pathogenic expressive styles and particular social-emotional difficulties in children is not understood. One possibility is modeling. Parents who express their anger in hostile and undercontrolled ways may implicitly teach their children to act out when they feel angry; whereas fathers who engage in conflict withdrawal may teach their children to express their feelings indirectly. Another possibility, from a family systems perspective, is that the children with externalizing difficulties may be trying to distract their mutually hostile parents from their intense conflict by drawing attention to themselves (Minuchin, 1974). What is clear is that qualitative aspects of parents' emotional communication influences children's expressive behavior, even when such emotional communication is not directed at the child.

EXPRESSIVE COACHING

"What would you look like, what would I see if I saw you angry? . . . What would be going on inside? What would you be feeling about being angry? What would you be thinking? . . . How does anger work in your life? What role does it play? . . . "

" . . . How do you react to (child's name) when (s)he's being angry? Can you tell that (s)he's angry? Can you tell subtle signs? . . . How do you respond? What do you think about the anger? What are your reactions, thoughts, feelings? What might you do? What would your goals be in this situation? . . . "

" . . . If you could sum it up, can you maybe describe a philosophy about the world of feelings, how to approach that, how to work with feelings, what they're for, what they're about?"

The questions above come from the Meta-Emotion Interview developed by Gottman and his colleagues (Gottman et al., 1996a, pp. 46–48). This semistructured interview pertains to parents' *meta-emotion philosophy*, that is, their thoughts and feelings about their own and their children's emotional reactions. These investigators contend that parents' meta-emotion philosophies influence how they respond to their children's expressions of emotion, which, in turn, influences children's ability to regulate their emotions. The idea of meta-emotion is quite similar to what we have described as the reflection component of emotion (see Chapter 2), although we find it conceptually clearer to separate thoughts about feelings (emotional reflection, e.g., "Anger is dangerous") and feelings about feelings (additional or subsequent emotional experience; e.g., "I am frightened of my anger").

Types of Parental Meta-Emotion Philosophies

Gottman and his colleagues (Gottman et al., 1996a, 1996b) believe that the optimal approach to parenting involves an *emotion-coaching* philosophy. Parents who describe this type of philosophy during the Meta-Emotion Interview value emotions. They are very aware of their own and their children's emotions. They talk about emotions comfortably, distinguishing between different types and intensities. These parents view their children's negative emotional responses as an opportunity for intimacy and teaching. They accept, empathize with, and respect their children's feelings, but beyond that, they also attempt to educate their children about emotions by helping the children to label their feelings verbally, stating rules concerning appropriate expression (e.g., "No hitting. If you're feeling angry, use your words."), and using a problem-solving approach to help the children identify goals and strategies for coping with the cause of their negative feelings. Gottman et al. (1996b) emphasize that emotion coaching is not the same as parental warmth. Parents can feel warmly toward their children and even express that affection without necessarily engaging in emotion coaching. There are very concerned, caring parents who are oblivious to their children's emotions or who do not attempt to actively work with their children to process and cope with negative emotions.

Based on responses to the Meta-Emotion Interview, Gottman and his colleagues (Gottman et al., 1996a, 1996b) also identify several other qualitatively different meta-emotion philosophies, in addition to the emotion-coaching philosophy. Parents with a meta-emotion philosophy involving *high acceptance/low coaching* are very caring and empathic toward their children, but they make no attempt to help their children understand or learn from their emotions. Their approach is more "hands off." They are accepting of their children's emotional expression, and may even espouse a belief that free expression is desirable, but they do not tend to follow up their acceptance with any particular teaching about emotion or problem solving. Essentially, they leave it up to their children to work out their negative emotional responses on their own.

In contrast to the benign but rather passive approach of high-acceptance/low-coaching parents, the three remaining meta-emotion philosophies are decidedly negative. Parents with a *dismissing* philosophy tend to ignore or deny the importance of their children's negative feelings. For instance, they may describe a child's anger as "cute" or "funny." They see negative feelings as something to get over quickly and not dwell on. They may use distraction or limited comforting efforts to help their children cope with negative feelings, but they are not interested in what their children are trying to communicate through their emotional expression, nor do they view emotional moments as opportunities for teaching or intimacy. Dismissing parents care about their children in the sense that they don't want them to be unhappy, but they tend to show little awareness or understanding of their children's feelings, and little interest in helping their children work with their feelings.

Still more negative toward their children's feelings are parents with a *disapproving* meta-emotion philosophy. These parents are noticeably critical and unempathic toward their children's feelings. They see negative feelings as something to be controlled. They are apt to punish their children for *any* expression of negative feelings, even if that expression does not involve misbehavior. Their goal seems to be to eradicate their children's negative feelings, which they view as unproductive. For instance, one mother reported that when her son got angry, she hit him to calm him down, because she didn't want him to grow up to have a bad temper like his father.

The final type of meta-emotion philosophy identified by Gottman and his colleagues involves *dysregulation* (Gottman et al., 1996a; Katz, Gottman, & Hooven, 1996). These parents feel out of control with respect to their own emotions, which interferes with their ability to help their children with their emotions. Dysregulated parents view negative feelings as dangerous. They report that their negative emotional responses are frequent, intense, problematic, and difficult to manage. They are acutely aware of their emotions, but they often respond in a derogatory way toward their children's expressions of negative feelings. It may be that these parents find negative emotions disorganizing, or perhaps they become overwhelmed because they are unable to achieve any psychological distance from their own or their children's emotions (see Cowan, 1996).

To summarize, the five meta-emotion philosophies identified by Gottman and his colleagues (1996a)—emotion coaching, high acceptance/low coaching, dismissing, disapproving, and dysregulation—involve different understandings of and reactions to children's emotional expression. Qualitative and quantitative research by these investigators indicates that these different philosophies translate into different parenting attitudes and behaviors. Eisenberg and her colleagues have observed similar varieties of parental approaches to children's emotions. For instance, Eisenberg and Fabes (1994) asked parents how they would respond to their children's negative emotions in everyday situations. Six categories of parental responses emerged: (1) parental distress, (2) minimizing or dismissing the child's emotions, (3) punishing the child or doing something to minimize the parent's own negative emotion, (4) comforting the child, (5) encouraging the expression of emotion, and (6) encouraging and helping the child to address the problem causing the negative emotion. The similarity of Eisenberg's categories to Gottman et al.'s (1996a) meta-emotion styles supports the validity of these distinctions, although the real test of the usefulness of these distinctions lies in their ability to predict child outcomes. In other words, does it matter how parents understand and respond to children's negative emotions?

Effects of Emotion Coaching

Gottman et al. (1996a, 1996b) report a remarkable set of findings showing that parental meta-emotion philosophy has long-term and multifaceted links to children's well-being. Parents' awareness of their own and their children's emotions and their tendency to use emotional coaching to help their children cope with negative emotions (all assessed using the Meta-Emotion Interview) were associated with better quality parent–child interaction during laboratory tasks. Specifically, parents with an emotional-coaching meta-emotion philosophy used more structuring and responsive praise and fewer derogatory comments while discussing a confusing story and playing a difficult video game with their children. Parental philosophies encompassing coaching and awareness were also associated with better regulatory physiology (i.e., higher vagal tone, increased vagal suppression) in children during these laboratory tasks. Gottman et al. (1996a, 1996b) interpret this to mean that an emotion-coaching approach to parenting is physiologically soothing to children. Most impressive are Gottman et al.'s (1996a, 1996b) findings that parents' emotion-coaching philosophy assessed when children were 5 years old predicted children's ability to self-soothe negative emotions as well as their level of academic achievement, quality of peer relationships (assessed by teacher reports), and physical health 3 *years later*. Gottman et al. (1996b) caution that these results should be considered preliminary, because their sample was relatively small and not racially or ethnically diverse. Moreover, only some of the meta-emotion philosophies have received empirical scrutiny (mainly emotion coaching and disapproving). However, the strength of the findings and the consistency of the patterns across settings, outcomes, and time all suggest that these results are meaningful.

What is it that children learn about emotional expression from emotion-coaching parents? Gottman et al. (1996b) insist that it is not a specific behavior. Emotion coaching doesn't lead children to become globally more (or less) expressive. Rather, it provides them with knowledge about the world of emotions that may allow them to more effectively regulate their feelings and more flexibly adapt their expressive behavior to current goals or circumstances. For school-age children, social competence often requires that they *not* express their feelings to their peers. Calling attention to oneself by openly communicating negative feelings is liable to elicit teasing and peer rejection in this age group (e.g., Putallaz & Gottman, 1981; Gottman & Parker, 1986). Although emotion-coaching parents encourage their children to talk about their feelings at home, these children do not then turn around and emote freely at the playground. Because emotion coaching is associated with better peer relations, somehow these children are able to discern what sort of emotional behavior is called for in social situations and to carry it out. Perhaps emotion-coaching parents' emphasis on understanding and coping with emotions means that their children are better able to regulate the level of their distress, so that they do not act impulsively. Perhaps these parents' behavioral limit-setting concerning acceptable and unacceptable forms of expression (e.g., talking rather than hitting) means that their children have had more practice discerning relevant social cues and adjusting their emotional behavior accordingly. Gottman et al. (1996b) suggest that emotion coaching provides children with "the tools to learn how to learn in emotionally challenging situations, even if that calls for inhibiting emotional responding" (p. 262).

Predictors of Emotion Coaching

Why is it that some parents have an emotion-coaching philosophy and others do not? At this point, there is no empirical answer to this question, although there are a number of possibilities. One obvious possibility is that parents' meta-emotion philosophies stem from what they learned about emotion in their own families of origin. Another, perhaps related, possibility is that parents' meta-emotion philosophies are an outgrowth of their abilities to cope with their own emotions. There are hints in the excerpts from actual Meta-Emotion Interviews quoted in Gottman et al. (1996a) that the roots of noncoaching philosophies lie in parents' fear of or discomfort with their own feelings. Eisenberg's research with children (e.g., Eisenberg, Fabes, Schaller, & Miller, 1989) suggests that they cannot feel empathy for another distressed child unless they are able to regulate the level of their own distress. Along this line of reasoning, parents who find their own feelings overwhelming may not be capable of responding in a helpful way to their children's emotions. Clinically, this means that helping parents to understand and regulate their emotional response may be a necessary first step before they can help their children learn about their emotions.

There is also some evidence that the child's characteristics may help determine whether or not parents adopt an emotion-coaching approach. Eisenberg and Fabes (1994) found that mothers who perceived their child's negative emotional reactions to be frequent and intense are more likely to report that they felt distressed by these reactions and that they tend to respond with minimization or punishment. Similar results were obtained by Eisenberg, Fabes, and Murphy (1996) with both mothers and fathers. Gottman et al. (1996b) did not find any effects of parents' perceptions of child temperament on parental coaching, but they did find that parents were more likely to use a coaching approach if their children had better-regulated physiological responses. It may be that it is easier for parents to coach children who are able to physiologically self-soothe. These children may be better able to focus their attention on and effectively use parental coaching instruction while they are emotionally aroused, which may in turn reinforce parents' coaching efforts (Katz et al., 1996).

Related research by Bugental (1991; Bugental, Blue, & Cruzcosa, 1989; Bugental, Blue, & Lewis, 1990; Bugental, Mantyla, & Lewis, 1989) looking at parental perceptions of control in interactions with their children provides a vivid picture of how characteristics of both the parent and the child contribute to the quality of their interactions. Bugental suggests that parents who perceive that they have a relatively high amount of control in interactions with their children tend to be confident and solution-oriented when interacting with a noncompliant child, which enables them to interact with that child in ways that encourage the desired behavior. In contrast, adults low in perceived control feel threatened and pessimistic when interacting with a noncompliant child, and they are less able to elicit desired responses from the child. In a series of studies, Bugental and her colleagues examined interactions of mothers with their own children as well as unfamiliar children. Mothers who reported that they believed they had little control over the outcomes of interactions with their children showed a pattern of interaction reflecting a "leakage of feelings of powerlessness," but only when they interacted with "difficult" children. Specifically, low-control mothers expressed increasing levels of facial and vocal sadness while interacting with noncompliant children. They also tended to send inconsistent or confusing emotional messages, such as combinations of reassurance and displeasure. Low-control mothers are also more likely to use abusive and coercive discipline strategies, such as slapping or biting. All of these maladaptive responses tend to increase negative and noncompliant behavior in children, which probably confirms low-control mothers' beliefs that they cannot influence their children. However, the maladaptive responses of low-control mothers were *not* evident when they interacted with easy, compliant children, only when they interacted with relatively difficult, unresponsive children.

Although Bugental's research involves child compliance with parental requests, it is easy to extrapolate from these findings to imagine how parental self-confidence and child difficulty might relate to emotion coaching. It seems likely that coaching efforts would be used most readily by parents who are more confident in their role, with children who have an easier time accepting and using parental input.

Summary

To summarize, parents' understanding of and responses to their children's expression of negative emotion influences children's' ability to regulate their own emotions and is linked to a variety of different measures of well-being. According to Gottman and his colleagues, the ideal response from parents involves a combination of empathic respect for the child's feelings coupled with active efforts to encourage the child's acquisition of emotion-related skills. These skills include labeling feelings, identifying causes, and problem solving to generate and implement constructive responses. The goal of this type of emotion coaching is *not* that children globally express more or less, but rather that children be attuned to their own emotional experience and be capable of flexibly adjusting their expressive behavior in adaptive ways. Effective emotion coaching requires that parents be aware of and be comfortable with their own emotional responses. Child characteristics may also influence the likelihood that parents adopt a coaching approach.

It strikes us that a coaching approach to emotions resembles an integration of experiential and cognitive-behavioral therapeutic perspectives. Like experiential therapists, emotion-coaching parents place a strong emphasis on exploring feelings and fleshing out their nuances and implications as a guide to adaptive coping. Like cognitive-behavioral therapists, emotion-coping parents also focus directly on their children's actual behavior, in terms of how they express their feelings and cope with the problems that elicit their distress.

So far we have considered how children's emotional behavior is shaped by the general expressive climate within their family as well as parents' specific responses to children's expressions of negative emotions. Still another perspective on family socialization of expression is attachment theory, which looks at the relationship between the quality of parent–child relationships and emotional behavior. The previous topics in this chapter start by observing some type of emotion socialization variable and then measuring outcomes such as expressive behavior and social relationships. Research on attachment theory typically takes the opposite approach: measuring patterns of expressive behavior and social relationships and hypothesizing about the socialization processes that created these patterns.

ATTACHMENT AND EXPRESSION

"I find it relatively easy to get close to others."
"I'm not very comfortable having to depend on others."
"I rarely worry about being abandoned by others."
"I'm nervous whenever anyone gets too close to me."
"I often want to merge completely with others, and this desire sometimes scares them away."

The statements above are from a questionnaire, developed by Simpson (1990), assessing attachment style. Attachment theory posits that people build mental models of themselves and others based on their relationship experiences, particularly their early interactions with caregivers. These mental models pertain to people's sense of self-worth and their expectations concerning how other people behave in relationships. People with a negative sense of self-worth tend to be anxious about relationships because they see themselves as unlovable and unworthy of support from others, so they fear that others will abandon them; people with a negative view of others tend to be uncomfortable with emotional closeness because they see others as untrustworthy and unreliable sources of support, so they avoid forming intimate relationships (see discussions by Bartholomew, 1990; Feeney, Noller, & Roberts, 1998).

Bartholomew (1990, 1993) describes four categories of attachment styles, reflecting the four possible combinations of positive versus negative views of self and others.[1] *Secures* have positive mental models of both themselves and others. They see themselves as likeable and other people as trustworthy. They have positive but realistic expectations of relationships. *Preoccupieds* have a negative view of themselves coupled with a positive view of others. They are anxiously concerned about relationships because they depend on others for self-validation. They tend to form clinging, possessive relationships. *Dismissive–Avoidants* have a positive view of themselves but a negative view of others. They pride themselves on their self-sufficiency. They view relationships as nonessential and are reluctant to get emotionally close to anyone. Finally, *Fearful–Avoidants* have negative mental models of both themselves and others. Social interaction makes them feel anxious. They fear rejection and emotional injury and therefore actively avoid forming intimate relationships. Not surprisingly, the Secure attachment style is associated with the most satisfied relationships and the greatest psychological well-being (Collins & Read, 1990; Feeney, Noller, & Callan, 1994; Fuller & Fincham, 1995; Simpson, 1990).

According to attachment theory, attachment styles evolve because of different sorts of experiences related to the expression of emotion in relationships, especially relationships with caregivers (see discussion by Feeney et al., 1998). Presumably because of different learning experiences involving emotional expression, different mental models of relationships emerge as attachment styles, which, in turn, are linked to different patterns of emotional behavior. Secure attachment is seen as the product of reasonably consistent, sensitive, and responsive caregiving, which allows individuals to express distress and receive comfort and support. Preoccupied (sometimes called Anxious/Ambivalent) attachment is hypothesized to be the result of insensitive or inconsistent caregiving, which leads individuals to express distress in a heightened way. Avoidant attachment is thought to develop because of distancing or rejecting responses by caregivers that teach individuals to restrict their expressions of distress and to avoid seeking support from others.

Assessment of Attachment Style in Children and Adults

Originally, attachment theory focused on young children's emotional reactions to separation from and reunion with their mother (e.g., Ainsworth, Blehar, Waters, & Wall, 1978; Bowlby, 1969, 1973). In toddlers, attachment style is usually assessed by observing their emotional behavior when their mother briefly leaves them in an unfamiliar setting and then returns. This procedure, developed by Ainsworth et al. (1978), is called the Strange Situation and was validated based on yearlong home observations. All young children tend to react with the same sequence of emotional responses (protest, despair, and detachment) when separated from caregivers, but there are qualitative differences in the responses of children with different attachment styles.

Secure children look to their attachment figure (usually their mother) as a secure base for exploration and a source of comfort. In the Strange Situation, they show signs of missing their mother when she leaves, greet her actively when she returns, and then resume playing with toys. They may or may not cry upon separation, but if they do, they are readily comforted by their mother when she returns. At home, Secure children show minimal anger or anxiety about minor separations. Mothers of Secure infants hold them tenderly and carefully. They are emotionally in sync with their children in that they demonstrate sensitivity to their babies' expressive signals and show contingent pacing in face-to-face interactions.

Avoidant children express extreme levels of detachment in the Strange Situation, through behavioral and emotional withdrawal. They focus on the toys, do not cry during separation, and ignore their mother when she returns. At home, these children show marked anger toward their mother and considerable anxiety concerning her whereabouts. Mothers of Avoidant children reject their children's efforts to be physically close to them, and they are especially uncomfortable with touching or being touched by their children.

Anxious children (analogous to Preoccupied adults), respond to separation in the Strange Situation with extreme levels of anger and protest or marked passivity. They appear preoccupied with their mother throughout the procedure and do not settle or resume playing with toys when their mother returns. These children also seem anxious at home. Mothers of anxiously attached children are not rejecting, but they are unpredictable. They appear inept at holding their babies and do not show contingent responses to their babies' expressive cues during face-to-face interaction.

More recently, investigators have considered the role of attachment in adolescent and adult relationships (e.g., Bartholomew, 1990, 1993; Hazan & Shaver, 1987; Shaver & Hazan, 1994). In these populations, attachment style is often assessed by asking direct questions concerning thoughts and feelings about relationships, like the ones quoted at the beginning of this section. In clinical studies, adult attachment style is usually assessed using the Adult Attachment Interview (AAI; George, Kaplan, & Main, 1985; Main & Goldwyn, 1991, in press). This semistructured interview, like questionnaire measures of attachment, asks adults to describe their relationship experiences and beliefs. In scoring the AAI, unlike questionnaire measures, *how* individuals respond is at least as important as what they say (Main, 1996). For instance, a woman might report that she had an "excellent" relationship with her mother, but then be unable to recall or describe any details or specific examples to illustrate this portrayal. Her attachment style would be classified by AAI criteria as Avoidant. A Preoccupied attachment style might be evident from confused responses, childlike speech, unusually long or irrelevant responses, or striking lack of collaboration with the interview. A Secure attachment style is evidenced by specific, coherent and collaborative descriptions of relationship experiences. The AAI is not so much a measure of attachment history, but rather a way of understanding adults' current understanding of their own childhood experiences (Main, 1995).

Although assessments of attachment styles in children and adults are based on very different types of behavior (i.e., seeking out mother vs. endorsing certain relationship beliefs or using a particular style of discourse), longitudinal studies suggest that they correspond (see review by Main, 1996). Two studies, conducted in different laboratories, found that roughly three-quarters of individuals are classified the same way in infant assessments and in the AAI assessments given more than 15 years later (Hamilton, 1995; Waters, Crowell, Treboux, Merrick, & Albersheim, 1995). These findings suggest that adult measures of attachment are not merely a function of retrospective memory biases.

Difference in Expressive Behavior
across Adult Attachment Styles

In young children, expressive behaviors comprise the defining features of different attachment styles. In adults, attachment-style assessments emphasize more cognitive aspects, such as beliefs, memories, or expectations, but quite a bit of research documents differences in emotional expression across attachment styles in adults. In terms of overall expressiveness and interpersonal warmth, Bartholomew and Horowitz (1991) found that Preoccupieds show the highest levels of expressiveness and warmth, Secures show moderate levels of these, Dismissive–Avoidants are relatively inexpressive and interpersonally cold, and Fearful–Avoidants show very low levels of expressiveness and neutral emotional tone (neither warm nor cold).

A more detailed picture of attachment–expression links emerges when we look at expression of positive versus negative emotion. In terms of positive emotions, observers report that, compared to the two Avoidant groups, Secures and Preoccupieds are more vocally and facially pleasant, showing more nonverbal intimacy and positive affect during short conversations with their romantic partners (Guerrero, 1996). As for negative emotions, Andersen and Guerrero (1998) suggest that the pattern of data across several self-report studies indicates that people with all three insecure attachment styles want to limit their expression of negative emotions, but that Preoccupieds have difficulty suppressing their negative feelings, perhaps because their intense involvement in relationships leads to correspondingly intense feelings. (This pattern suggests that Preoccupieds may experience ambivalence over expression. See Chapter 4.)

In a related vein, different attachment styles are associated with different styles of coping with negative emotions. In an experimental study, Simpson, Rholes, and Nelligan (1992) surreptitiously videotaped couples while they waited for the woman to participate in a stressful laboratory procedure. Secure women actively sought support from their romantic partners, whereas Avoidant women did not seek support from their partner. These coping patterns were more marked when the women were more anxious. Other research suggests that Preoccupieds tend to cope with negative affect by dwelling on it and seeking social support in a "hypervigilant manner" (Simpson & Rholes, 1994, p. 183). Both of the avoidant attachment styles involve a lack of social support seeking. However, reflecting the distinction we drew in Chapters 1 and 3 between nonexpression due to lack of awareness of emotion and nonexpression due to conscious suppression, Dismissive–Avoidants tend to exclude negative emotions from their conscious awareness, denying that they experience any distress, whereas Fearful–Avoidants experience high levels of distress but deliberately refrain from expressing it to others for fear of alienating them (Bartholomew, 1990).

Feeney et al. (1998) argue that a full picture of the attachment–expression relationship requires that we consider not just expression of negative versus positive emotions, but also expression of specific emotions. In particular, they argue that although Preoccupieds tend to be extremely expressive of their negative emotions in general, anger may represent a special case because of its potential threat to a relationship. In other words, Preoccupieds may specifically inhibit their expression of anger because they fear that this emotion, more so than say sadness or anxiety, may lead to abandonment. In a self-report study, Feeney (1995) found that Secures said they usually express anger directly by talking it out and negotiating with their partner, whereas Preoccupieds said they generally used indirect tactics, such as pouting, to express their anger. Predictably, Dismissive–Avoidants said they use avoidant strategies. Surprisingly, Fearful–Avoidants reported that they usually use aggressive tactics to express anger. P. A. Andersen and Guerrero (1998) report a somewhat different pattern for anger expression, more consistent with general negative emotional expression strategies for each attachment style: In their study, Preoccupieds said they favor aggressive strategies such as yelling or slamming doors, whereas Fearful–Avoidants said they tend to keep angry feelings inside and to use passive–aggressive strategies such as ignoring their partner. Observational and/or diary studies could help clarify how people with different attachment styles actually express different emotions.

Attachment Style and Interpretations of Expressive Behavior

Collins and Read (1994) suggest that different attachment styles are associated not only with different likelihoods of experiencing and expressing particular emotions, but also with different interpretations of other people's expressive behavior. For instance, suppose a woman receives a brief hug from a coworker after finding out that she did not receive an expected promotion. If that woman has a Secure attachment style, she probably interprets this hug as a gesture of affection and comfort. If she has a Preoccupied attachment style, she might experience the hug as frustratingly brief and unsatisfying. If she has a Dismissive–Avoidant style, she probably sees the hug as unnecessary or even condescending. Finally, if she has a Fearful–Avoidant attachment style, she is likely to experience the hug as threatening and anxiety-provoking. The obvious and critically important clinical implication of this is that therapists' usual expressions of warmth and empathy can carry strikingly different meanings for clients with different attachment styles. (See also Dozier, Cue, & Barnett, 1994, concerning how therapists' effectiveness can vary based on the therapist's own attachment style.)

Modification of Attachment Styles

So far in this section, we have described research and theory suggesting that early experiences involving emotional expression with attachment figures leads to the development of working models concerning oneself and others in relationships. These models shape individuals' subsequent emotional behavior and influence their understanding and expectations of social interactions. The working models underlying attachment styles tend to operate outside conscious awareness, so they are resistant to change (Bretherton, 1985).

However, many theorists have emphasized that attachment styles are not immutable (e.g., Barbee, Rowatt, & Cunningham, 1998; Berman & Sperling, 1994; Fox, 1995; Kobak & Hazan, 1991). Although the mental models of themselves and others that people bring to relationships undoubtedly shape relationships, the partner's behavior can also influence mental models. Repeated experience with a particular type of interaction may confirm and reinforce an existing model or it may lead people to revise their models of relationships. This reasoning is consistent with the idea of therapeutic interaction as a means of providing corrective emotional experiences that allow clients to update their views of themselves and others (cf. Safran, 1990a, 1990b). For instance, Barbee et al. (1998) speculate that the impact of a particular support-seeking interaction on attachment style depends on whether (1) the support seeker perceives a positive response from the support provider and (2) the support seeker perceives that his or her need for support has been satisfied. When both of these conditions are met, the interaction is likely to reinforce or enhance a secure attachment within this relationship. When neither condition is met, negative views of the self and the partner are evoked, and Fearful-Avoidant attachment is increased. Preoccupied attachment can increase if support is given only intermittently or if support is given in a desirable way, yet the support seeker still feels unable to cope. Either scenario could result in a positive view of others coupled with a negative view of the self. Finally, Dismissive–Avoidant attachment is enhanced when support responses are disappointing yet the support seeker manages to cope anyway.

CONCLUSION

In this chapter, we described three approaches to family socialization of emotional expression. The first approach looks at implicit teaching about emotional behavior through matching of quantitative and qualitative aspects of family expressiveness. The second approach considers explicit teaching about emotional behavior through emotional coaching. The third approach considers a combination of implicit and explicit teaching about emotional behavior through attachment relationships.

To us, the most interesting aspect of family socialization of expression is that it influences not only what and how people express, but also the meaning that expression carries for individuals. Family experiences involving expression help determine what people view as normal or typical or desirable concerning emotional behavior in themselves and others. These experiences influence what level of expression people find most comfortable. They affect the extent to which people value or dismiss expression. They determine people's expectations concerning how others will respond to emotional expression.

Clinically, helping clients to recognize patterns of expressive behavior in past or current family interactions and to articulate the values and interpretations they draw from these interactions can provide a powerful means of understanding and perhaps modifying emotional behavior. For example, reconsidering past expressive socialization experiences in light of current circumstances may shed new light for clients on how they usually express their feelings and how they want to express their feelings. A therapist's accepting response to clients' expressions of distress may allow clients to revise their beliefs that such expressions are unimportant, undesirable, or intolerable. Within a marital or family therapy context, explicating beliefs and past experiences concerning expression may help partners to reframe each others' emotional behavior so that they understand it in more compassionate terms. Identifying patterns and interpretations of emotional behavior within current interactions can help clients to interact in new ways, for instance, by expressing their feelings more directly or in a less blaming way.

NOTE

1. Griffin and Bartholomew (1994) point out that very few adults conform perfectly to a single attachment style. These styles are more accurately understood as continuous rather than categorical variables, with certain individuals having stronger tendencies than others toward particular attachment styles.

6

Men, Women, and the Language of Love

INTRODUCTION

Generations of mothers have warned their daughters that men are "only interested in One Thing." In his best-seller *Mars and Venus in the Bedroom,* Gray (1995) argues that men want sex whereas women want romance. Drawing mainly from anecdotal evidence, he contends, "It is sex that allows a man to feel his needs for love, while it is receiving love that helps a woman to feel her hunger for sex" (p. 2). In 1985, in a nationwide survey that drew responses from more than 90,000 women, Ann Landers found that 72% said they would be content to live without sex in favor of being held tenderly. In response to that survey, Art Buchwald quipped that before he was married, he met all 62,000 women who preferred cuddling to sex (survey and response cited in Hatfield & Rapson, 1987).

The stereotypes are quite clear. According to popular wisdom, when it comes to love, women and men speak different languages and have different goals. Women care about intimacy and emotional closeness. Men just want to have sex. Women want to share their feelings and talk about the relationship. Men just want to have sex. Like many stereotypes, the stereotypes about men and women and expressions of love have a small grain of truth in them, but vastly overstate between-group differences, understate within-group differences, overlook situational influences, and underestimate the complexity of the phenomena in question (cf. Aries, 1996; Deaux & Major, 1987; Eagley & Wood, 1991).

Clinical Relevance of Love

Understanding love is critically important from a clinical perspective. For the majority of people, close, loving relationships are the most important

135

thing in their lives (e.g., S. Brehm, 1985). Many clients present with difficulties involving love, such as trying to find someone to love or trying to improve a faltering love affair. Even when they feel love, they may be reluctant to express it because they fear exposure, rejection, loss of control, or loss of identity (Hatfield, 1984; see also Baxter, 1988). Expressing love is essential for creating close relationships, but "coming on too strong" by expressing too much too fast can drive potential partners away (Derlega et al., 1993). Even in established relationships, people may have difficulty communicating love in a way that their partner understands and appreciates (e.g., Marston & Hecht, 1994; Sternberg, 1986).

Research on marital interaction suggests that negative emotional behavior is more important than positive emotional behavior for distinguishing between distressed and nondistressed couples and for predicting day-to-day marital satisfaction for distressed couples (e.g., Gottman, 1979; Jacobson, Waldron, & Moore, 1980). However, this does *not* mean that expressions of love are unimportant. Positive behaviors are better than negative behaviors for predicting marital satisfaction among generally happy couples (Jacobson et al., 1980). Moreover, declines from high to moderate levels of marital satisfaction are associated with low levels of positive behavior (Filsinger & Thoma, 1988). Taken together, these studies suggest that expressions of love don't necessarily compensate for problems in a relationship, but in the absence of severe problems, expressions of love bring joy, zest, and even meaning to relationships. For example, the protestations of love by a husband who regularly beats his wife are unlikely to make up for the beatings. However, in a happily married couple, a husband who surprises his wife by bringing her flowers or scrubbing the bathroom when it isn't even his turn is likely to find that his wife is delighted and eager to reciprocate his expression of love (see Canary, Emmers-Sommer, & Faulkner, 1997, for discussion of couples' division of household chores).

In order to help clients have truly satisfying relationships, clinicians need to understand clients' wishes and fears concerning expressions of love. They need to know how clients express love as well as how these expressions fit into the relationship context and how they are viewed by potential or actual partners. The clinical importance of love requires that we move beyond crude stereotypes toward a more dynamic, interpersonal, and multifaceted view that encompasses individual beliefs, relationship context, and changes over time in women's and men's expressions of love.

What Is Love?

Before we can talk about expressions of love, we need to consider what we mean by love. In our view, the core of love is a feeling that involves a strong desire to be with a specific other person. However, different cultures and historical periods are characterized by different perspectives on love and different scripts for how to express it (e.g., Averill & Nunley, 1992; Contreras, Hendrick, & Hendrick, 1996; Stearns, 1993). For instance, Stearns (1993) notes that, in the 17th century, suitors in Wales urinated on their fiancées' robes as a sign of affection. Modern women are unlikely to appreciate such a gesture. Moreover, each person experiences love differently, and even the same person may experience love in different ways at different times or with different partners. The way we love can change as a result of time, age, developmental stage, or relationship context. Love can be passionate or tender or comforting. It can bring anguish or elation (Baumeister & Wotman, 1992). As S. S. Hendrick and Hendrick (1992) point out, love is one of life's supreme values, but it is also integral to the mundane experiences, like rubbing elbows and chatting about nothing, that make up everyday life (cf. Duck, 1994). Not surprisingly, psychologists have offered numerous possible definitions of love (e.g., Aron & Aron, 1991; Berscheid & Walster, 1978; Fehr, 1988; Hatfield & Sprecher, 1986; Hazan & Shaver, 1987; C. Hendrick & Hendrick, 1986; Z. Rubin, 1973). Most of these definitions have focused on describing components of love and/or different types of love relationships.

It is doubtful that any one definition can truly capture the complexity of love, but one particularly useful view is Sternberg's (1986) triangular theory of love. Sternberg argues that love is composed of three components: *passion,* which involves psychological and physical arousal and sexual desire, *intimacy,* which involves emotional closeness, and *commitment,* which involves a recognition that one loves the other person and a decision to be together. These components vary across different types of intimate relationships. For instance, intimacy is central to many close relationships, such as loving a parent, a friend, or a mate. Passion is generally reserved for mates. Commitment is usually prominent in love for one's children, but perhaps less so in love for a friend. The three components also vary within intimate relationships, as people or relationships change. Sternberg (1986) identifies a number of different types of love that entail different proportions of the three components—passion, intimacy, and commitment. These are summarized in Table 6.1. For example, *empty love* is characterized solely by commitment. Partners feel no sense of desire for each other, nor do they feel connected at an emotional level, but they are determined to stay together, perhaps out of moral, practical, or child-rearing concerns, or perhaps out of simple habit. *Romantic love* occurs when partners desire each other (passion), and feel a sense of emotional closeness (intimacy), but have not made any serious decision to stay together long term. *Consummate love* involves all three components. An example of this would be a couple in which the partners have been together for 15 years, are enthusiastic lovers, consider themselves each other's best friend, and are committed to weathering life's ups and downs together.

Sternberg's distinctions among the components of love are conceptu-

TABLE 6.1. Types of Love

Type of love	Components		
	Passion	Intimacy	Commitment
Nonlove	—	—	—
Liking	—	Yes	—
Infatuated love	Yes	—	—
Empty love	—	—	Yes
Romantic love	Yes	Yes	—
Companionate love	—	Yes	Yes
Fatuous love	Yes	—	Yes
Consummate love	Yes	Yes	Yes

Note. Based on Sternberg (1986).

ally useful as a way of understanding different types of love and changes in a particular loving relationship. However, he notes that the three components are interactive rather than independent phenomena. In real relationships, passion, intimacy, and commitment tend to be strongly correlated, mutually influencing, and intricately woven.

The strength of Sternberg's triangular theory of love is that it is elegantly simple and flexible. It encompasses many of the definitions of love offered by other psychologists. Moreover, for our purposes, it provides an excellent backdrop for understanding the role of emotional expression in love.

Chapter Overview

In this chapter, we look at research concerning men, women, and the language of love. We examine the role of emotional expression in the development and maintenance of close, heterosexual relationships. (We confine our discussion to heterosexual relationships because of the dearth of research on expressions of love in homosexual relationships.) We describe how women and men tell each other the messages that are the crux of these relationships: "I want you," "I care for you," "I love you." Following Sternberg's triangular theory, we first discuss expressions of sexual interest and desire, which pertain to the *passion* component of love. We then look at expressions of trust, understanding, and closeness, which are central to the *intimacy* component. Finally, we turn to expressions of affection, which are relevant to the *commitment* component. A key theme that emerges from our discussion is that to understand the impact of emotional behavior on relationships, we need to consider not only what and how individuals express, but also how partners interpret that expression. Because it seems heartless to talk about love without poetry, rather than providing illustrative anecdotes, in this chapter we complement our discussion of research and theory with several vividly evocative poems concerning expressions of love.

PASSION: EXPRESSIONS OF SEXUAL
INTEREST AND DESIRE

O Blush Not So! O Blush Not So!

O blush not so! O blush not so!
 Or I shall think you knowing;
And if you blush and smile the while,
 Then maidenheads are going.

There's a blush for won't, and a blush for shan't,
 And a blush for having done it;
There's a blush for thought, and a blush for nought,
 And a blush for just begun it.

O sigh not so! O sigh not so!
 For it sounds of Eve's sweet pippin;
By those loosen'd hips, you have tasted the pips,
 And fought in an amorous nipping. . . .

There's a sigh for yes, and a sigh for no,
 And a sigh for I can't bear it!
O what can be done? Shall we stay or run?
 O cut the sweet apple and share it!
 —JOHN KEATS, 1795–1821

This early 19th-century poem alludes to many features of the expression of sexual interest and desire[1] that have been documented by late 20th-century research. In particular it highlights the importance of a woman's nonverbal sexual signaling in the initiation of sexual interaction. This signaling is often subtle and requires interpretation. In the poem, the man carefully observes the woman's blushes, sighs, and hip movements in an effort to deduce their meaning. The line asking "Shall we stay or run?" alludes to ambivalence about sexual contact that partners often experience and sometimes express, particularly early in a relationship.

Having sex is complicated—more so than participants might realize. Ethologists' descriptions of human courtship and mating document intricate choreographies involving specific sequences of behaviors. For instance, Birdwhistell (1970) identifies 24 steps between initial contact and full sexual intimacy in female–male relationships. Morris (1971) spells out 12 steps: (1) eye to body, (2) eye to eye, (3) voice to voice, (4) hand to hand, (5) arm to shoulder, (6) arm to waist, (7) mouth to mouth, (8) hand to head, (9) hand to body, (10) mouth to breast, (11) hand to genitals, and (12) genitals to genitals or mouth to genitals. These steps usually occur in this order. A person who skips steps may be perceived as "fast," whereas someone who fails to respond to a step may be seen as "slow." Negotiating these complicated sexual sequences requires that partners engage in a great deal of signaling and responding. Directly and indirectly, sexual partners express to each other their desire to start, to stop, to continue, to proceed, to move an awkward elbow, etc. Thus, a full understanding of sexual interaction requires that we have a clear picture of the emotional expressions that initiate and regulate sexual activity.

Simon and Gagnon (1987) suggest that what may appear to be a spontaneous sexual interaction is actually a confluence of three levels of scripts regarding sexual behavior: (1) The *intrapsychic sexual script* reflects an individual's understanding of what should be done to create, sustain, and maximize his or her sexual arousal and satisfaction; (2) the *interpersonal sexual script* involves an individual's understanding of what behaviors will lead to the fulfillment of the intrapsychic script with another person; and (3) the *cultural sexual script* reflects societal meanings and messages regarding sexual behavior. Together, these sexual scripts constitute norms and expectations that guide the expression, interpretation, and negotiation of sexual feelings.

Stereotypical Sexual Roles

In Western culture, traditional sexual scripts dictate that the man is the sexual aggressor, while the reluctant woman fends off his advances (see discussions by McCormick, 1979; Perper & Weis, 1987; and historical perspective by Cate & Lloyd, 1992). Consistent with this script, men report initiating sex more often than women (e.g., Spitz, Gold, & Adams, 1975). Both men and women view strategies aimed at having sex as used mostly by men and strategies aimed at avoiding sex as used mostly by women. These same expectations are voiced by students with traditional sex-role values as well as those with profeminist views (McCormick, 1979).

A recent meta-analytic[2] review of gender differences in sexuality (Oliver & Hyde, 1993) found that men have more permissive attitudes toward sex and they masturbate substantially more than women. Gender differences in reports of other sexual behaviors were only in the small-to-moderate range, albeit in the expected direction: Men report a slightly higher incidence of sexual intercourse, a somewhat younger age of first intercourse, and a slightly greater number of sexual partners. The fact that men's more permissive sexual attitudes don't necessarily translate into more sexual behavior with a partner is consistent with the socially proscribed roles of men as the sexual initiators and women as the sexual restrictors.

Theorists have proposed numerous possible explanations for stereotypical sexual roles (see Oliver & Hyde, 1993, for a review). Some theorists point to society at large. They argue that society creates a double standard for men's and women's sexual behavior, and it rewards role-consistent behavior and ignores or punishes role-inconsistent behavior (e.g., Mischel,

1966). Other theorists focus on individual experience, suggesting that men's sexual arousal is more obvious, more intense, and more distracting than women's arousal. This leads men to have a more body-centered perspective on sexuality, whereas women tend to have a more person-centered perspective (DeLamater, 1987). Some theorists suggest that the roots of these roles lie in men's and women's differential investment in child bearing and child rearing (e.g., D. M. Buss & Schmitt, 1993). They suggest that, from an evolutionary perspective, it makes sense for men to mate widely, while women mate wisely (Hinde, 1984). Other theorists suggest that differential sexual roles arise in early childhood, because little boys' development emphasizes autonomy and breaking away from their mothers, whereas little girls are taught to define themselves in relational terms, and never completely separate from their mothers (e.g., Chodorow, 1978; Gilligan, 1982). Still other theorists (Gagnon & Simon, 1973) point to early adolescent experiences that lead to different meanings of sexual behavior for men and women. During this period, boys typically engage in a great deal of masturbation, usually alone and in secret. Girls are much less likely to masturbate during this period and are more likely to focus on attracting male attention. Girls' first sexual experiences occur later and usually with a partner, rather than alone. These theorists suggest that the outgrowth of these experiences is that, for males, the meaning of sexuality is more closely linked to individual pleasure, whereas for females, sexuality reflects the quality of a relationship.

Many of these theories concerning the origins of sexual roles are difficult to either refute or verify. The more sweeping ones, focusing on evolution or early childhood experiences, have a harder time accommodating cultural differences and historical changes in sexuality (e.g., the sexual revolution, AIDS paranoia). We are dubious of theories that try to explain the "true" nature of women's or men's sexuality. Along these lines, it is important to note that, although current theorists focus on explaining women's relatively more restrained sexuality, from a historical perspective, it wasn't too long ago that theorists warned against women's uncontrollable sexuality or denied that women are sexual at all (see discussions of historical perspectives by Cate & Lloyd, 1992, and S. S. Hendrick & Hendrick, 1992). If we had to pick a favorite, it would be Gagnon and Simon's (1973) theory focusing on early adolescent experiences. This theory fits well with survey and observational data concerning actual sexual behavior of young men and women (cf. Moore, 1995; Oliver & Hyde, 1993). Because it emphasizes learning, this theory is also able to accommodate overlap in men's and women's sexual behavior as well as changes in sexuality as women and men gain more experience and mature from young adults to older adults. However, in addition to individual experience, we also think it is important to take into account the impact of prevailing cultural proscriptions concerning appropriate sexual roles.

We now turn from general sexual stereotypes to specific studies looking at women's and men's expressions of sexual interest and desire. As we shall see, these expressions are less rigidly sex-segregated and more changeable over time than stereotypes suggest.

Courtship Signaling

Women's Expressions of Sexual Interest

The stereotypical view of women as sexually reluctant is contradicted by data showing that women often initiate and escalate sexual encounters. When asked, women are able to provide explicit descriptions of numerous verbal and nonverbal cues that they use to indicate sexual interest in a man (e.g., Jesser, 1978; McCormick, 1979; Perper, 1985; Remoff, 1984).

Perper and Weis (1987) investigated proceptive and rejective strategies used by college women. They define proceptivity as "any behavior pattern a woman employs to express interest to a man, to arouse him sexually, or to maintain her sociosexual interaction with him." These behaviors are important in the transition between presexual and sexual behaviors. Rejective behaviors, on the other hand, are used to limit sexual contact. They suggest that proceptivity and rejectivity represent complementary strategies that women use to balance their sexual interest and their sexual hesitancy, as well as to evaluate their partners' interest.

In order to elicit descriptions of proceptive strategies involved in initial sexual encounters, Perper and Weis (1987) asked college women to imagine that they were on a second date with a man. "So far, there hasn't been any kind of sex between the two of you. . . . You feel really turned on by him. How would you influence this person to have sex with you? (Of course, we mean going only as far as you want to.)" The women responded to this question with open-ended essays. The most commonly reported proceptive strategies were (1) *talking*, which includes nonsexual conversation, laughing, complimenting the man, sexual talk, and explicitly asking the man to engage in sexual activity; (2) *environmental signaling*, which involves dressing seductively, creating or seeking out an intimate ambiance, and playing music or dancing; (3) *touching*, such as holding hands, offering to rub his back or read his palm, caressing his hair; and (4) *kissing*, which ranged from friendly to passionate. Interestingly, there was no evidence that either the number or type of proceptive strategies was related to the liberalism or conservatism of the women's sexual values. In other words, both conservative and liberal women report that they can and would express sexual interest in men.

Nevertheless, the essays provide an important perspective on the initiation of sexual activity between women and men: These women see themselves as taking the initiative. Perper and Weis (1987) comment, the essayists "see the beginning of sexual interaction not in the man's first overt sexual act (e.g., he touches her breasts) but in the prior proceptive interaction between the man and the woman. In the proceptive script, the woman sees his action as a response to her behavior, not as self-initiated by him and him alone" (p. 475).

Do women really do all these things? The fact that the Perper and Weis essays are based on hypothetical scenarios raises the possibility that the college women are merely reporting sexual scripts involving a "femme fatale." Maybe they read about how to entice men in a romance novel or *Cosmopolitan* magazine, but wouldn't actually use any of these behaviors themselves.

Observational studies indicate that women do all of these things and then some. For instance, Moore (1985) defined courtship behaviors as nonverbal signals that (1) were commonly observed in courtship settings but rarely seen in noncourtship settings and (2) consistently elicited or maintained male attention. Based on her observations of over 200 women in singles' bars, restaurants, and parties, she derived an entertaining list of 52 female courtship behaviors, detailing how women flirt. The list includes numerous signals involving a woman's face and head, such as giving a man short, darting glances, running fingers through her hair, licking her lips, and tilting her head to expose her neck. It also includes broader gestures, involving other parts of a woman's body, such as briefly showing her palm, caressing an object, hiking her skirt to reveal more of her leg, parading across the room while swaying her hips, and touching a man with her knee, thigh, or breast. Observations of these behaviors in 20 target women showed that women in courtship settings are very busy flirting: They perform an average of 44.6 courtship behaviors per hour, eliciting an average of about two approaches by men per hour. Moore and Butler (1989) found that the frequency of women's courtship signaling is more important than physical attractiveness in predicting the number of approaches by men.

In a follow-up study, Moore (1995) observed courtship behavior by young teenaged girls at shopping malls, roller rinks, and other "hangouts." The girls used many of the same flirting behaviors that she had identified in her earlier observations of women, but they also showed some intriguing differences compared to women. First, girls were less serious about flirting. They used considerably more silly flirting, such as playful teasing, and were much less likely to use overtly sexual behaviors. Second, girls were less skilled at flirting. For instance, when women toss their heads and stroke their hair, their gestures are graceful: noticeable, but subtle. When girls do the same thing, their gestures are less refined: They use broad, exaggerated movements and take longer doing them. Third, girls flirt in herds. If two women are together in a courtship setting, they tend to use different signals and to do them at different times. For instance, if one woman strokes her hair, her friend might smooth her clothing some time later. Women seem to try to distinguish themselves, but girls mimic each other. So, if the lead girl in a group fluffs her hair, all the other girls do, too. Finally, girls' flirting was less frequent and less effective. Girls did an average of 7.6 courtship signals per hour (about one-sixth the frequency for women) and elicited only 0.3 approaches by boys per hour. Moore (1995) argues that, taken together, these observations suggest that the girls she observed are just practicing flirting. Although they talk about boys a lot, these girls aren't seriously interested in attracting boys. Most of their attention is focused on their same-sex friends. She suggests that this practicing has adaptive significance because it allows girls to refine their flirting skills so that, by the time they are interested in finding lifetime mates and fathers for their children, they have efficient courtship signaling systems.

Women's Expressions of Sexual Reluctance

So far, we have only talked about women's "come hither" signals. However, sexual stereotypes suggest that women are in charge of limiting sexual contact, so it's also important to look at expressions signaling a desire to stop or avoid sexual contact. To elicit descriptions of rejective strategies, Perper and Weis (1987) presented the women with the same second-date scenario, but specified, "While he is really turned on by you, you know you are not interested. How would you influence this person to avoid having sex?" Essays written in response to this scenario often mentioned explicitly saying "No," making excuses, and providing diversions and distractions. These and other behaviors occurred in the context of two broad types of rejective strategies: (1) *Avoid Proceptivity,* which involves ignoring the man's signals of sexual interest and trying to avoid doing anything that might signal interest on the woman's part (e.g., don't touch him; stick to mundane conversation topics, like the weather), and (2) *Incomplete Rejection,* which involves trying to avoid further sexual involvement for the time being while continuing the relationship. This latter strategy is characterized by a mixture of positive and negative expressions. For example, the woman expresses concern about the man's feelings, but states that she will not see him unless he respects her desire not to have intercourse. She might tell him she needs more time or more emotional closeness before she becomes more sexually involved, suggesting that this is a future possibility.

Comparing Men's and Women's Courtship Signals

What about men? How do they signal interest in sexual activity and how do their sexual expressions compare to women's? Fichten, Taglakis, Judd, Wright, and Amsel (1992) used structured interviews to ask men and women how they express interest or disinterest in a potential dating partner. They found no significant gender differences in reported use of interest cues. Both men and women were able to describe a wide variety of cues for expressing interest, including verbal, visual, and paralinguistic signals. They described interest cues more specifically than disinterest cues. Most of the cues related to expressing romantic interest, rather than simple conversational interest, were nonverbal.

McCormick (1979) asked over 100 male and female unmarried college students to imagine that they were alone with someone of the opposite sex with whom they had "necked" but had not yet had sexual intercourse. They were then asked to write essays explaining (1) how they might try to influence their partner to have sexual intercourse, and (2) what they would do to avoid having intercourse with a "turned on" partner. Raters then coded these responses into 10 strategies. Both men and women reported using indirect strategies to have sex and direct strategies to avoid sex. Indirect strategies included body language and subtle hinting through manipulations of one's appearance or the setting. Direct strategies included directly informing a partner whether or not sex was desired, discussing the relationship, or logically reasoning with the partner. This suggests that when men and women have the same goals in courtship situations, their behavior is similar.

Despite men's and women's similar reliance on nonverbal expressions of sexual interest, in relatively new relationships men may be responsible for initiating more overtly sexual behavior. Perper and Weis (1987) found that women in their study were able to describe their early courtship signals, but they had difficulty depicting their later behaviors involving moving toward sexual intercourse. Similarly, Peplau, Rubin, and Hill (1977) found that it was quite unusual among dating couples for the woman to actively initiate the couple's first intercourse. Men usually took the initiative, but women controlled the onset and timing of intercourse.

Wouldn't it be easier, instead of all this subtle signaling, to express sexual interest by asking directly? If they want to have sex, why don't people just say to their partners, "So, would you like to make wild, passionate love with me?" Sometimes they do. Jesser (1978) conducted a survey of over 150 college students enrolled in a course on sex roles, asking them about sexual initiations, responses, and attitudes. Consistent with the studies we have already described, he found that the most commonly used strategies for signaling sexual interest were nonverbal: Over 70% of both men and women in this sample reported that they persuaded a partner to have sex by using the strategies of "touching (snuggling, kissing, etc.)" and "allow hands to wander." However, the next most common strategy was "ask directly," which was endorsed by almost 60% of both the men and the women. Comparing the women who do versus do not report asking directly for sex indicates that the former group tended to have partners who also asked directly for sex. Unfortunately, Jesser's study contains no information about the length or seriousness of relationships, which (as we discuss below) might affect the likelihood of using direct requests for sex. Direct expressions of sexual desire carry the risk of direct rejections, thus they seem most likely to be used either when the initiator is reasonably confident that a partner will respond positively or when the initiator is not concerned about being rejected.

Sexual Expressions in Established Relationships

So far we have discussed signaling of sexual interest and initiation of sexual activity in the early stages of relationships. What happens in more established relationships? As relationships become more established and more intimate, the rules governing interactions tend to become more idiosyncratic of the dyad and less reflecting of general cultural scripts (Knapp, 1984). There is some evidence that men in married and cohabiting couples initiate sex more frequently than women (e.g., M. Brown & Auerback, 1981; Byers & Heinlein, 1989), but M. Brown and Auerback (1981) suggest that the discrepancy in husbands' and wives' rates of initiation decreases over time. In their survey of 50 middle-class couples who had been married from 2 to 35 years, spouses reported that in the first year of marriage the average ratio of husband versus wife initiations was 75:25, but in later years the average ratio changed to 60:40. Moreover, O'Brien (1981) notes that multiple periodic interviews indicate that women's sexual initiatives are more common than they appear to be based on retrospective reports. In established relationships, women may feel more free to express sexual desire because they don't fear negative reactions from their partner (e.g., O'Sullivan & Byers, 1993; Roche, 1986).

Byers and Heinlein (1989) studied initiations and refusals of sexual activities in married and cohabiting heterosexual couples, using a self-monitoring methodology. They asked 22 men and 55 women to keep ongoing records of sexual interest, initiations, and responses to initiations. Although male partners initiated sex and thought about initiating sex more often than female partners did, when the number of initiations was statistically controlled, there were no sex differences in responses to sexual initiations. Contrary to sex-role stereotypes of women as sexual restrictors, in these couples, on average, both men and women responded positively to sexual initiations 75% of the time. This means that for a given sexual initiation, male and female partners are equally likely to respond positively. However, because men initiate more often, women are more often in the position of reacting to initiations. This means that, over time, women will respond, both negatively and positively, more often than men. Byers and Heinlein (1989) speculate that retrospective studies that have characterized women as sexual restrictors (e.g., Blumstein & Schwartz, 1983) may be based on individuals' perceptions of the total number of rejections rather than the number of positive responses or the percentage of positive responses. Alternatively, these retrospective studies may simply reflect cultural stereotypes.

Consistent with research on less-established couples, Byers and Heinlein (1989) found that among married couples both men and women tended to respond positively to sexual initiations and to indicate their responses in similar ways. Positive responses usually involved nonverbal behaviors, starting or continuing the sexual interaction, whereas negative responses tended to be verbal. These direct rejections offer the opportunity to protect the initiators' feelings by providing an account (e.g., "I'm really tired tonight"), arranging to have sex at another time, or just agreeing to disagree.

Women's expressions of sexual interest may become increasingly important in established relationships. For instance, Huston and Vangelisti (1991) found that women's expressions of sexual interest were related to men's marital satisfaction in couples who had been married for 2 years, but not at earlier points in the marriage. However, we agree with Canary et al. (1997) who argue that to understand sexuality we cannot focus exclusively on intercourse. They note that gender differences in sexual desire may be apparent if we consider only desire for coitus, but including a broader spectrum of activity in our understanding of sexuality may erase these gender differences.

In that vein, we noticed that although there are many studies on the role of emotional expression in initiating or avoiding sexual interactions, we were unable to find any research on the role of expression during or immediately after sexual interactions. This exclusive focus on outcome and neglect of process seems like a curious omission to us. Expressions involved in initiating or refusing sex no doubt influence whether or not sexual activity occurs, but later expressions are likely to be critically important in determining the meaning of sexual activity for the couple. Particularly in established sexual relationships, it seems likely that the important issue is not simply "Who did what?" or even "How often do they do it?" but rather "How was it?"

Imagine two men who express sexual interest to their partners. Both men's partners respond positively initially, in that they agree to have sex. However, the first man's partner's response is lukewarm, at best ("If you must . . . "), and her expressions during and after their sexual interaction range from merely tolerant to disinterested. In contrast, the second man's partner expresses considerable enthusiasm during their sexual interaction ("Yes! Yes!") and afterward ("That was incredible!"). It is entirely conceivable that the second couple couldn't care less who started what, since both partners thoroughly enjoyed themselves. Their similar, warm, eager expressions color their interaction with mutuality and pleasure. In contrast, the mismatched expressions of the first couple give their interaction the ugly taint of a passive–aggressive power play.

To summarize, we have described expressions of sexual interest and reluctance by men and women, in beginning and established relationships. In the early stages of a relationship, individuals attempt to meet multiple goals, including impression management and relationship definition (Cupach & Metts, 1991). Because partners don't know each other very well, they tend to rely on generalized cultural scripts as guides for how they should behave and how the relationship ought to proceed. This means that early in a relationship partners are more likely to follow sexual stereotypes with the man initiating sexual activity while the woman controls its occurrence. We have noted that although men may take the lead more often in overt sexual behaviors, women are anything but passive in expressing sexual interest. Their proceptive cues are important triggers of men's sexual initiatives in courtship relationships and probably in established relationships as well.

The research we reviewed shows quite a bit of overlap in women's and men's sexual expressions. When men and women have similar sexual goals, they behave similarly. In both courtship and established relationships, women and men are most likely to use indirect expressions to signal sexual interest and direct expressions to signal sexual reluctance. In established relationships, women's direct expressions of sexual interest become increasingly likely. Rather than relying on stereotypical proscriptions to guide their behavior, established couples tend to create their own sexual scripts. One of the best predictors of women asking directly for sex is having a partner who also asks directly for sex.

We now turn from describing how men and women express sexual interest or reluctance to examine how these expressions are understood by partners. How do partners interpret each others' sexual expressions?

Interpretations of Sexual Expressions

Interpreting sexual expressions is by no means a straightforward process. For effective sexual communication to occur, partners need to notice and correctly interpret the intended meaning of each other's expressions (cf. Perper & Weis, 1987). Cupach and Metts (1991) insist that sexual interaction is not just a matter of wanting sex, expressing that desire, and having a partner comply or not. Instead, sexual interaction is more like a negotiation, as both partners use multiple (often subtle) behaviors to communicate multiple (not necessarily shared) goals, which are interpreted in the light of individual experience, and relational and cultural context. Thus different people may understand the same sexual signal in different ways.

The fact that expressions of sexual interest are frequently subtle and indirect means that often partners are just plain guessing what the other person means. Was that quick kiss meant as a sign of affection or a prelude to intercourse? Similarly, subtle expressions of sexual reluctance may be misread or overlooked.

The women in Perper and Weis's (1987) study mention in both the proceptive and rejective essays that men might not "get the hint," which suggests that sexual signaling is not always understood. Many of the behaviors described by the women are ambiguous. For example, laughing was mentioned as a proceptive signal, but, obviously, women don't always mean "I want to have sex with you" when they laugh. Indirect rejective strategies seem particularly open to the possibility of miscommunication. With the Avoid Proceptivity strategy, the man has to recognize that the woman would be sitting closer to him or talking about different topics if she were interested. With the Incomplete Rejection strategy, which involves mixed signals, the man may discount the negative cues in favor of the positive. Either strategy might lead a man to believe that he should try harder rather than back off in his sexual overtures.

Misunderstandings stemming from ambiguous expressions are one source of variability in interpretations of sexual expressions. However, differences in interpretation can also arise from more global differences in perceptions, goals, and values concerning sexual behavior. Below, we describe research concerning differences in the meaning assigned to sexual expressions for men and women and for different couples.

Male–Female Differences in Perceptions of Sexual Expressions

Some researchers have suggested that men wear "sex-colored glasses" (Cupach & Metts, 1991). Men tend to perceive sexual interest in both males and females to a greater extent than women do (Abbey & Melby, 1986; Koeppel, Montagne-Miller, O'Hair, & Cody, 1993; Shotland & Craig, 1988). Although both men and women make distinctions between friendly and sexually interested behavior, men have a much lower threshold for perceiving sexual interest (Shotland & Craig, 1988). However, in established, monogamously dating couples, gender differences in perceptions of sexual interest are not evident: Women are just as likely as men to misperceive their partners' intent (Frandsen, 1989).

A great deal of research shows that, in general, young men take sex a lot less seriously than do young women. As we mentioned earlier, based on their meta-analysis, Oliver and Hyde (1993) conclude that men are substantially more permissive than women in their attitudes toward sex, especially casual sex. A study by R. D. Clark and Hatfield (1989) vividly illustrates men's greater receptivity to casual sex. These investigators had a male or female confederate of average attractiveness approach strangers of the opposite sex with one of three requests: (1) Would you like to go out tonight? (2) Will you come over to my apartment? or (3) Would you go to bed with me? The great majority of men approached with this last request said that they were willing to have sex. Not one of the women approached with this request agreed to have sex. A similar experiment by R. D. Clark

(1990) also showed that men were more willing than women to go to the apartment of someone they had just met to engage in casual sex. Compared to women, men tend to have more permissive and instrumental attitudes toward sex (S. S. Hendrick, Hendrick, Slapion-Foote, & Foote, 1985). Men are more apt to see sex as merely a bodily function, like eating, whereas women tend to see it in more emotionally laden terms, like the communion of two souls (S. S. Hendrick & Hendrick, 1987; see also Brigman & Knox, 1992).

Some researchers suggest that the old double standard specifying that only men are allowed to be sexual has been replaced by a new, conditional double standard saying that casual sex is fine for men, but women are only allowed to be sexual in the context of a serious relationship (Sprecher & McKinney, 1993). Consistent with this view is evidence showing that interpretations of touch vary depending on the relational context in which they occur. For instance, Nguyen, Heslin, and Nguyen (1976) asked married and unmarried women how they would react to sexual touching. The unmarried women said they would react negatively, whereas the married women said their reactions would be strongly positive. When asked to rate the relational commitment entailed in different types of romantic touch, ranging in intimacy from holding hands to having intercourse, both men and women viewed the more explicitly sexual forms of touch as entailing more commitment (K. Johnson & Edwards, 1991). Women were somewhat more likely to ascribe greater commitment than men to the more intimate types of touch. However, these gender differences were small compared to the effect for type of touch.

Substantiating the existence of this new double standard is evidence showing that young women are concerned about violating it, and young men look askance at women who do violate it. It is noteworthy that even in Jesser's (1978) young, sexually experienced, presumably liberal sample, 35% of the women and 16% of the men endorsed the belief that men are turned off by women who are too sexually aggressive. Oliver and Sedikides's (1992) study of preferences for dating and marriage partners showed that young men consider a woman who has engaged in a great deal of sexual activity to be the most desirable dating partner, but they judged a woman who was low in sexual permissiveness to be an acceptable marriage partner. L. B. Rubin (1990) suggests that differing expectations regarding men's and women's sexual behavior prompts many women to conceal or understate their sexual activity.

Muehlenhard (1988) notes that sexual scripts specifying that "nice women don't say yes" and "real men don't say no" may lead some men to believe that a woman doesn't really mean it when she rejects his sexual advances. These men may believe that the woman wants sexual involvement but says "No" only because she doesn't want to appear promiscuous. This misunderstanding is compounded by the fact that women are likely to express their sexual reluctance politely and indirectly, in consideration of the man's feelings (cf. Falbo & Peplau, 1980; Lewin, 1985). Moreover, Muehlenhard and Hollabaugh (1988) found disturbing evidence that some women occasionally do offer only token resistance to sexual advances (i.e., they say "No" when they mean "Yes").

Reliance on stereotyped sexual roles early in a relationship may stem to some extent from uncertainty and anxiety. Relationships in general and sexual relationships in particular can be anxiety provoking, especially in the early stages (see discussion by DeLamater, 1991). As Reiss (1989) points out, "Experiencing [and expressing] intense physical pleasure in the presence of another person reveals parts of oneself which are not generally known even by one's close friends" (p. 10). A person in a new sexual relationship may feel anxious because of fear of intimacy, fear of rejection, concern about the partner's degree of commitment, uncertainty about a partner's expectations and intentions, and concerns about the mechanics of initiating and engaging in sexual activity. In more established relationships, partners will have created interpersonal and sexual scripts that may lessen at least some of these concerns.

However, the extent to which stereotypical gender differences in interpretations of sexual behavior persist in established relationships is not clear. It is doubtful that married women or women in established cohabiting relationships would be concerned that their partners might perceive them as "easy" if they express too much sexual interest. Nevertheless, there is some evidence that women in established relationships continue to take sex more seriously than do men. For instance, Metts and Cupach (1987) asked married couples to describe their sexual relationship. The wives were more likely than the husbands to describe emotional themes involving comfort, responsiveness, specialness, and communication. The husbands were more likely to focus on physical characteristics of the interactions, such as frequency and arousal.

On the other hand, gender differences in the meaning attributed to sexual activity may lessen with age. Sprague and Quadagno (1989) examined volunteers' ratings of the importance of physical release and love as motives for intercourse. Consistent with sexual stereotypes, young men, aged 22 to 35, rated physical release as more important than did young women, while young women rated love as more important than did young men. However, among individuals over 35 years of age, men and women gave similar ratings to love as a motivation for intercourse. Furthermore, among individuals over 45 years of age, women saw physical release as a more important motivation for sex than men did.

Between-Couple Differences in the Meaning of Sexual Expressions

In addition to male–female differences in the interpretation of sexual behavior, there are also differences between couples in the meanings they assign to sexual interactions (Christopher & Cate, 1985; Peplau et al., 1977). For instance, Christopher and Cate (1985) identified five types of couples:

1. *Rapid-involvement couples* had intercourse on their first date and reported being motivated to do so by feelings of physical arousal.
2. At the other extreme, *low-involvement couples* endorsed traditional values concerning sexuality, wanting to save intercourse for marriage.
3. *Gradual-involvement couples* had intercourse when they were considering becoming a couple; for these couples, sexual interaction was a means of judging whether to move toward monogamy.
4. Finally, *delayed-involvement couples* engaged in low levels of sexual activity in the early stages of their relationship, but became much more sexually involved once they had made a commitment to a monogamous relationship. For these couples, intercourse was a sign of commitment.

These different couple types show that a single expression of sexual desire—intercourse—can have multiple meanings or symbolic functions. For some couples it is a means of developing intimacy, for others it is a sign of established intimacy or commitment.

Direct versus Indirect Sexual Expressions

Based on our discussion so far, sexual expression seems to involve a lot of fumbling around in the dark (physically and metaphorically). When we consider the complexity of cultural proscriptions, the multiplicity of interpersonal goals, the subtlety of sexual cues, the variety of relationship histories, and the fluidity of partners' perceptions and interpretations of sexual expressions, it seems miraculous that anyone ever establishes a mutually satisfying sexual relationship.

There is a good reason why sexual signaling is often subtle or indirect: It is safer that way. Ambiguous sexual expressions can allow partners to avoid overt rejection. Through subtle signs of sexual interest a person may gain sexual access without risking direct rejection. If a partner responds favorably to these subtle initiations, then both partners can move on to more direct sexual activity. On the other hand, if a partner does not respond positively, both partners can simply ignore these subtle signals. No direct refusal or rejection is necessary. Similarly, subtle signals of sexual reluctance may protect partners' feelings. Research indicates that unwanted sexual advances in dating situations are most likely to be stopped by strong, direct, persistent refusals (Byers, 1988; Christopher & Frandsen, 1990; Murnen, Perot, & Byrne, 1989). However, such vigorous refusals are likely to be used only as a last resort, since they pose considerable threat to the continuation of the relationship. Moreover, ambiguous sexual expressions may be a subtle means of gathering information about a potential partner without asking embarrassing or threatening questions. Perper and Weis (1987) speculate that the Incomplete Rejection strategy is a subtle kind of test for men: Only men who are sufficiently sensitive to and respectful of the woman's expressions of sexual reluctance pass this test. A man who persists in his sexual advances in the face of incomplete rejection shows that he fails to recognize or respect the woman's feelings and is therefore rejected by the woman as a long-term partner.

Nevertheless, talking directly about sexual feelings is critically important to fostering understanding between partners. Earlier we mentioned that couples do sometimes ask directly for sex (Jesser, 1978). However, cultivating understanding in sexual communication involves more than just saying "Let's do it!" Talking directly to each other about sexual feelings can help partners align their meanings for sexual behavior, clarify which behaviors are most satisfying, and negotiate the implications of sexual interactions for the relationship (Cupach & Metts, 1991). Because men and women are not equally aroused by the same sexual behaviors (Geer & Broussard, 1990) and because individual preferences may vary, people need to be able to clearly express their needs and desires and to communicate to their partner when they are enjoying a particular sexual activity. They also need to be able to solicit, understand, and accept these types of expressions from their partner (D'Augelli & D'Augelli, 1985; Metts, Sprecher, & Regan, 1998).

Direct emotional expression can play an important role in managing a sexual relationship over the long haul. Both the frequency and the quality with which couples talk about sex are strongly related to their level of satisfaction with their sex lives and their relationship in general (Cupach & Comstock, 1990; Metts & Cupach, 1989). Tavris and Sadd (1978) found that 50% of women who said they always discussed their sexual feelings with their husband were very satisfied. In contrast, only 9% of women who said they never discussed sexual feelings with their husband were very satisfied. Cupach and Metts (1991) emphasize that talking about sex makes it possible for partners to communicate about their desires and preferences, to coordinate inferred meanings of sexual behaviors, and to negotiate the timing and form of sexual interactions.

However, talking about sex doesn't have to be dire and serious. For instance, Adelman (1989) noted that expressions of humor can also be helpful in sexual communication. She observed safe-sex talk in simulated discussions among college students and found several instances in which humor eased the inherent awkwardness of the situation. One young man told his partner that a friend had given him condoms with "those Goodyear radial ribs on them that will drive you *wild*." Adelman comments that this remark not only addressed the practical task of negotiating birth control, but it turned a tense moment into a playful one and served as a kind of verbal foreplay, hinting at upcoming pleasures.

Summary

To summarize, differences between men and women in expressions of sexual interest are most apparent at the early stages of a relationship, when social scripts and sexual stereotypes are likely to be most salient. There is considerable evidence that young men have more permissive attitudes toward sex, whereas young women tend to take sex more seriously. However, the idea that men are solely in charge of initiating sexual contact whereas women seek only to restrict it is just plain wrong. Women have a vast array of cues that they use to signal sexual interest. They spend years practicing and refining these cues.

In established relationships, interactions tend to be more equitable. Concerns about following sexual stereotypes become less important as partners know each other better and establish their own patterns of sexual communication. In general, women tend to feel more comfortable about sex in established relationships, but there is considerable variability across couples in the role that sexual behavior plays in relationship development. For instance, some couples use sex as a means of establishing closeness, others use it only after they are involved in a committed relationship. For many couples, talking directly about sexual feelings is an important way of clarifying meanings of sexual expressions for each partner and for the relationship.

Overall, research concerning expressions of sexual interest and desire shows considerable overlap in the behavior of men and women. Both men and women want to have sex and express this desire to their partners. Both men and women sometimes reject their partner's sexual initiatives. Both men and women share concerns, especially early in a relationship, about being rejected. Consequently, both men and women tend to initiate sexual activity in nonverbal ways, although men may be responsible for initiating more overtly sexual activity. As Moore (1995) notes, "Neither gender dominates in a successful flirtation. Each person takes a turn at influencing the partner and at signaling that the other's influence attempts are welcome" (p. 320).

INTIMACY: EXPRESSIONS OF TRUST, COMFORT, AND CLOSENESS

I Want to Breathe
you in I'm not talking about
perfume or even the sweet o-

dour of your skin but of the
air itself I want to share

your air inhaling what you
exhale I'd like to be that

close two of us breathing
each other as one as that.
—JAMES LAUGHLIN, b. 1914

The central feature of intimacy is feelings of emotional closeness. Intimacy involves a deep sense of being known by and connected to another person (cf. Reis & Shaver, 1988; Sternberg, 1986). In the sensual poem above, intimacy is described as a kind of merging of two people. It involves sharing at a very basic level. It is as elemental as breathing. The partners' reciprocal inhaling and exhaling points to the mutuality of intimacy. Perhaps the most striking feature of this poem is the way the pairs of lines flow together, suggesting that intimacy involves continuity and synchrony between partners.

According to cultural stereotypes, intimacy is women's domain; men find intimacy either bewildering or frightening. The stereotypes about men and women and expressions of intimacy are consistent with the ideas of theorists who argue that the developmental roots of gender differences in communication behavior lie in girls' and boys' experiences growing up in different subcultures (see reviews by Gottman & Carrere, 1994; Maccoby, 1990). From a very young age, most children prefer to interact with other children of their own sex. This leads to sex segregation, which persists even into adulthood. Moreover, when they interact with their own sex, girls and boys play differently. Girls interact in small groups or pairs. Their interaction is cooperative, and their speech involves efforts to acknowledge and support each other. In contrast, boys' interactions occur in larger groups and are more competitive. Their speech is likely to involve verbal challenge and attempts to establish and protect their position in the group hierarchy. Thus, according to the separate subcultures theory, boys and girls learn different ways of relating and different rules for communicating, with the result that confusion and misunderstanding prevail when adult men and women interact.

However, based on her extensive review of women's and men's communication, Aries (1996) presents a number of cogent arguments against the separate subcultures theory:

1. The assumption that boys and girls grow up in separate cultures might be unwarranted. Children interact with people of both sexes in their immediate and extended families and in their community. Moreover, depictions of rigidly sex-segregated peer environments overemphasize the coher-

ence of these groups and are based primarily on observations of dominant or popular children (Thorne, 1993).

2. Not all men and women have trouble communicating with each other. Research on marital communication documents the existence of happily married couples who are quite able to express their feelings and accurately interpret each other's nonverbal communication. Even unhappily married couples are capable of communicating well with people other than their spouse. Many unhappy couples are also able to communicate well with each other in a laboratory situation, when they are asked to "fake" good communication (see Fitzpatrick, 1988, p. 38).

3. Many of the empirical observations of gender differences in communication fail to recognize situational influences, especially those involving power differences. In more similar situations, with more similar roles, men and women behave more similarly.

4. There is enormous overlap in men's and women's communication behavior. Aries notes that in most studies, gender accounts for less than 10% of the variance in behavior. Moreover, the largest differences observed between men and women in communication are only of moderate effect size—which translates to an overlap of 67% in the distributions of men and women. Many of the observed communication differences involve only small effect sizes—meaning there is an 85% overlap in the behavior of men and women.

Taken together, Aries's arguments suggest that polarizing men's and women's communication behavior or styles of relating creates a false dichotomy. It makes more sense to ask, under what circumstances are these differences more or less apparent?

A close look at the research on expressions of intimacy shows that they take many forms. While women may have some advantage in certain circumstances, it is not at all accurate to say that intimacy is solely women's purview. Below, we look at three forms expressions of intimacy that have received considerable research attention: self-disclosure, accuracy of emotional communication, and rapport.

Self-Disclosure

Unlike the very visceral portrayal of intimacy in the poem at the beginning of this section, psychologists' operationalizations of intimacy tend to be quite cerebral. In particular, researchers and theorists have often conceptualized intimacy as involving increasing levels of self-disclosure (Altman & Taylor, 1973; Derlega & Berg, 1987; Derlega, Metts, Petronio, & Margulis, 1993). Derlega et al. (1993) define self-disclosure as the verbal revealing of one's thoughts, feelings, and experiences. (Thus the term *self-disclosure* is more specific than our use of the term *emotional expression*, in that it specifies a verbal mode of communication, but it is broader than emotional expression in that it involves communicating thoughts as well as feelings.) A meta-analysis by Collins and Miller (1994) shows that self-disclosure and interpersonal liking are closely linked: We generally like people who disclose to us, we self-disclose more to people we like, and we tend to like others more after we have disclosed to them. These findings suggest that self-disclosure may be a means of expressing and enhancing feelings of intimacy.

Gender Differences in Self-Disclosure

Dindia and Allen (1992) conducted a meta-analysis of over 200 studies addressing gender differences in self-disclosure. Overall, aggregating across a variety of topics, relationships, and methodologies, they found that women self-disclose only slightly more than men. The direction of this difference was quite consistent across all comparisons: Women disclose more than men to women, to men, to same-sex partners, to opposite-sex partners, to strangers, and to people whom they know. However, Dindia and Allen state that it is debatable whether the magnitude of these differences is either theoretically meaningful or practically important. They end their review by stating vehemently, "It is time to stop perpetuating the myth that there are large sex differences in men's and women's self-disclosure" (p. 118).

The magnitude of gender differences in self-disclosure varies depending on the circumstances under which that disclosure takes place. In Dindia and Allen's (1992) review, gender differences in self-disclosure were more apparent in interactions with people participants know well than with strangers, and with same-sex partners than with opposite-sex partners. The largest gender differences in self-disclosure are seen when comparing same-sex friends: In general, female friends disclose more to each other than male friends do. These differences correspond to a moderate effect size.

Other theorists have argued that it is not so much the total *amount* of self-disclosure that distinguishes men's and women's communication behavior, but rather the *intimacy* of those disclosures (see discussion by Aries, 1996; C. J. Hill & Stull, 1987). Numerous studies show on the basis of self-reports, diary records, and observer ratings that, compared to men, women talk to each other about more personal topics and feelings. Talking intimately also seems to be more important to women's friendships than men's (e.g., Baxter & Wilmot, 1986; Caldwell & Peplau, 1982).

However, Aries (1996) cautions that these findings do not mean that men never have intimate conversations with their male friends or are incapable of discussing intimate topics, rather they just have these types of conversations less often. Consistent with this view, F. Johnson and Aries (1983) found that nearly half of the men in their college-age sample reported that they spoke frequently with their best friends about doubts and fears (46%), personal problems (46%), and intimate relationships (51%). In contrast, 75% of women talked about these topics frequently with their best friends. These gender differences are statistically significant, but they are nowhere near indicating that men are completely inexpressive concerning intimate topics. In another study, Reis, Senchak, and Solomon (1985) asked men and women to come into the laboratory and have a "meaningful" conversation with their same-sex best friend. They instructed volunteers to discuss something important and reveal their thoughts, feelings, and emotions. The men were just as capable as the women at sharing their intimate feelings. There were no gender differences in either their objectively rated level of self-disclosure or in volunteers' perceptions of the meaningfulness of the conversations.

Self-Disclosure in Male–Female Interactions

What about when women and men interact with each other? Earlier reviews suggested that men and women disclose to each other at an intermediate level—less than in female–female interactions but more than in male–male interactions (e.g., C. T. Hill & Stull, 1987). In one study, Wheeler, Reis, and Nezlek (1983) had college students record every interaction they had lasting more than 10 minutes over a 2-week period. They found that men's interactions with other men were less intimate and involved less self-disclosure and other-disclosure compared to women's same-sex interactions. However, when men and women interacted, their intimacy and self-disclosure rates were equal and comparable in level to women's same-sex interactions. Hill and Stull (1987) suggest that reciprocity is important in establishing couples' levels of self-disclosure. They speculate that women's high rates of self-disclosure elicit more self-disclosure from their male partners, whereas men's lower rates of self-disclosure lead their female partners to disclose less. The result is that both partners settle on an intermediate level of disclosure.

On the other hand, Dindia and Allen's review suggests that in opposite-sex interactions, women don't settle on an intermediate level of self-disclosure—they clam up. Specifically, Dindia and Allen found that although women disclose slightly more than men in opposite-sex interactions, and female-to-male disclosure was significantly less than female-to-female disclosure, female-to-male disclosure was *not* significantly greater than male-to-male disclosure. Citing Rosenfeld's (1979) research showing that women avoid self-disclosure in an effort to avoid being hurt or hurting their relationship, they speculate that women may inhibit their self-disclosure when they are interacting with men because they feel threatened. Women may perceive that they are more likely to be emotionally hurt by confiding in men than by confiding in other women.

How do we reconcile these inconsistent depictions of self-disclosure in opposite-sex interactions? Are these interactions characterized more by reciprocity or reticence? One possibility is that patterns of self-disclosure change over time as relationships develop.

Variability in Self-Disclosure across Relationship Stages

Dindia and Allen's meta-analysis shows that women self-disclose more than men do both with strangers and with people they know. Curiously, the evidence for women's greater self-disclosure with strangers is only evident from observational data. In self-reports, women claim they disclose less than men do with strangers. Dindia and Allen note that almost all of the observational studies of self-disclosure between strangers involve people who are brought into a laboratory with no expectation that they will ever see each other again. The relevance of this type of interaction for relationship formation is dubious. Women's self-reports of initial guardedness may be an accurate description of their efforts to test the water before jumping into a potential relationship.

There is some evidence that women approach relationships more cautiously than men do. Shaffer and his colleagues (Shaffer & Ogden, 1986; Shaffer, Smith, & Tomarelli, 1982) found that even in same-sex interactions with strangers, the prospect of future interaction led men to disclose more intimately and women to disclose less intimately. In the earliest stage of a romantic relationship, men may actually self-disclose *more* than women in an effort to initiate the development of intimacy (J. D. Davis, 1978; Derlega, Winstead, Wong, & Hunter, 1985; Stokes, Childs, & Fuehrer, 1981). For instance, J. D. Davis (1978) had opposite-sex partners meet for the first time and take turns selecting prescaled conversation topics of high, medium, or low intimacy. The men selected more intimate topics to talk about than did the women who were their partners. The men also disclosed more than women in same-sex interactions. Women tended to reciprocate their partners' level of self-disclosure, but they enjoyed the exercise most when it involved a same-sex partner who stuck to low-intimacy topics. Men, on the other hand, seemed to like getting their opposite-sex partners to disclose more. Their enjoyment of the exercise was positively related to the level of intimacy of their female partner's disclosure. Consistent with this pattern of women's initial guardedness, Adams and Shea (1981) observed in a longitudinal study that for men self-disclosure precedes romantic feelings, whereas for women, romantic feelings precede self-disclosure.

Men's greater self-disclosure at the beginning of a relationship may stem from their desire to take an active role in starting the relationship, or perhaps from traditional male role prescriptions specifying that men should be the initiators in romantic relationships. Alternatively, men's early self-disclosure may stem from subtle or not so subtle cues from women encouraging them to do so. In social interactions, women smile and laugh more than men do, and they tend to be more expressive in both their faces and their bodies (Hall, 1984). Women rate themselves as better than men at eliciting self-disclosure from others (Miller et al., 1983), and, as C. T. Hill and Stull (1987) note, many women are taught by their mothers that men like to talk about themselves, so they should ask questions and express interest in order to encourage this. Encouraging a man's self-disclosure in this way is not just a means of pleasing him, but also a means of obtaining information about his suitability as a romantic partner.

As relationships intensify, reciprocity may guide interactions, as both men and women seek to get to know each other better and confide in each other. Both men and women see self-disclosure as central to developing intimacy (Monsour, 1992; see also discussion of intimacy motivation by M. S. Clark & Reis, 1988). In fact, men are even more likely than women to mention expressing emotions as being important to intimacy in cross-sex relationships (Monsour, 1992). In a study of dating couples, Z. Rubin, Hill, Peplau, and Dunkel-Schetter (1980) found that across various topic areas, there were no significant differences between men and women in their self-reported self-disclosure. These researchers suggest that an "ethic of openness" encourages the majority of couples to engage in high levels of self-disclosure. In their study, 58% of women and 57% of men reported that they disclosed "fully" to their partners. A number of participants specifically noted that they valued open communication in their relationship. However, many couples also indicated that self-disclosure was easier for the woman than the man.

In established relationships, gender differences in self-disclosure may be less apparent. For instance, men and women in cross-sex friendships report self-disclosing to one another with the same degree of frequency (Monsour, 1988). The day-to-day emotional disclosures of husbands and wives are also similar: In naturally occurring conversations, men and women do not differ in the overall frequency with which they refer to feelings (Shimanoff, 1983).

There is some evidence that self-disclosure is less important in established relationships than it is in beginning relationships. Couples who have been married 1 year disclose less to each other about their wants and concerns and talk less about the relationship than they did as newlyweds (Huston, McHale, & Crouter, 1986). Similarly, S. S. Hendrick (1981) observed that although disclosure is a good predictor of marital satisfaction, it is negatively correlated with years of marriage. It may be that self-disclosure is less critical when partners have been together for a long time, know each other well, and are generally satisfied with their relationship.

Early models of relationship development (e.g., Altman & Taylor, 1973) assumed that relationships gradually become emotionally closer as partners increasingly confide in each other concerning more intimate topics and a broader range of topics. However, later research has shown that intimacy doesn't necessarily grow in an orderly, gradually increasing way (see Derlega et al., 1993, for a review). Sometimes partners "click" immediately, showing a rapid rise in self-disclosure within weeks of meeting each other. Studies by Hays (1984, 1985) found that amounts of self-disclosure level off as early as 6 weeks into a new relationship. Also inconsistent with the gradual increases model of self-disclosure is evidence that partners in established relationships may show either a quick drop (Huston et al., 1986) or a gradual decline (S. S. Hendrick, 1981) in self-disclosure. Moreover, self-disclosure is sometimes used as a means of ending relationships (Baumeister & Wotman, 1992; Baxter, 1987; Dindia, 1994). Thus, it is *not* accurate to say that self-disclosure always leads to relationship development, or, conversely, that relationship development always leads to self-disclosure.

Interpretations of Self-Disclosure

The impact of self-disclosure on a relationship depends largely on the meaning that the recipient infers from that self-disclosure. Self-disclosure, by definition, conveys information about the sender. However, recipients do not react only to the content of self-disclosures. They also use self-disclosures to infer the sender's intentions, the sender's view of the recipient, and the sender's view of the relationship. One person holding forth doesn't necessarily lead to intimacy. Based on their review of the literature, Derlega et al. (1993) note that self-disclosure elicits greater liking only when it entails an expression of trust or special regard for the recipient. Under these circumstances, it is more likely to be reciprocated. When disclosure is indiscriminately offered or when it is too early, too negative, or outside the context of a positive relationship, it does not lead to greater liking of the discloser. For instance, Prager (1986) found that individuals who were involved in intimate relationships disclose more personal information to their closest friend than to a stranger, whereas individuals who had *not* been able to attain an intimate relationship disclosed equally and extensively to both friends and strangers. People who reveal too much too soon about themselves elicit negative evaluations from both interaction partners and observers (e.g., Wortman, Adesman, Herman, & Greenberg, 1976; see also Cappella, 1981, for a review).

It's important to note that couples do not always seek to share their feelings fully with each other. In fact, sometimes they actively avoid disclosing feelings to each other. For instance, Baxter and Wilmot (1985) found that virtually all relationships have at least one taboo topic. Moreover, men and women generally do not differ in either the type or number of taboo topics that they report. The most frequent taboo topic is metacommunication about the relationship. Based on her clinical observations, Hatfield

(1984) outlines a number of dangers of intimacy that lead most people to be at least somewhat wary of intimate encounters. In deciding how intimate they dare to be with friends or lovers, Hatfield suggests that individuals weigh their desire to deeply know and be known by another person against their fears of intimacy. These fears may include fear of exposure, fear of abandonment, fear of angry attacks, fear of loss of control, fear of one's own destructive impulses, and fear of losing one's individuality or of being engulfed. Similarly, Baxter (1988, 1990) notes that even in established relationships partners vacillate in their desire for connection versus autonomy.

In summary, research on self-disclosure shows that under most circumstances women disclose more than men do. However, men are by no means incapable of self-disclosure, and the relative use of self-disclosure by men and women varies across different stages of relationship development. Both men and women report that they value self-disclosure as a means of developing intimacy, but men may find it more difficult than women. The impact of self-disclosure on a relationship depends on the meaning with which partners construe it.

After reviewing the enormous body of research on self-disclosure, we are left with the sense that self-disclosure is definitely not the whole picture when it comes to expressions of intimacy. Self-disclosure is clearly important in relationship development. Intuitively, it makes sense that getting to know each other is a necessary step in establishing intimacy. But, the idea that self-disclosure ought to continue at very high levels over the long haul seems implausible. How many innermost feelings can any one person have? Moreover, merely tallying the number of self-disclosures or even the number of intimate self-disclosures seems an artificial way of understanding intimacy. It doesn't capture the flow and comfort of intimacy, or its interactive nature. This is readily apparent when we contrast self-disclosure research with the depiction of intimacy in the poem at the beginning of this section. Self-disclosure is deliberate, even effortful, but the poem above describes intimacy as a process as natural as breathing. Also, counting each partner's self-disclosures addresses the matching of partners' behavior in a crude, static, aggregate way. In contrast, the poem emphasizes ongoing coordination in partners' behavior underlying the give and take of intimacy.

Our hunch that self-disclosure is only one small part of expressions of intimacy in male–female relationships is consistent with several lines of data. First, naturalistic studies show that in real life, outside the laboratory, deeply meaningful self-disclosure just doesn't happen that much (e.g., Duck, Rutt, Hurst, & Strejc, 1991). As we mentioned earlier, self-disclosure seems to be more important in developing relationships than it is in established relationships. Moreover, self-disclosure may be more important in relationships other than romantic ones. We noted above that self-disclosure is especially important in women's friendships with other women. At least among college students, both men and women rate conversations with lovers as being of lesser quality than conversations with relatives, best friends, and friends (Duck et al., 1991).

Finally, verbal self-disclosure is not the only way or even necessarily the best way for partners to understand each other's feelings. Sillars, Pike, Jones, and Murphy (1984) had married couples discuss 10 potential conflict areas and then rate their own and their spouse's feelings about these areas. In inferring their spouse's feelings, partners tended to rely first on their own feelings, and second on their spouse's nonverbal behavior during the discussion. At least in this scenario, partners' verbal descriptions of feelings contributed little to understanding. Consistent with these findings, Montgomery (1988) argues that nonverbal emotional expression is more closely related than verbal expression to the quality of relationships. Perhaps because nonverbal communication seems more spontaneous, observers often view it as more honest and less strategic than verbal communication. Experimental investigations suggest that somewhere between 60% and 90% of the information gleaned in social interactions stems from nonverbal cues (Burgoon, 1985; Mehrabian & Wiener, 1967).

Perhaps it is not so much the *quantity* of self-disclosure that is important for establishing and maintaining intimacy. Rather, the critical factor for intimacy may be *effectiveness* of emotional communication: When people express their feelings, how well are they understood within the context of particular relationships?

Effectiveness of Emotional Communication

Effective emotional communication depends on the skills of both senders and receivers. Senders have to express their feelings clearly, and receivers have to interpret those expressions correctly. A great deal of research has been done on accuracy of emotional communication, measured as the degree of matching between the intended versus the actual impact of couples' emotional expressions.

Male–Female Differences in Communication Accuracy

Many studies indicate that women are more skilled than men at emotional communication. Laboratory studies consistently show that women are better at both sending and receiving messages nonverbally (Hall, 1984, 1987). Women also claim to be more empathic than men, although this difference is less evident when physiological or nonverbal indicators of empathy are used (see review by Aries, 1996).

Other researchers have argued that the relationship context influences accuracy of sending and receiving emotional communications. In general, knowing and liking the sender leads receivers to be more accurate in interpreting emotional expressions. This is particularly true for male receivers. Zuckerman, Lipets, Koivumaki, and Rosenthal (1975) found that men are more accurate at receiving emotional communications from people with whom they already have a relationship. Noller (1978) also found that husbands who reported greater marital satisfaction sent clearer emotional messages and made fewer receiving errors than husbands with low marital satisfaction. No relationship was found for wives between communication skills and marital satisfaction. Montgomery (1988) also notes that dissatisfied partners show more discrepancies between the intent and the impact of their emotional communications, and they are especially likely to misinterpret positive or neutral messages as having negative intent. More alarming is Noller and Venardos's (1986) finding that unhappy couples are not only more likely to misinterpret each others' intent, but they are also more confident in their interpretations.

In a recent study of on-line empathic accuracy, G. Thomas, Fletcher, and Lange (1997) videotaped married couples during a problem-solving discussion. They then had these couples watch the videotape of their interaction and report their own and their partner's thoughts and feelings. An important feature of this study is that they controlled for partner similarity, which means that accuracy ratings were not clouded by projection of a partner's own feelings onto the spouse. These investigators found *no* evidence of gender differences in empathic accuracy (see also review by T. Graham & Ickes, 1997). However, greater empathic accuracy was related to being more educated (particularly for husbands) and being married for a shorter time. This suggests that in established relationships, communication skills and motivation are more important than gender differences in establishing effective emotional communication.

Noller (1984), on the basis of her research on nonverbal communication between married couples, argues that gender differences in nonverbal emotional communication are most evident when looking at positive messages. Both wives and husbands are able to communicate negative emotional messages to each other clearly. However, wives are noticeably clearer than husbands in sending positive emotional expressions. She suggests that expressions of positive feelings should be a particular target of clinical intervention.

Overall, research on accuracy of emotional communication suggests that, compared to men, women have some advantage in this area initially, but that these differences become less noticeable in established relationships and in happy relationships. However, husbands may have more difficulty than wives in recognizing positive nonverbal expressions. It is important to note that the research we have just described refers only to *accuracy* of emotional communication—how well people get their messages across. It says nothing about *styles* of emotional communication—the way in which people express their feelings. There is substantial evidence that men and women tend to communicate their negative feelings in different ways. We discuss expressions of distress in marital relationships in detail in Chapter 7.

Between-Couple Differences in Emotional Communication Skills and Values

How important is effective emotional communication? "Good relationships require good communication" is such a truism in Western culture that it is hard to imagine anyone disagreeing with this statement. However, Burleson and Samter (1994) offer an important caution against psychologists' frequent assumption that skilled emotional communication is essential for relationship satisfaction. Their research looking at individual differences in communication skills suggests that rather than wanting as much verbal intimacy as possible, people are most comfortable relating to other people with a similar level of communication skill to their own. For instance, dating couples are most satisfied with and committed to their relationship when partners have similar levels of communication skills (Burleson, Birch, & Kunkel, 1993). In a study of married couples, Burleson and Denton (1992) looked at three indices of communication skill that are very relevant to emotional expression: accuracy in perceiving another's intentions, accuracy in predicting the emotional impact of one's messages, and effectiveness at achieving intended communication outcomes. Spouses' levels on these communication skills were highly correlated. Moreover, partners with similarly low levels on the skills were no less satisfied with their marriage than partners with similarly high levels on the skills. There was also a trend for happier couples to have more similar skill levels.

These findings suggest that communication skill similarity may be more important than absolute level of skillfulness in predicting relationship satisfaction. In other words, rather than there being an optimal style of relating (i.e., the highly emotionally self-disclosing style usually espoused by psychologists) the important issue may be that partners agree on a style of relating to each other. In fact, Burleson and Samter (1994) insist, "There may be substantial segments of the population for whom achieving accurate and sensitive understandings through verbal interaction just is not that important. Further, the highly skilled individual's concern with validating the other's view of self and the world, with exploring the feelings and motivations of the other, with working out disagreements by developing greater mutual understanding, with soothing upset and distress by helping the other articulate and elaborate his or her feelings, and so forth, may be seen as obsessive, boring, and intrusive by 'less skilled' individuals" (p. 85). For these couples, doing things together may be a more important expression of intimacy than sitting around talking about their feelings.

Burleson and Samter's observations are consistent with Fitzpatrick's

(1987) findings that married couples are characterized by different patterns of relating. In particular, she identified three types of couples: At one extreme are *Independent* couples who disclose substantially more to their partners than other couples. They value open communication and confrontation, and they readily disclose both positive and negative emotions to their partners. Their relationships tend to be intense but conflict ridden, and they report less marital satisfaction than other couples. At the other extreme are *Separate* couples, who value autonomy, privacy, and emotional distance. They avoid self-disclosure and tend to be dissatisfied with their marriages. Between the two extremes are *Traditional* couples, who value emotional communication but tend to limit their expressions to positive feelings and topics about the partner and the relationship. These couples tend to have high levels of marital satisfaction, but this satisfaction does not seem to be mediated through open communication. Fitzpatrick suggests that neither extreme openness nor extreme reserve leads to positive outcomes in marriage. Rather moderation in the degree and kind of self-disclosure leads to greater marital satisfaction. She further cautions that therapists need to have a pluralistic view of what constitutes "good communication." Often, couples seeking therapy are urged to adopt the communication style of Independents, regardless of their own values. She speculates that psychologists themselves tend to have this type of relationship. However, Fitzpatrick notes that the emotionally confrontive communication style of Independents is not the only possible style, nor is it necessarily the most satisfying.

These statements by Burleson and Samter and by Fitzpatrick fly in the face of a great deal of clinical practice that involves encouraging couples to express their feelings clearly and openly. We believe that expression can and often does play an important role in therapy and in relationships, particularly when other styles of relating are not working, but we recognize the important challenge that these researchers' perspectives present to clinicians. Specifically, clinicians need to understand and respect clients' values concerning emotional expression (see Chapter 4, concerning individual differences in expressive goals, beliefs, and values). Urging clients to express their feelings more clearly and openly is not always appropriate. Some clients may genuinely prefer other styles of relating involving greater emotional distance. Furthermore, greater clarity in emotional communication is not always the answer to relationship difficulties. No doubt more skilled sending and receiving of emotional communications leads to fewer misunderstandings. However, as Sillars et al. (1984) point out, there is no guarantee that accurate emotional communication leads to greater relationship satisfaction—it depends *what* partners express to each other. Two people who hate each other may be quite adept at telling each other about their hatred clearly and openly, but their skill at this type of emotional communication is unlikely to enhance their relationship. All of this suggests that understanding expressions of intimacy requires a more multifaceted view than is obtainable from either counting deliberate verbal disclosures or testing the accuracy with which couples send and receive emotional communications.

Rapport

One of the most sophisticated and comprehensive views of expressions of intimacy is Tickle-Degnen and Rosenthal's (1990) discussion of the nonverbal correlates of rapport. They explain that rapport is characteristic of interactions rather than individuals. Although some people may be especially adept at developing rapport with others, the experience of rapport emerges from the behavior of each individual in the interaction. Broadly, rapport involves positive interaction and a subjective sense of union or cohesiveness. Colloquially, it is often described as "clicking" or having "good chemistry." More specifically, Tickle-Degnen and Rosenthal (1990) describe three essential components of rapport:

1. *Mutual attentiveness* involves intense mutual interest in and focus on what the other person is saying or doing. It is expressed nonverbally through closer interpersonal distances and bodily postures involving features such as a forward lean and direct body orientation. These expressions of attentiveness both provide and signal communication accessibility.

2. *Positivity* involves feelings of mutual friendliness and caring. It is expressed nonverbally through behaviors such as smiling and head nodding. These expressions indicate that participants like and approve of each other.

3. *Coordination* involves mutual responsiveness and a sense of being "in sync" with the other person. Unlike the other components of rapport, coordination is not expressed through any single behavior. Rather, it involves a meshing of partners' patterns of behavior, so that they interact smoothly as a unit. Coordination is evident through postural mirroring (e.g., LaFrance, 1979, 1985), well-regulated turn taking in speaking and listening roles (e.g., Duncan & Fiske, 1977), and general interactional synchrony (Bernieri, Resnick, & Rosenthal, 1988).

Tickle-Degnen and Rosenthal note that rapport is dynamic because it varies over time. Although feelings and behaviors reflecting mutual attention, positivity, and coordination are present to some degree in initial encounters as well as in later interactions involving rapport, the relative importance of these components for the experience and expression of rapport changes as relationships develop. Tickle-Degnen and Rosenthal offer a number of specific hypotheses concerning how the meaning of components of rapport might change as a relationship develops:

1. They suggest that early in a relationship, partners' judgments of rapport are determined mainly by feelings and expressions of positivity. Partners would expect their interactions to involve a certain amount of awkwardness just because they do not know each other very well. Although some coordination may be present in their early interactions because of partners' knowledge of societal conventions such as politeness, their general social skills, or their shared interaction styles, this coordination would not be maximized. In later interactions, however, the relative importance of positivity and coordination is likely to reverse. Because partners who know each other well have developed stable perceptions of each other, they are less constrained by impression management concerns. Thus, positivity, while still necessary, becomes less central to the experience and expression of rapport in established relationships.

2. In contrast, established partners are likely to expect considerable interactional coordination. As partners get to know each other, they become more able to adopt each other's perspectives, they develop their own communication conventions, they are able to communicate in more diverse ways, and they have fewer misunderstandings, all of which enable them to have smooth, efficient interactions. Awkward pauses or frequently interrupting each other are likely to be seen by partners in an established relationship as evidence of a lack of rapport and indications that they are not functioning as a relational unit. Tickle-Degnen and Rosenthal note that because coordination cues are complex and less available to conscious control, they are difficult to fake. This suggests that, once established, coordination might be an especially sensitive barometer of relationship quality.

3. Tickle-Degnen and Rosenthal speculate that the other component of rapport, attention, does not change in the magnitude of its importance as relationships develop, but it does change in its experiential quality. They hypothesize that partners would expect a high degree of attention from each other both early on and later in the relationship, but the meaning of that attention changes. Initially, expressions of attention may signal interest, which is a precondition for establishing a relationship. Later, once partners know each other well, expressions of attention may indicate unity and mutuality of goals.

Tickle-Degnen and Rosenthal's model of rapport is specific, flexible, integrative, dynamic, and empirically testable. Although individual components of the model have received research attention, the most interesting parts of the model, involving the interaction of components and changes over time, have not yet been studied. To our knowledge, there has also been no research concerning sex differences or similarities in rapport. Moreover, these theorists note that very little research has been done concerning expressions of rapport in established relationships, which is surely where it is most important. Nevertheless, their model is conceptually useful and emphasizes the importance of understanding intimacy as an emerging and interpersonal process. Unlike the other views of expressions of intimacy that we have discussed, rapport involves less deliberate expression. It depicts intimacy as a pattern of interaction expressing comfort and connection, rather than discrete instances of emotional communication. To us, the view of intimacy entailed in rapport seems quite similar to the one evoked by the poem at the beginning of this section.

COMMITMENT: EXPRESSIONS OF AFFECTION

A Red, Red Rose
. . . As fair art thou, my bonnie lass,
   So deep in love am I;
And I will love thee still, my Dear,
   Till a' the seas gang dry.—
Till a' the seas gang dry, my dear,
   And the rocks melt wi' the sun:
O I will luve thee still, my dear,
   While the sands o' life shall run.
   —ROBERT BURNS, 1759–1796

This poem declares, "I'll love you forever!" The poet expresses to his bonnie lass not only the depth of his affection but also his commitment that his love will endure. Sternberg (1986) remarks that the third component of love, commitment, may seem less interesting or dramatic than either passion or intimacy, but it is nonetheless important. He notes that it is commitment that enables couples to stay together and work through difficulties that might arise with either passion or intimacy.

Expressions of affection and commitment are closely connected. D. M. Buss (1988) argues that "love acts," such as giving gifts or demonstrating fidelity, have two functions: (1) mutual display of resources, to aid in mate selection, and (2) maintaining exclusivity and commitment in an established relationship, to aid in raising offspring. In this section we describe expressions of affection that enable men and women to move relationships toward more serious commitment and to reaffirm commitment in existing relationships. We describe four broad categories of expressions of affection, which we have labeled *formal, presentational, dyadic,* and *declarative.* We then consider how expressions of affection change over the course of relationship development.

Formal Expressions of Affection

Formal expressions of affection are the big steps, such as asking someone out or proposing marriage, that carry strong implications for the level of involvement or commitment in a relationship. These expressions directly define relationships in formal ways that are generally recognizable (e.g., "We're dating"; "We're engaged"; "We're married."). Stereotyped courtship scripts depict the male as the initiator of these formal expressions of affection that define increasing levels of commitment, as the relationship progresses smoothly and harmoniously toward marriage.

However, accounts from actual couples show considerable variability in the form and development of relationship commitments (Surra, Batchelder, & Hughes, 1995). For instance, in a study of dating couples, Surra and Hughes (1997) found that about 43% of couples described their commitment to their relationship as developing smoothly and positively. In contrast, 57% of couples described their commitment as developing in more dramatic ways with many reversals involving sudden bursts of commitment or retreats from involvement. Interestingly, several studies suggest that relationships in which commitment develops in a less volatile way are more apt to thrive (see discussion by Surra et al., 1995).

Orbuch, Vernoff, and Holmberg (1993) also found variability in partners' responsibility for formal expressions of affection. They asked married couples to recount which partner initiated the relationship and which partner proposed marriage. About half of the couples reported that the man initiated the courtship (e.g., by asking the woman out), while the remaining couples stated that both partners, the wife, or a third party initiated the relationship. Only one-third of the couples indicated that they had followed the traditional script with the husband proposing marriage. For one-fifth of the couples, the wife proposed. For the remaining couples the marriage proposal was the result of both partners' efforts.

Overall, these studies suggest that neither men nor women generally dominate in formal expressions of affection. Instead, different couples show different patterns in the way they take formal steps in commitment.

Public Presentational Expressions of Affection

Expressions of affection sometimes serve a public presentational function (Goffman, 1972; Patterson, 1991; Scheflen, 1974). Rather than merely reflecting felt emotion, expressions of affection are sometimes used to communicate a pair identity to some audience. For instance, Goffman (1972) uses the term *tie-signs* to describe behaviors such as standing close, touching, or holding hands that relationship partners use to announce not only to each other but also to those around them, "We are a couple." Many of the same behaviors that are used in private to express intimacy can be used in public to serve a social presentational function, creating an identity or image for observers (e.g., Patterson, 1988). Such public expressions of affection are a means of establishing legitimacy and obtaining support for the couple from the social network. By recognizing these cues and responding to the couple as a single social unit, others acknowledge and affirm the couple's relationship identity. Interestingly, tie-signs are sometimes initiated in response to a potential threat to the relationship. Fine, Stitt, and Finch (1984) had male or female interviewers ask the female member of couples waiting in line for a movie either intimate questions about childhood memories or impersonal questions about preferences in music, art, and cities. They expected the most threatening condition to involve a male interviewer asking personal questions, and this condition did in fact elicit the greatest number of tie-signs from the male partner.

The amount of public touching varies across different stages of relationships. Guerrero and Andersen (1991) observed opposite-sex couples standing in lines at the zoo or movie theater, then asked couples to characterize their relational stage. They found a curvilinear relationship between touching and relational stage, with less touching by casually dating and married couples compared to seriously dating couples. In a follow-up study (Guerrero & Andersen, 1994), they found a greater degree of matching in partner's amount of touching in married couples than in dating couples. It may be that in dating relationships public touching is a means of expressing an increasing desire for commitment, whereas in more established relationships public touching reflects existing mutual comfort and bondedness.

Observational studies of couples in public places also indicate that while both men and women engage in similar amounts of public expressions of affection, there are some gender differences in the form of these expressions. Men are more likely to initiate touch in casual dating relationships. Men and women initiate touch at similar rates in serious dating relationships, but women are more likely to initiate touch in married relationships (Guerrero & Andersen, 1994). Also, men are more likely to put their arms around the shoulders of a woman, and women are more likely to link their arm through a man's arm (Hall & Veccia, 1990). Some theorists have interpreted this pattern of differential touching as reflecting social dominance by men (e.g., Henley, 1977). However, there are no conclusive data showing that women generally interpret a shoulder hug as domineering. A simpler explanation of these differences in the form of public expressions of affection is that they reflect average height differences: Because men are generally taller than women, they are more likely to touch their partners higher up.

Dyadic Expressions of Affection

So far, we have described formal expressions of affection, which involve big steps in commitment, and presentational expressions, which involve public announcements of the relationship. Both of these types of expression can be important to relationship development, and they may even influence relationship satisfaction. However, dyadic expressions of affection are likely to be much more closely linked to satisfaction.

Dyadic expressions of affection refer to all the ways that partners express their caring for each other to each other. Although they don't define relationships in the strict way that formal expressions do, they are an important means by which partners communicate to each other, "You are special; this relationship is special." Private expressions of affection may also be important in defining a relationship as romantic rather than just friendly.

Stereotypes are mixed regarding roles for men and women in dyadic expressions of affection. On the one hand, many of the cultural scripts regarding romantic acts involve things that generally men, but not women, are supposed to do (e.g., sending flowers, singing under balconies, writing poems hailing a partner's beauty). In fact, men generally endorse more romantic beliefs than women. For example, men are more likely than women to believe in love at first sight, that love conquers all, and that there is only one true love for each person (Sprecher & Metts, 1989). On the other hand, dyadic expressions of affection are supposed to be more important to women than to men. "Mushy stuff" is women's domain; men are supposed to be tough and independent (e.g., Snell, 1986). These gender roles concerning dyadic expressions of affection may be learned through the experiences of young children with their parents. Noller (1978) observed parents leaving their children at preschool and noticed differences in the way mothers and fathers interacted with their children. Fathers were less likely than mothers to express affection, and the least affection was shown between fathers and sons. Noller interprets this to mean that little boys learn through both observation and experience that males express less affection than females.

In several studies investigators have asked volunteers to specify which behaviors they consider to be romantic. For instance, R. K. Tucker, Vivian, and Marvin (1992) asked a sample of adults, ranging in age from 19 to 79 years, to describe up to 12 different "romantic acts." There was considerable overlap in responses concerning what constitutes a romantic act. The most popular responses were: kissing, giving or receiving flowers, having a special dinner together, talking, holding hands, hugging, sharing outdoor leisure activities (e.g., picnic, beach, walk), giving gifts, walking, and touching. In another study, which involved talking, in a seminar context, to hundreds of workers of various ages and occupations, R. K. Tucker and Yuhas Byers (1992) obtained a similar list of romantic acts plus several additional responses: saying "I love you," leaving notes, keeping in touch, and doing little favors. In still another study, R. K. Tucker, Marvin, and Vivian (1991) observed that college men and women tend to report very similar lists of romantic acts, although one noteworthy difference is that, across all three studies, only college men consider making love to be a romantic act. Taken together, these studies indicate that dyadic expressions of affection are governed by highly specific and widely agreed upon scripts. Unfortunately, these studies only reflect knowledge of romantic acts. They do not indicate whether women and men actually do these things to the same extent.

In addition to the conventional forms of dyadic expressions of affection entailed in romantic acts, couples sometimes invent their own idiosyncratic expressions of affection. These expressions may function to create a sense of the relationship partners as a unique and special unit—a sense of "we-ness" relative to the rest of the world. For instance, in an entertaining article entitled "Did You Bring the Yarmulke for the Cabbage Patch Kid?", Bell, Buerkel-Rothfuss, and Gore (1987) note that couples often establish personal idioms that serve as a sign of their felt connection. Examples of such idioms include nicknames, such as "Fifi" or "Special K," unique words or phrases like "huggle" or "you're a mouthful" to say "I love you," and idiosyncratic sexual referents, such as saying "Wanna do a load of laundry?" to initiate sexual encounters. The number of such idioms that a couple reported for expressing affection, initiating sexual encounters, and referring to sexual matters was positively associated with both partners' feelings of love, commitment, and closeness. Interestingly, men, rather than women, were most often the inventors of these personal idioms.

Declarative Expressions of Affection

Declarative expressions of affection involve directly telling a partner "I love you." These are perhaps the cardinal form of expression of affection in romantic relationships. The first time that members of a couple say they love each other is a milestone (C. E. King & Christensen, 1983). It often marks a transition toward a more intimate, committed relationship.

Owen (1987) conducted a qualitative study of young couples saying "I love you." He asked college students to keep daily diaries for 4 to 5 months, in which they recorded, in an open-ended format, what was said and done on their dates, and the relational implications of these events. Of the 92 diaries collected, those from 9 men and 9 women described instances of the individual or a partner saying "I love you" and reflected a movement from "dating" to a "serious" relationship. Conclusions from these data must be considered tentative because of the small sample size and the young age of the participants. However, the richness of the descriptions provided by these 18 students is compelling and informative of how people understand and interpret this critical communication event. In all but one case, the man said "I love you" first. Based on thematic analyses of these diaries, Owen offers several possible explanations for men's initiative and women's reticence in first declarations of love.

1. *Men may say "I love you" strategically, as a means of eliciting greater commitment from women.* When someone says, "I love you," the

only acceptable response is "I love you, too." Because there is such a strong reciprocity script governing love, any other response ("Oh," "Thank you," "How nice," "Uhhhh . . . ") is at best very awkward, at worst extremely painful to both parties (see Baumeister & Wotman's [1992] descriptions of unrequited love). One woman in Owen's study wrote that she felt like her partner was trying to "push me into a relationship" by declaring his love. She even quoted her partner saying, "You can tell me that you love me whenever you want to." Another man in Owen's study decided to tell his partner how much he loved her because he felt her slipping away.

2. *Men may say "I love you" impulsively; They may be less able than women to refrain from expressing felt love.* Both the men's and the women's diaries contained instances of declarations of love bursting forth from men. One man reported, "I said I love you before I knew what I was doing! . . . It was like I was . . . a dog foaming at the mouth out of control!" A woman wrote about her partner, "He said 'I love you' today. . . . He said he couldn't wait any longer and that it was like a 'cork in a bottle.' Saying he loved me lifted that cork out." In contrast, the women often described feeling love but deliberately refraining from expressing it. One woman wrote, "I dare not tell him I love him first."

3. *Women may be less likely to say "I love you" first because they make clearer distinctions between loving, liking, and lusting.* Men in Owen's study expressed confusion concerning their feelings, whereas the women seemed quite clear about how they felt and focused on distinguishing love from related feelings. One woman wrote that she was so shocked when her partner said he loved her that she told him, "How can you *love* me after only *two* weeks?!" She later wrote, "I'm not going to admit I *love* him when I *like* him. I mean I *care* for him, but I wouldn't call it *love*."

4. *Women may be less likely to say "I love you" first because courtship scripts dictate that the man should take the lead.* Both men and women in the study indicated that they considered it to be the man's job to take the lead in saying "I love you." The women expressed fear that they would be evaluated negatively or push men away if they failed to let men initiate declarations of love. Following this script was sometimes difficult, as it was for one woman who stated, "I know I love Henry, but I don't know how much longer I can hold out telling him." Even the one woman in the study who said "I love you" before her partner did voiced knowledge of this script and concerns about the repercussions of not following it. Her partner was surprised by her declaration of love. She wrote in her diary, "I wish I'd just waited longer. I really should've just kept my mouth shut and sat on my feelings. My mother was right—always let the man lead!"

To summarize, we have described four broad categories of expressions of affection: formal, presentational, dyadic, and declarative. Overall, there is no clear pattern of gender differences in expressions of affection. Data concerning formal expressions of affection, involving major steps in relationship commitment, show that in some couples men take the initiative, in other couples women take the initiative, and in still other couples men and women share this responsibility. Observational studies show that both women and men engage in presentational expressions of affection, announcing their relationship status to people around them. However, the specific form of these expressions may vary across gender. Dyadic expressions of affection, in which partners inform each other that they care for each other, are probably the most important for ongoing relationship satisfaction. Men and women agree as to what constitutes conventional expressions of affection, but we do not know to what extent they actually engage in these behaviors. Men may be more likely to initiate unique forms of dyadic expressions of affection. Finally, declarative expressions of affection involve telling a partner directly "I love you." Although couples consider the first declaration of love to be an important milestone, there is very little research about this. One small study suggests that women are more comfortable if men take the lead in first saying "I love you." Very little is known about declarative expressions of love in established relationships.

We now turn from describing expressions of affection to considering how they change over the course of relationship development. Most of the research described in the next section focuses on dyadic and declarative expressions of affection.

Changes in Expressions of Affection over the Course of Relationship Development

Expressions of affection are important at all stages of a relationship. In her review of relationship maintenance strategies, Dindia (1994) notes that verbal and nonverbal expressions of affection are used to initiate, escalate, and maintain relationships.

However, expressions of affection are especially important as a means of intensifying relationships. Tolhuizen (1989) found that verbal expression of affection is one of the strategies that dating couples report using most frequently to intensify their relationships. Similarly, Guerrero, Eloy, and Wabnik (1993), in a longitudinal study of dating couples, found that couples who perceived an increase in their partners' assurances of love and commitment over an 8-week period also perceived that their relationship escalated over this time period. As partners become more seriously involved, expressions of affection become more direct. Stafford and Canary (1991) found that, compared to recently dating couples, seriously dating, engaged, and married couples perceived that their partners offered more assurances of affection.

In contrast to the escalation in expressions of affection that characterizes developing relationships, the frequency of expressions of affection seems to decline over time in established relationships. For instance, Huston et al. (1986) found that after only 1 year of marriage, both partners were less physically affectionate and said "I love you" less often. This decrease in expressions of affection occurred even though the couples were still very satisfied overall with their relationships. Does this mean that our poet's expressions of affection are doomed to disappear well before the seas gang dry? Not necessarily.

First of all, there is considerable variability across established couples in the degree to which they express affection. Dickson's (1995) interviews with couples who have been married for at least 50 years contain touching examples of expressions of affection, which demonstrate clearly that such expressions can continue even in very long-term couples. One husband, describing his wife of 52 years, declares, "Look at this jewel I still have. Pretty, smart . . . sexy." Another long-term couple laugh together over a recent adventure: They decided they wanted lobster for dinner, so they spontaneously packed up the car and drove from Rochester to Maine. They ate lobster 3 nights in a row and then drove home.

Husbands' behavior is particularly important in establishing couples' patterns of affectionate expressions over the long run. Huston and Vangelisti (1991) looked at affectionate behavior in newly married couples over a period of 2 years. They conducted yearly face-to-face interviews to assess marital satisfaction, with the first one occurring approximately 2 months after the couple was married. These yearly interviews were each followed by three telephone interviews in which spouses reported whether various social-emotional behaviors had occurred in the past 24 hours. The results point to the importance of expressions of affection to marital satisfaction—especially husband's expressions. Receiving more affection is associated with greater concurrent satisfaction for both partners, but giving affection is more strongly and consistently related to husbands concurrent satisfaction. Analyses of longitudinal data indicate that husbands' who express more affection early on have wives who are more affectionate later in the marriage. Wives' early affection does not predict husbands' later behavior.

It is also possible that the apparent decline in expressions of affection in established relationships actually involves a change in the form and function of these expressions rather than a general decrease in such expressions.

In terms of form, perhaps because they know each other well, established couples may rely more on subtle or indirect expressions of affection than on direct ones. Evidence consistent with this possibility comes from two studies examining married couples' self-reported strategies for relationship maintenance and repair (Canary & Stafford, 1992; Dindia & Baxter, 1987). In discussing these two studies, Wilmot (1994) notes that specific relationship enhancement strategies can be grouped into two general approaches: *Implicit relational moves* involve indirect signs such as behavioral changes, rituals, spontaneity, or positivity by which partners signal their desire to continue or improve the relationship. *Explicit relational talk* involves direct verbal communication about the relationship. It includes strategies such as openness, assurances, communication, and metacommunication. In general, the married couples in these studies reported that they are more likely to use implicit strategies that show their affection and commitment rather than explicit strategies that involve talking about their feelings. Moreover, Dindia and Baxter (1987) found that relationship satisfaction was not related to maintenance strategy preference.

Subtle signs of affection may be at least as important as grand gestures. Duck (1994) argues that in studying close relationships, researchers have focused almost exclusively on The Significant and have therefore overlooked the routine daily interactions that appear trivial by themselves but collectively are critically important to building and maintaining relationships. He notes (Duck, 1991) that relationships are predominantly and inevitably (but not exclusively) negotiated through everyday talk and mundane daily relational communication. Based in diary data, Duck et al. (1991) demonstrate that the mere occurrence of conversation is more important than the topic of conversation for maintaining a relationship. Silly insignificant conversations, telling jokes, commenting on passersby, complaining about coworkers, suggesting what to eat for lunch—all of these reify, sustain, define, and produce relationships. This apparently idle chatter demonstrates and creates a symbolic union between partners, subtly and implicitly sustaining the relationship (Duck, 1994).

Changes in expressions of affection over time may also involve changes in the function of these expressions. Early on, expressions of affection or commitment are critical to defining and creating a relationship. In established relationships, expressions of affection may be more important for maintaining or positively managing the relationship. Cartensen, Gottman, and Levenson (1995) conducted an observational study comparing the communication of married couples in their 40s with that of couples in the 60s. Compared to the middle-aged couples, the older couples expressed significantly more affection for each other and less negativity while discussing marital problems. These differences were evident even after statistically controlling for the severity of the problem discussed. Cartensen et al. argue that these findings are consistent with other evidence showing improvements in emotional understanding (Labouvie-Vief & DeVoe, 1991), emotional control (Lawton, Kleban, Rajagopal, & Dean, 1992), and marital satisfaction (Levenson, Cartensen, & Gottman, 1993) as individuals enter old age. Older people may be especially likely to manage social interactions in a way that maximizes emotional benefits (Cartensen, 1993). Cartensen et al. (1995) did observe gender differences in the emotional expression of husbands and wives in both the middle-aged and older couples. Compared to the husbands, the wives were more expressive overall, and they expressed more of several specific emotions, including anger, contempt, sadness, and joy. Wives were also especially likely to reciprocate positive affect. However, there were no gender differences in expressions of affection, which suggests that high levels of affection expressed by the older couples reflects the mutual efforts of both partners.

We have noted that expressions of affection can take many forms and that they can change in both form and function as relationships develop. In our discussion of expressions pertaining to passion and intimacy, we stated that how partners interpret such expressions determines their impact on the relationship. The same is true for expressions of affection.

Interpretations of Expressions of Affection

The key issue when it comes to expressions of affection is that partners understand and appreciate the particular form these expressions take in their particular relationships. Based on interviews of over 260 adults of varying ages, Marston and Hecht and their colleagues (Hecht, Marston, & Larkey, 1994; Marston, Hecht, & Robers, 1987) developed a list of seven common "love ways" that refer to different ways of experiencing and expressing love. According to their typology, *collaborative love* is expressed through mutual support and negotiation; *active love* is expressed through doing things together; *intuitive love* is expressed nonverbally through facial expressions, sex, and physical contact; *committed love* is expressed by making a commitment, discussing the future, and spending time together; *secure love* is expressed through the discussion of intimate topics; *expressive love* is expressed by doing things for the other and saying "I love you"; *traditional romantic love* is expressed through togetherness and commitment. These different love ways often occur in combination. Some of Marston and Hecht's love ways are difficult to differentiate (e.g., committed love and traditional romantic love). Moreover, like most of the data on relational maintenance, the list of love ways was obtained based on single interviews rather than observer ratings or even careful self-monitoring over a period of time. Thus, it is not clear to what extent they translate into actual behavior. Nevertheless, the love ways are important because they suggest the variety of ways of expressing affection. The most interesting part of Marston and Hecht's work is their discussion of interactions between different love ways.

Marston and Hecht (1994) argue persuasively that understanding how the love ways of two partners in a relationship do or do not mesh is essential for understanding their pattern of interaction. The most obvious matching occurs when two lovers rely on the same love ways, such as two committed lovers making mutual commitments. However, love ways can also mesh if they are complementary, as when a collaborative lover supports and cares for a secure lover who believes love involves being cared for. It is also possible for love ways to be functionally linked, such that one partner's loving behavior evokes the other partner's loving behavior. Thus a commitment from one partner might evoke a commitment from the other partner, or an inexperienced lover may learn to give and receive love sexually from a sexually expressive lover.

On the other hand, what Marston and Hecht refer to as "love problematics" arise when partners' ways of loving do not mesh. Partners may overvalue symmetry in love ways, expecting the other person to express love in exactly the same way they do. Because partners are likely to differ at least somewhat in their love ways, this expectation can lead to disappointment and interfere with the enjoyment of an otherwise satisfying relationship. Problems can also arise when partners overvalue a particular form of loving. For instance, one partner might insist, "If you really loved me you would. . . . " This "test" of love devalues other expressions of love that might contribute to a satisfying relationship. Alternatively, overemphasizing a single way of loving may prevent partners from addressing real problems in the relationship, as when a partner blindly insists, "As long as we are honest with each other, everything will work out."

Clinically, Marston and Hecht (1994) emphasize the importance of helping clients to have a multifaceted view of expressions of affection. Either extreme of ignoring specific problematic incompatibilities or generalizing from a single problematic element to the entire relationship should be avoided. Marston and Hecht also note that it may be useful for clients to understand their priorities when it comes to love ways. Given that it is unlikely that they will find a partner who is absolutely compatible at all times, they may need to acknowledge and accept incompatibility in elements that are less central to their experience and expression of love.

Marston and Hecht do not specifically mention this, but it also seems essential that partners communicate to each other about their preferences for expressing and receiving love. Ideally, this should be done with openness and acceptance rather than coercion. The key message needs to be "I like . . . " rather than "You must. . . . " Suppose, for example, that a woman enjoys receiving mushy, sentimental cards. These type of cards may do nothing for her partner. In fact he may even think they are silly or embarrassing. But suppose he knows that she likes them, and so he sends her one. She is thrilled to receive it. Not only did he express his affection for her, but his gesture shows that he went to the effort to express it in a way she appreciates.

CONCLUSION

Our review of research concerning expressions of the three components of love (passion, intimacy, and commitment) shows that there is a kernel of truth to the stereotypes about men and women and love, particularly in new relationships, when partners do not know each other well and gender roles are most salient. However, overall, our review suggests that men and women are more similar than different in their expressions of love (cf. Aries, 1996; Canary et al., 1997; S. S. Hendrick & Hendrick, 1995).

In terms of passion, in general, men take the initiative in overt expressions of sexual interest, particularly in the early stages of a relationship. Although cultural scripts discourage women from overt expressions of sexual desire, women are by no means passive in expressing passion. Surveys and observational studies indicate that women have a vast array of strategies for expressing sexual interest. Moreover, in established relationships, cultural scripts become less important, and women are more likely to take the initiative sexually. Expressions of sexual desire are best understood as an interactive process involving both partners.

In terms of intimacy, in opposite-sex interactions, women self-disclose slightly more than men overall, but there is evidence that the magnitude and direction of these differences varies across relationship stages. Women are somewhat better than men at accurately sending and receiving emotional communications, but, again, these differences are less apparent in established relationships. A true understanding of intimacy does not involve static assessments of quantity or skillfulness of communication. Intimacy is a dynamic interpersonal process in which both partners attend to each other, respond warmly, and relate in a synchronous manner.

Finally, in terms of commitment, we found no clear pattern of either gender dominating expressions of affection, except for some evidence suggesting that women prefer men to say "I love you" first. Instead, we noted that expressions of affection take many forms and can vary between individuals, across couples, and over time, as relationships develop.

In all three of the main sections of this chapter, we noted that interpretations of expressions of love determine the impact of these expressions on relationships. No emotional expression has an invariant social meaning (Patterson, 1983; Reis & Shaver, 1988; Scherer & Ekman, 1982). A smile may reflect feelings of warmth or anxiety. Eye contact may indicate interest or hostility. A touch may be perceived as spontaneous or manipulative, affectionate or sexist; and intimate self-disclosure may be construed as welcome or presumptuous. Interpretations are especially important because many expressions of love are subtle or indirect. As Baxter (1987) points out, "The typical relationship process is not dominated by open, direct relationship communication, but rather involves the construction of a web of ambiguity by which parties signal their relationship indirectly" (p. 194). How expressions of love are interpreted depends on numerous factors including communication partners' relationship goals and beliefs, and their individual and joint history. Clinically, helping partners to reconcile different styles and interpretations of expressions of passion, intimacy, or commitment can be an important step toward enhanced relationship satisfaction.

For conceptual clarity, we talked about passion, intimacy, and commitment separately in this chapter. However, in real life they are often closely interrelated. For instance, DeLamater and MacCorquodale (1979) showed that the best predictor of a couple's level of sexual intimacy is their degree of emotional intimacy. Affection and commitment may follow sexual interaction and emotional sharing or precede them (e.g., Christopher & Cate, 1985). Understanding love requires that we look at all three components and their interrelationships.

In conclusion, emotional expression is central to love because it helps create, define, and maintain close relationships. Emotional expression is the basic link connecting two people's subjective experience of love. This expression may be verbal or nonverbal, intentional or unintentional, public or private (cf. Marston & Hecht, 1994). Through expression, partners signal to each other, "Are we friends or are we lovers?" "Is this a casual relationship or a serious one?" "Are we growing closer or farther apart?" Partners also use expressions of love to enhance or intensify their relationships. As Sternberg (1986) remarks, "Without expression, even the greatest of loves can die" (p. 132).

NOTES

1. Various theorists have offered their opinions as to how sexual desire is related to love and whether or not sexual desire qualifies as emotional experience (see discussions by Aron & Aron, 1991; Metts et al., 1998). Our perspective is that sexual desire constitutes one possible component of love, and that it is a form of emotional experience, involving a subjective feeling that is distinguishable from but often accompanies sexual arousal and sexual behavior.

2. Meta-analysis is a technique for quantitatively reviewing research. It is used to infer statistically the size of the relationship between variables across a large number of studies. Meta-analysis has the advantages of being systematic and objective, and it is especially useful when the number of relevant studies is so overwhelmingly large that narrative review techniques become unwieldy.

7

Telling One's Troubles: Expression of Distress in Intimate Relationships

INTRODUCTION

Although we may chuckle to ourselves while thinking of an amusing incident or shed tears alone during a private moment of sadness, usually emotional expression is a social occurrence: We express our feelings *to others*. Social expression of emotion is extremely common. An overwhelming majority of people report that they discuss their emotions with others, particularly their significant others. They communicate their feelings shortly after the emotion-eliciting event, and they talk about the same emotional experience repeatedly (Rimé et al., 1991). Most people consider talking over their feelings with a friend to be a useful strategy for coping with distress (Parker & Brown, 1982; Rippere, 1977). The perceived opportunity to share feelings is related to well-being and is a defining feature of close relationships (Derlega et al., 1993).

Chapter Overview

In this chapter, we focus on a particular kind of social expression of emotion: the expression of distress in intimate relationships. In Chapter 6, we considered how the expression of positive emotions can lead to the formation of relationships and the development of intimacy. This chapter examines the opposite side of the coin: how the expression of negative emotions affects existing close relationships.

Most clients seek psychotherapy because they feel distressed. If therapists only consider individual clients and their feelings, they have a very limited picture of clients' distress. A fuller understanding requires that therapists also consider whether and how clients express their distress in the context of their close relationships and what sort of responses their distress expression elicits. Helping clients to recognize and perhaps modify their interpersonal patterns of distress expression can improve their relationships and enable them to elicit the social support they need in their daily lives.

As background to our discussion of distress expression in close relationships, we first consider the possible benefits and risks of distress expression. We also explain how patterns of emotional communication emerge in close relationships, in the form of cognitive-interpersonal cycles. We then describe three married couples who illustrate prototypical and empirically documented maladaptive patterns of distress expression. We address how people interpret expressions of distress and how these interpretations influence their responses to distress expression. We conclude this chapter by offering some clinical guidelines concerning expressions of distress in close relationships.

Possible Benefits and Risks of Distress Expression

The ubiquitousness of distress communication is not surprising given its many potential benefits. In addition to the intrapersonal benefits described in previous chapters, such as distress resolution or self-understanding, there are also interpersonal benefits that can occur when negative emotions are expressed to another person (e.g., Coates & Winston, 1987; Derlega et al., 1993; Rimé et al., 1991; Wills, 1985). One such benefit is practical support. Communicating distress is a means of eliciting tangible aid or new information that can enhance coping efforts. We're more likely to get help from others if they know we need help.

Another possible benefit of social expression is bolstering self-esteem through validation. An accepting response from others to distress disclosures can improve self-esteem and decrease distress. Experiencing intense negative emotions can be frightening. Sometimes people who are feeling extremely distressed wonder if they are crazy, or falling apart, or just unable to handle things the way most people can (Thoits, 1985). Talking about feelings of distress with others may prompt them to offer reassurances of their love and acceptance or to relate similar experiences. Either of these responses to distress expression can relieve self-doubts.

A third possible benefit of distress communication is improved interpersonal relationships. Emotional expression can redefine a relationship by influencing intimacy or status. Revealing our feelings to others fosters intimacy (1) by communicating that we trust them and want an intimate relationship with them, (2) by allowing them to get to know us better, and (3) by creating a normative demand or expectation that they will reciprocate this self-revelation, thereby allowing us to get to know them. The type of emotion expressed affects the relative status of relationship partners. Expressing fear or sadness is a sign of vulnerability, which tends to disarm and elicit compassion, whereas expressing anger or disgust is a sign of strength, which tends to assert independence and delineate interpersonal boundaries (L. S. Greenberg & Johnson, 1990).

Despite the potential benefits of emotional communication, people sometimes *avoid* revealing their negative feelings to others. Daily stress is one possible cause of avoidance of expression. In several studies, Repetti (see Repetti, 1992, for a summary) found that exposure to stressors at work, such as having a particularly high workload or having negative interactions with supervisors or coworkers, subsequently leads people to withdraw temporarily from social contact, avoiding expression and interaction with others at home (Repetti, 1992). Repetti suggests that this temporary social withdrawal can be a useful short-term coping response. It can be a means of "refueling" by giving stressed individuals time and space to remedy their negative affect, decrease their stress-related arousal, and lessen their fatigue.

Other times avoidance of expression is a response to the many possible risks entailed in emotional communication (e.g., Derlega et al., 1993; Fisher, Goff, Nadler, & Chinsky, 1988; see also related discussion by Kelly & McKillop, 1996, concerning the risks of confiding personal secrets). If recipients of emotional expression respond negatively, the person expressing may feel rejected, misunderstood, embarrassed, or betrayed. Even when recipients respond positively, seeking support can threaten expressers' self-esteem by making them feel inferior, inadequate, or dependent because they can't manage on their own. Although the perceived availability of support is related to better well-being, having sought or received support is associated with poorer well-being (J. C. Coyne & Downey, 1991). This finding could indicate simply that more distressed people are more likely to seek help. Alternatively, it may reflect the costs to self-esteem of receiving help, or the inadequacy of the help received. People may also avoid expressing negative feelings out of a desire to protect others. For instance, in a study of Holocaust survivors, Pennebaker et al. (1989) found that only 30% of survivors had ever talked with anyone about their war experiences. One of the most common reasons survivors gave for avoiding expression was not wanting to upset their family or friends.

So far, our discussion suggests that distress expression is a phenomenon riddled with paradoxes and complexities. People seek out opportunities to express their negative feelings to others, but they also avoid doing so. Sharing one's feelings with others is essential for eliciting support or building intimacy, but it also carries the risk of rejection or loss of self-esteem. To know whether a particular instance of distress expression is likely to have positive or negative consequences, we need to understand the interpersonal context in which it occurs. In the next section, we describe how patterns of emotional behavior emerge in interpersonal relationships. These patterns involve cognitive-interpersonal cycles that determine what type of emotional behavior occurs and what type of response it elicits.

Cognitive-Interpersonal Cycles and Emotional Behavior

Safran and his colleagues (e.g., Muran & Safran, 1993; Safran, 1984, 1990a; Safran & Segal, 1990) posit that patterns of social interactions can often be described in terms of *cognitive-interpersonal cycles*. Specifically, they suggest that individuals' understanding of their social context is guided by their *interpersonal schemas*. These schemas are cognitive representations of generalized self–other relationships, drawn from past experience. They are prototypes or working models containing information about how relationships generally work and how one must act in order to connect with others. Interpersonal schemas shape perceptions of social interactions, and they lead to behaviors consistent with these perceptions. These behaviors then evoke complementary responses from other people, which tend to confirm interpersonal schemas. In other words, our beliefs guide our behavior, and our behavior tends to elicit consequences that confirm our beliefs. (Social psychologists refer to this process as "behavioral confirmation" or "self-fulfilling prophecy"; e.g., Snyder, Tanke, & Berscheid, 1977.)

According to Safran and his colleagues, all people show some degree of consistency in how they think and act in a social context, but individuals with interpersonal difficulties tend to have overly rigid, negative beliefs about relationships and a restricted range of interpersonal behaviors. Their limited behavioral repertoire means they are more likely to behave the same way with everyone. Because other people find their typical behavior aversive, all of their relationships tend to turn out the same unhappy way. So, their negative interpersonal schemas are repeatedly confirmed by the interpersonal consequences of their own problematic behavior. This results in a self-perpetuating, maladaptive cognitive-interpersonal cycle. For example, someone who believes that other people are generally hostile and hurtful in relationships is likely to behave in a hostile manner toward others, simply for self-protection. This hostile behavior is likely to evoke hostile responses from others, confirming the original belief about others' hurtfulness. (See Horowitz, 1991, for descriptions of related psychodynamic perspectives on maladaptive interpersonal relationship patterns.)

Safran's model of cognitive-interpersonal cycles refers to social behavior in general, but it seems especially relevant for describing emotional behavior in close relationships. This model highlights several themes concerning social interactions that are important for understanding the consequences of emotional expression in general and distress expression in particular. First, the model describes the *reciprocal influence* of partners' emotional behavior. When two people interact, each person's expressive behavior is both a cause and a consequence of the other's behavior. Second, it points to the importance of *interpretation* in the development of interpersonal patterns. Our response to someone else's emotional behavior depends on how we construe that behavior—what meaning we infer from it. Third, although this is not explicitly stated, the model also suggests a theme of *transformation* over time. Both the idea of interpersonal schemas as working models derived from experience and the cyclical nature of interactions suggest that interpersonal patterns can evolve over the course of multiple transactions, moving in either an improving direction or in a deteriorating, ultimately stagnating, direction. This suggests that, long term, distress expression can have the effect of bringing partners together or driving them apart.

MALADAPTIVE PATTERNS OF EMOTIONAL BEHAVIOR IN CLOSE RELATIONSHIPS

In order to understand the implications of distress expression in intimate relationships more fully, let's take a look at the interactions of three imaginary married couples. These couples illustrate specific, empirically documented, maladaptive patterns of emotional behavior in close relationships. We focus on maladaptive patterns because of their theoretical and clinical importance. For each couple, we describe the pattern and the underlying processes that produce and maintain it. We also discuss how these patterns might be avoided or remedied. Although the specific patterns illustrated by each of the couples are distinct, drawing from disparate research areas, the interpersonal processes involved are quite similar. All three couples show destructive reciprocal influence, hostile interpretations, and deteriorating transformation of interactions. And, for all three couples, the expression of distress precipitates a cycle of thoughts and behaviors that ultimately results in both partners feeling more miserable and less connected with each other.

The Distressed–Caregiver Couple: Dan and Claire

Dan has been out of work for 6 months because of a back injury. Claire comes home from a particularly frantic day at work to find that the house is a mess and Dan is lying on the couch watching television. She is exhausted and annoyed, but she takes a deep breath and tries to seem cheerful as she greets Dan.

CLAIRE: Hi, honey. How are you feeling?
DAN: Terrible. My back is killing me.

CLAIRE: I'm sorry to hear that. Did you do your exercises?

DAN: No, I didn't do my exercises! I just told you: I'm in pain.

CLAIRE: I'm only reminding you for your own good. The doctor said you need to do the exercises to get better.

DAN: You just don't get it! My back hurts. A lot. All the time. It's ruining my life. I'm miserable, and all you do is nag me.

CLAIRE: It's ruining *your* life?! I work hard all day and then I come home and have to cater to you and pick up after you while you just lie there and complain. You're not even trying to get better!

DAN: Nag! Nag! Nag! That's all you ever do. Why can't you understand that I'm in pain?

Dan and Claire illustrate an unhappy pattern of distressed–caregiver interaction. Both partners express strong negative feelings, but this interaction is only nominally "communication." Neither partner acknowledges anything the other person says. Claire's response to Dan saying he is miserable seems perfunctory, while Dan completely ignores Claire's statements about feeling overburdened. Neither partner feels understood. They are locked into a maladaptive pattern of interaction: The more Dan says he is suffering, the more Claire demands that he get better; the more Claire demands that he get better, the more Dan insists he is suffering. Their interaction leaves both partners brimming with frustration, hostility, and resentment.

Dan's and Claire's reactions are guided by the meaning that they infer from their spouse's emotional communication. Both partners in the anecdote above make negative interpretations of the other's expressions. Dan interprets Claire's expressions of concern as insincere and controlling, while Claire interprets Dan's expressions of distress as contrary, unappreciative, self-centered, and self-indulgent. These interpretations of the spouse's emotional behavior are a reaction to both overt communication and more subtle, nonverbal emotional signs.

Nonverbal emotional leakage can alter the interpersonal meaning of emotional communication. As we noted in Chapter 1, control over expressive behavior is incomplete. Emotional responses have a way of "leaking out," even without our awareness or intention (Collier, 1985). When nonverbal and verbal emotional messages conflict, it is the nonverbal cues that have greater social impact. If our words are friendly, but our face, body, and tone of voice signal hostility, then recipients of our emotional communication perceive hostility. At least initially, Claire seemed to be trying to approach Dan positively. But, perhaps both Dan and Claire detected signs of resentment in the other, which colored their interpretations of the other's overt expressions and elicited negative reactions.

How did Claire and Dan get into such a negative pattern of emotional communication? Coyne and his colleagues (Coyne et al., 1988) have described a process of miscarried helping in which well-intentioned support efforts deteriorate into hostile and coercive exchanges. In attempting to reduce and control another's distress, caretakers may unwittingly exacerbate and perpetuate that distress. This process evolves over extended interactions between the caretaker and the distressed person, in which each person's behavior is a stimulus for and a response to the other's behavior.

1. In the initial stage of this process, the distressed person's expressions of suffering are met with expressions of support and affection by the caregiver. These support expressions are gratefully acknowledged by the distressed person. The partners may feel a special closeness during this "honeymoon" period, as they resolve to put other concerns on hold and cope with the stressor together.

2. The second stage of this process is characterized by inhibited or conflicted expression by one or both partners. As the partner's distress continues, the caregiver begins to feel the strain of continued support efforts. The practical burdens of being responsible for another person and the unavailability of the distressed person as a source of support may lead the caretaker to feel emotionally drained, trapped, or resentful. Yet, the caregiver feels unable to express his or her own needs directly—it seems crass or selfish to further burden the distressed partner. The caregiver continues to express support and reassurance, but these expressions are less wholehearted and may be colored by impatience, frustration, or worry.

The distressed partner becomes aware of the strain on the caregiver through the caregiver's increasingly ambivalent and ambiguous communications. At the same time, the distressed partner becomes aware of the costs of receiving help. He or she may feel guilty, inadequate, or resentful at being "babied." Moreover, the distressed partner may feel pressure to improve for the caregiver's sake. The distressed partner is faced with a dilemma: Continuing to express distress adds to the caregiver's strain and elicits ambivalent feedback, but adopting a more stoic self-presentation sets up unrealistically positive expectations in the caregiver and raises doubts about the legitimacy of subsequent difficulties.

3. The third stage is characterized by increasingly negative emotional communications by both partners. This is the stage illustrated by Dan and Claire. As the distressed partner's condition continues to fail to improve, the caregiver feels increasingly frustrated and even rejected because support efforts have been ineffective. He or she begins to blame the distressed partner for not trying hard enough. By now, the caregiver is highly invested in producing improvement in the distressed partner. He or she monitors progress intensively, offering advice and making explicit demands. The distressed partner responds by expressing more distress, partly in an effort to elicit sympathy and decrease the caregiver's demands, partly as a counter-

reaction to what is perceived as intrusive surveillance, and partly out of a sense of failure and helplessness in the face of enduring distress. If the distressed partner also expresses anger about his or her loss of functioning or about the caregiver's humiliating intrusiveness, this further angers and alienates the caregiver (C. Lane & Hobfoll, 1992).

4. In the final stage of the miscarried helping process, the couple becomes entrenched in a coercive stalemate characterized by direct and indirect expressions of hostility. Each partner tries to influence the other's behavior by being as aversive as possible. The distressed partner shows deliberate ineptness or lack of improvement in order to diminish the caregiver's demands. The caregiver is increasingly critical and demanding in order to diminish the distressed partner's complaints. This pattern becomes self-perpetuating as both partners feel increasingly unwilling to do what the other wants, inviting further attempts at coercive control. The couple's original goals and commitments are long forgotten, as they focus only on controlling the other and avoiding being controlled.

The best evidence for Coyne's model of miscarried helping would be a longitudinal study, documenting changes in distressed–caregiver couples' perceptions of each other and emotional behavior over time. To our knowledge, this has not been done. However, considerable evidence substantiates components of the model, including the strain on caregivers (e.g., Folkman, Chesney, Cooke, Boccellari, & Collette, 1994; E. H. Thompson & Doll, 1982), the occurrence of rejecting or clearly unsupportive responses from support providers (e.g., Piening, 1984; see Marcus & Nardone, 1992, and Segrin & Abramson, 1994, for reviews), and the negative effects on the distressed partner of a hostile or overinvolved caregiver (e.g., Hooley, Orley, & Teasdale, 1986). Moreover, Hops and his colleagues (1987) have documented the reciprocal and coercive pattern of expressive behavior in families in which one member is depressed: Family members express aggression in order to decrease the depressed person's expressions of distress, while the depressed person expresses distress in order to decrease family member's aggressiveness. Biglan and Thorensen (1987) have described a similar pattern between chronic pain patients and their spouses.

The importance of Coyne's model for our purposes is that it is a vivid description of the process of reciprocal influence and transformation in emotional communication and the mediating role of interpretations of other's behavior. Each partner's emotional expression is both a cause and a consequence of the other's reaction. The meaning of a particular expression changes over time with evolving interactions. Initially, expressions of distress and concern are interpreted as bids for emotional closeness. By the end of the process, ostensibly identical emotional behaviors are interpreted as criticism and rejection.

This downward spiral in the relationship between the distressed partner and the caregiver is not inevitable. For example, sometimes the distressed partner improves, which removes much of the strain on the couple. A positive outcome allows the distressed partner to feel more competent and less needy, and it allows the caregiver to feel rewarded for helping efforts as well as less obligated to take care of the distressed partner. A positive outcome may also foster emotional closeness between the partners, if they view the ordeal as something they managed together successfully.

In the absence of a positive outcome, the maladaptive pattern might still be avoided if objective evidence or external corroboration of impairment is available. This evidence helps to resolve ambiguity concerning expectations for the distressed partner's level of functioning. Caregivers are less likely to respond with rejection or criticism when they consider the distressed person's behavior to be appropriate (Revenson & Majerovitz, 1990).

Finally, the deteriorating cycle might be halted if the couple is able to communicate openly and constructively about their interactions. Sometimes each partner is able to acknowledge the other's point of view and recognize his or her own contribution to interactions. This understanding diffuses hostility and tempers negative interpretations, allowing more positive interactions.

The Bereaved Couple: Bob and Brenda

A bit over a year ago, Bob and Brenda's 9-month-old daughter died inexplicably in her sleep. Bob is sitting in the kitchen reading the newspaper. Brenda approaches him, carrying a small pile of photographs. Her eyes look red from crying.

BRENDA: I came across those photos from when we took the baby to the beach. Remember that?

BOB: (*not looking up from the paper*) Yeah.

BRENDA: She's wearing that hat your mother bought for her—you know, the one with the ruffles.

BOB: (*still not looking up*) Hmmm.

BRENDA: Do you want to see the photos?

BOB: No. (*He turns the page of the newspaper abruptly and scans it aimlessly.*)

BRENDA: (*She watches him silently. Tears start running down her face. Finally, she blurts:*) I don't understand you. She was our baby! Don't you miss her? Don't you care?

BOB: (*gruffly*) Of course I miss her! I just don't want to talk about it. (*He closes the newspaper and walks out of the room.*)

Bob and Brenda are coping with a shared stressor. Both partners have to manage their own distress and also serve as a potential source of support for the other. To further complicate matters, they have incompatible preferences for emotional expression: She wants to talk about her feelings; he prefers to avoid focusing on his feelings. Actually, both partners express distress in this interaction: Brenda's expressions are overt communications of profound sadness, while Bob's expressions involve more subtle, nonverbal signals of anxiety and discomfort with the discussion. Under other circumstances, Bob and Brenda could probably accommodate the mismatch in their preferred coping styles. But, the loss of their daughter is so intensely painful that it is hard for either of them to be helpful to the other.

Both partners' emotional behavior contributes to an escalating cycle: The more Brenda tries to get Bob to talk about feelings, the more he withdraws; the more Bob avoids dealing with feelings, the more Brenda tries to draw him out by expressing her feelings. This escalation is fueled by the negative interpretations each partner makes for the other's emotional behavior. Brenda sees Bob's lack of expression of sadness as uncaring; Bob views Brenda's expressivity as overwhelming, demanding, and intrusive. At the end of their interaction, both partners feel resentful, and neither partner feels understood.

K. R. Gilbert (1989) conducted semistructured interviews with married couples who had experienced infant or fetal death. The couples provided some intriguing qualitative data regarding variables they perceived to be related to low conflict versus high conflict and estrangement. The low-conflict variables identified by the bereaved couples involve authentic communication, understanding, and a sense of connection between the partners. Among the positive variables they mentioned were expressing their feelings together, validating each other's views, nonverbal communication about the loss, and sensitivity to each other's needs.

In contrast, the high-conflict variables identified by the bereaved couples entail a lack of understanding and either disconnection or destructive connection between the partners. Key among these high-conflict variables was disparate views about appropriate emotional behavior for grieving, like those illustrated by Bob and Brenda. Having experienced a shared trauma, the couples expected to respond similarly and were often disconcerted when this was not the case. For example, the partners sometimes differed in their views about appropriate private versus public grieving behaviors or the speed at which they came to terms with their grief. Frequently, they were just "out of sync" with each other: One partner might feel a bit better while the other partner experienced a period of intensified grief, making it hard for either partner to relate to the other's experience. Interestingly, the couples reported that they often deliberately tried to influence each other to grieve in the "best" or "right" way (see also Gottlieb & Wagner, 1991). These attempts occurred partly out of a desire to be helpful to the other, partly as a means of validating their own way of coping, and partly out of a need to increase their sense of control by having an impact on the other partner.

The bereaved couples in Gilbert's study also mentioned a phenomenon of "resonating grief." One partner expressing his or her feelings sometimes had the effect of making the other feel worse, "pulling" the other down. And sometimes, expression precipitated a competition in which each partner tried to "prove" that he or she had suffered more. Gilbert's data should be regarded as preliminary, since they are based on retrospective self-reports. However, they describe some vivid and intriguing examples of the reciprocal influence of spouses' emotional behavior.

In keeping with the idea of resonating grief, there is accumulating evidence that emotions are contagious. We tend to "catch" the feelings of those around us because their emotional expression elicits similar or complementary emotional reactions in us. This emotional contagion (Hatfield, Cacioppo, & Rapson, 1992) can occur without conscious awareness. It is most likely to occur when the other person is someone we care about, and when that person is expressing strong emotions. Thus, emotional contagion is likely to be particularly problematic in the case of a shared trauma, like Bob and Brenda's, in which partners have to manage their own distress but also feel responsible for helping each other. Bob found it unbearable to see Brenda's distress. Perhaps her expression intensified his own feelings of grief to the point that he could not be helpful to her. This possibility is consistent with developmental research showing that the ability to moderate one's own level of distress is a prerequisite to responding empathically to another's distress (Eisenberg & Fabes, 1992).

Alternatively, perhaps seeing Brenda's suffering evoked Bob's empathy, but also made him feel inadequate for being unable to help her. Individuals experiencing traumatic events are often discouraged by significant others from expressing their feelings (Coates & Winston, 1987; Wortman & Dunkel-Schetter, 1979). This emotional avoidance by significant others occurs for several reasons. It is distressing for others to see someone they care about suffering. In particular, the intensity of the trauma victim's distress may be alarming for others and may lead them to conclude that talking about the trauma just makes things worse. Moreover, others may feel confused or helpless about how to respond to such intense distress. Thus avoidance of feelings can stem from both other-protective and self-protective motives (DeLongis, Wortman, Silver, & O'Brien, 1991): Significant others may want to protect the bereaved person from experiencing distress, and they may want to protect themselves from experiencing upsetting interactions with the bereaved person.

Bob and Brenda's interactions also fit what marital researchers call the *demand–withdraw* pattern (e.g., Christensen & Heavey, 1990; Fruzzetti & Jacobson, 1990). This pattern is characterized by differential engagement or desire for intimacy. One partner, usually the woman, desires greater closeness, sharing, and emotional intensity and pursues these goals through greater emotional expression, while the other partner, usually the male, prefers greater separateness, autonomy, and emotional distance and pursues these goals through avoidance and withdrawal. An escalating and conflictual cycle is established: The more one partner withdraws, the more intensely the other partner demands intimacy; the more intensely the other partner seeks intimacy, the more urgently the first partner seeks separateness. Evidence for the existence of the demand–withdraw pattern comes from self-reports, partner reports, and observer ratings. The frequent occurrence of this pattern is strongly associated with marital dissatisfaction.

What causes the demand–withdraw pattern, and why do the roles tend to be gender-linked? One explanation concerns males' greater physiological reactivity to stress (Gottman & Levenson, 1988; Notarius & Johnson, 1982). Males may withdraw from conflict or other intense emotional communication because they find it uncomfortably arousing. Alternatively, this pattern may stem from the different socialization of males and females (Gilligan, 1982). According to this view, women are raised to value relationships and fear rejection or abandonment, whereas men are raised to value autonomy and fear engulfment or intrusion. Still another possible explanation concerns social structure (Jacobson, 1983, 1989; Thibaut & Kelley, 1959). The less powerful and less satisfied partner (usually the wife) is more likely to seek discussion and change, whereas the more powerful and more satisfied partner (usually the husband) has a vested interest in not changing. Moreover, the husband's withdrawal has the effect of underscoring the power differential in a couple. Men can achieve the autonomy they desire unilaterally, but women must depend on their partners' cooperation to achieve the intimacy they desire (Christensen & Heavey, 1990).

Clearly, not all couples are characterized by the demand–withdraw pattern. Satisfied couples are able to achieve a communication compromise that strikes a balance between their needs for emotional closeness and separateness (Blechman, 1990; Derlega et al., 1993). Precisely how such a compromise is achieved is not clear. However, the compromise is likely to entail strategies that make emotional discussions more palatable or at least less threatening to the potentially withdrawing partner. These strategies might include easing in gently to emotional communication (Petronio, 1991) or dividing responsibility such that "one partner schedules and manages hot discussions and the other partner embeds hot discussions in a stream of cool activities" (Blechman, 1990, p. 218). Still another possible compromise might involve having the more expressive partner do some expressing with other people. For instance, if a wife is able to talk over her feelings with her women friends, she may feel less need to talk about them with her husband. If the wife's discussions of her feelings then become less intense or less frequent, the husband may be better able to respond positively.

Some evidence suggests that if one partner adopts a nonexpressive style, over time the other partner will become similarly nonexpressive. In an interview study of married couples with a seriously ill child, Gottlieb and Wagner (1991) found that husbands preferred a rational coping style and pressured their wives to behave more stoically, whereas wives preferred an emotion-focused coping style and pressured their husbands to express their feelings openly. Over time, at least some wives reported that they tended to hide their feelings, in keeping with their husbands' coping preferences, in order not to lose their support. Another study (J. J. Stern & Pascale, 1979) found that husbands who used denial to cope with their myocardial infarction had wives who engaged in excessive worrying. One possible explanation for these findings is that the husbands' avoidant coping strategy limited their wives' opportunity to express their feelings openly, which resulted in the wives' silent rumination. We suspect that some compromise position, in which the expression of emotion within the couple is allowed but contained, would be associated with the most adaptive outcomes.

The Angry Couple: Adam and Ana

Adam and Ana have just left a dinner party at a friend's house. During the 15-minute drive home, Ana sits silently fuming. Adam doesn't know why she's mad at him, but he dreads the argument that he knows is coming. By the time they get home, Ana is seething with resentment, and Adam is irritated with her for being mad at him.

ANA: (*snidely*) Well, *you* certainly had a good time at the party.

ADAM: What's that supposed to mean?

ANA: Just that you spent an awful lot of time talking to that Susan.

ADAM: You're imagining things.

ANA: You talked to her all through dinner!

ADAM: She was sitting next to me—what was I supposed to do? There you go again, blowing things completely out of proportion. At least Susan was friendly and pleasant to talk to instead of constantly complaining, like you.

ANA: You know, I was really looking forward to tonight. We never go out anymore, so I thought this party was going to be a real treat. But you had to ruin it for me by flirting with some woman.

ADAM: We never go out anymore because we never have any money. We never have any money because you're always spending it. Like yesterday: What was that big credit card receipt I saw?

ANA: I never spend money on myself—just on the kids. Both boys needed new shoes for soccer. Not that you would know this, since you're never around. It's amazing that the kids even recognize you.

A great deal of communication took place during the 15-minute car ride in which neither Ana nor Adam said a word. Nonverbal emotional expression is particularly important in conflicts (Gottman, Markman, & Notarius, 1977; D. A. Newton & Burgoon, 1990). Ana and Adam's silent communication negatively colored their later verbal discussion. By the time they got home, both partners were stewing for a fight and ready to interpret everything the other person said in the most hostile light. The discussion started out with an intensely negative and antagonistic tone that never abated.

Adam and Ana's interaction fits a pattern that marital researchers call *cross-complaining* and *negative escalation* (Gottman, 1979; Gottman & Levenson, 1986). In just a few short exchanges, they managed to bring up half a dozen issues and resolve none of them. Each comment only intensifies their negative feelings toward each other and precipitates an even more negative comment in response. Adam's and Ana's comments are aimed at hurting each other rather than understanding or resolving any issues. Negative escalation cycles are very effective discriminators between satisfied and dissatisfied couples and powerful predictors of future distress (Gottman & Levenson, 1986; Julien, Markman, & Lindahl, 1989).

Virtually all close relationships experience conflict at some point. The question becomes, then, how is this conflict managed? The tendency to reciprocate negative expressions of emotion is very strong (Cahn, 1990; Gaelick, Bodenhausen, & Wyer, 1985; Gottman et al., 1977). However, most couples don't argue continuously, so there must be ways of disengaging from conflict.

One strategy of conflict disengagement is for both partners to simply withdraw. Kahn, Coyne, and Margolin (1985) have described a cycle of hostility–inhibition–more hostility among distressed couples. Intensely negative and unproductive conflicts lead couples to try to avoid further conflict by inhibiting their expression of negative feelings. However, during this avoidance, chronic tension simmers as previously unresolved issues continue and new issues arise. When overt conflict does occur, it is often noncontingent: A minor incident brings forth a stormy expression of accumulated resentment and hostility. This new conflict is likely to be even more intensely painful and unconstructive, which leads to further inhibition. We suspect that this pattern applies to Ana and Adam. Listening to their interactions, one gets the feeling that the same issues have been raised many times before and that this particular conflict will end in a stalemate.

Another conflict disengagement strategy focuses on the man's behavior. Gaelick and her colleagues (Gaelick et al., 1985) videotaped problem discussions by married or cohabitating couples. They then had both partners in each couple review their videotape and rate significant communications according to the feelings the speaker intended to convey, the feelings the speaker expected to elicit, and the recipient's actual reaction. As expected, Gaelick et al. found that expressions of hostility tended to be reciprocated, fueling an escalation cycle. Partners were less accurate in perceiving expressions of love and therefore less likely to reciprocate these positive expressions. However, an interesting asymmetry emerged in partners' interpretations of each other's behavior. The absence of an expression of love was interpreted by men, but not women, as a hostile response from the partner. The absence of an expression of hostility was interpreted by women, but not men, as a loving response from the partner. Based on this finding, Gaelick and her colleagues conclude that women's behavior is likely to play a crucial role in escalating conflict, because they can elicit hostility from men by either expressing hostility or failing to express love. In contrast, men's behavior is likely to be important in deescalating conflict, because they can elicit love from women by simply not responding with hostility. This study underscores the critical importance of interpretations of emotional communication.

Gottman (1979) argues on the basis of observational data that how deescalation of conflict occurs depends on the intensity of the conflict as well as general marital satisfaction. In satisfied marriages, men tend to deescalate low-conflict discussions, whereas women are responsible for defusing high-conflict discussions. Satisfied wives are likely to regulate conflict intensity by limiting the beginning of a negative escalation cycle (Notarius, Benson, Sloane, Vanzetti, & Hornyak, 1989). Deescalation tends to take the form of a "contract" cycle, in which partners alternate suggesting solutions to the problem and responding with agreement. In contrast, in dissatisfied relationships, neither spouse takes responsibility for deescalation. Suggested problem solutions, if they occur, are met with counterproposals, rather than with agreement (Gottman et al., 1977). Moreover, dissatisfied partners' physiological arousal levels tend to be linked (Levenson & Gottman, 1983). When one partner is highly upset, so is the other. Neither partner is able to step back and break out of the cycle of negative affective reciprocity.

Over time, how conflict is managed has a tremendous effect not only on future behavior and partners' individual satisfaction but also on couples' shared definition of their relationship. Notarius and Vanzetti (1983) describe a sense of "relational efficacy" that some couples develop. This term refers to a belief that they can cope with conflict together and a confidence that engaging in conflict will lead to positive resolution. The key to developing this sense of relational efficacy is sharing a history of positively resolved conflicts. Perhaps this explains Gottman and Krokoff's (1989) finding that the expression of negative affect is associated with less concurrent marital satisfaction but improved marital satisfaction at a 3-year follow-up (see also Menaghan, 1982; however, see Woody & Costanzo, 1990, for a skeptical view of this finding).

How do couples acquire a history of positive conflict resolution? The crucial element is the ability to regulate the intensity of negative emotional expression (Blechman, 1990; Fruzzetti & Jacobson, 1990; Lindahl & Markman, 1990). Engaging in "tolerable doses" of expression of negative emotions toward a spouse is less arousing for both self and spouse than more intense expression (see Chapter 2). For this reason, it has a number of potential advantages. First, moderately intense expression is less aversive, which makes it more likely that partners will continue to engage in the discussion until a solution is achieved, rather than disengaging prematurely. Second, moderate expression makes it more likely that partners will be able to think constructively and come up with solutions, rather than experiencing cognitive deficits due to excessive arousal (e.g., being so mad they can't think straight). Third, tolerable expression makes it more likely that partners will be able to assimilate new information and develop better understanding of each other, which is linked to satisfaction in long-term relationships (Cahn, 1990). Finally, when negative expression is only moderately intense, and especially when it leads to positive resolution, then subsequent conflicts are likely to be approached with less dread or anticipatory anxiety. Thus, successful regulation of expression facilitates conflict resolution, which precipitates future successful regulation and resolution.

Couples with a sense of relational efficacy, who are able to moderate the intensity of their negative emotional expression, are likely to view the expression of distress as unpleasant but not unbearable and to see it as a possible means of enhancing understanding and intimacy. In contrast, negative emotional expression is likely to have a very different meaning for couples like Adam and Ana, who experience it as intensely painful and out of control.

Similarities among the Three Couples

The three patterns of distress communication illustrated by the couples in our anecdotes are drawn from diverse research literatures, but they reflect similar interpersonal processes. The couples' interactions involve patterns of reciprocal influence, in which one partner's emotional expression is both a response to and a cause of the other partner's behavior. To understand these patterns, we need to see how they transform over time. For example, looking only at the angry couple's brief interaction might lead one to think that they are intensely engaged with each other, but a more extensive view of their interactions over time shows that their pattern involves alternations between intense negative engagement followed by disengagement. Similarly, an extended view reveals the "out-of-sync" grieving patterns of the bereaved couple and the building resentment and coercion of the distressed–caregiver couple.

The couples are also similar in the outcomes of their distress communication. The interactions of all three couples are maladaptive because they leave partners feeling more miserable and less connected with their spouse. None of the couples is able to resolve any difficulties or even respond empathically to each other's distress expression.

At the beginning of this chapter, we identified a number of possible benefits of expressing distress to others, such as evoking concrete assistance, bolstering self-worth, and positively altering existing relationships. However, all of these possible benefits require that the receivers of distress communication comprehend it and react positively.

At the most basic level, we express our negative feelings to others because we want to be heard and understood. In other words, we hope that our distress communications will be met with responsiveness. Miller and Berg (1984) define responsiveness as "the extent to which and the way in which one participant's actions address the previous actions, communications, needs, or wishes of another participant in the interaction" (p. 191). They distinguish between "conversational responsiveness," which involves behaviors indicating interest in and understanding of another person's communication, and "relational responsiveness," which involves behaviors addressing another person's needs.

Both types of responsiveness are in short supply among the couples in our anecdotes. They talk at each other or past each other, but never to each other. The spouses fail to acknowledge their partner's communication and also feel unheard themselves. The lack of responsiveness leaves everyone feeling frustrated, resentful, and rejected.

What determines whether or not distress expression is met with responsiveness? In describing the couples in our anecdotes, we argued that partners' reactions depend on the meaning that they construe from their spouses' emotional behavior. This suggests that we need to look more closely at possible meanings of distress communication.

In the next section, we discuss how partners interpret expressions of distress in close relationships. For the sake of clarity, we will refer to one partner as the receiver and the other partner as the expresser. However, it is important to remember that the process of reciprocal influence means that, in most couples, *both* partners actually play *both* roles.

INTERPRETATIONS OF DISTRESS EXPRESSION

We believe that the key factor determining receivers' responses to a particular expression of distress expression is the extent to which they view that expression as personally threatening. The more threatening they find it, the less likely they are to respond warmly or empathically.

Below, we describe four threat-related interpretations that influence the receivers' responses to their partners' expressions of distress. These interpretations focus on the implications of the distress expression for receivers' personal worth and freedom, as well as judgments of expressers' intent and the receivers' coping capacity. These threat-related interpretations involve receivers' conscious or preconscious construal of expressers' emotional behavior. They are responses to expressers' nonverbal as well as verbal communication.

Receivers' Personal Worth

One interpretation that receivers of distress communication make involves asking themselves, "What does this say about me, as a person?" To some extent, everyone has a basic desire for social recognition and approval. This desire can only be satisfied by other people's actions (P. Brown & Levinson, 1978; Segrin & Abramson, 1994). Having the approval of people who play important roles in our lives seems especially important. So, receivers' responses to their partners' expression of distress is determined in part by whether they interpret this expression as conveying a positive or negative view of themselves.

It is easier to respond warmly when someone tells us "I'm mad at him" than when he or she says "I'm mad at you." The first message is flattering. It means the expresser is confiding in us and views us as a trusted ally. The second message is threatening. It suggests there is something unlikeable about us. Shimanoff (1987) presented married couples with scenarios involving disclosures of negative emotions directed at either the spouse or some other person (e.g., friend, coworker). When spouses received distress disclosures about other people, they felt more intimate with their partner. When the distress disclosures were about themselves, spouses felt less intimate.

Among our three couples, distress expression was construed by receivers as personal criticism and rejection. The criticism is quite overt in the angry couple, as they hurl insults at each other. The mismatched coping styles of the bereaved couple also imply criticism of the partner for not coping the "right" way. In the distressed–caregiver couple, Claire sees Dan's continued distress as rejecting and unappreciative of her helping efforts, while Dan interprets Claire's feelings of being overwhelmed as criticism of his lack of improvement. Perceiving their partners' distress expression as personal criticism raises receivers' hackles: It makes them more concerned with defending themselves than understanding what is going on with their partners.

On the other hand, tempering the criticism implied in distress communication can elicit more positive reactions from receivers. With all three of our couples, we noted that validation of the partners' perspective can play a key role in halting maladaptive expressive cycles. For example, if Dan can tell Claire that he truly appreciates her efforts, it will be easier for Claire to listen to his distress.

Receivers' Freedom

A second type of threat-related interpretation that receivers of distress expression make involves asking themselves, "Do I have a free choice in how I respond?" People do not like to have their sense of personal freedom impeded or imposed upon by others (Brown & Levinson, 1978; Segrin & Abramson, 1994). Threats to one's ability to think or act freely induce a negative arousal state called *reactance* (J. W. Brehm, 1972) and a strong desire to be rid of that external control. If we help someone in distress, we want it to be because we choose to do so, not because we are manipulated into it. When distress expression is interpreted by receivers as a demand rather than a request for help, when it evokes a sense of obligation rather than choice, it is perceived as more threatening and it is less likely to evoke a warm response. Under these conditions, any help that receivers offer is given grudgingly.

Among our couples, distress expression is used as a means of coercive control, and it is therefore threatening to the receivers' sense of personal freedom. The spouses behave in aversive ways toward each other in an attempt to make their partners behave in a certain way. In the distressed–caregiver couple, Dan expresses pain in order to reduce Claire's demands for improvement, while Claire expresses feelings of being overburdened in order to induce him to function better. In the angry couple, Ana snarls at Adam to try to get him to pay attention to her, while Adam snarls at Ana to try to get her to stop criticizing him. In the bereaved couple, Brenda repeatedly tries to draw Bob out by expressing her feelings of loss. The harder she tries to get him to express, the more he resists. When and if receivers give in to their partners' efforts to influence them, they do so with great resentment, and they are even less willing to cooperate next time.

For receivers to respond positively to distress expression, they need to feel that they have some say over what happens—some influence over the nature of the couple's interactions. For example, with the bereaved couple, we noted that a communication compromise that lessens the unpleasantness of emotional discussions for the withdrawing partner is one way of avoiding the maladaptive demand–withdraw cycle.

Expressers' Intent

The third type of interpretation that receivers make in determining the degree of threat entailed in distress communication involves asking themselves, "*Why* is this person expressing this distress to me?" When receivers perceive that the intent behind distress expression is malicious, they feel more threatened and are less likely to respond positively.

All of the people in our anecdotes perceive that the intent behind their partners' distress expression is to be deliberately hurtful. So, their reactions to their partners' emotional behavior look more like efforts to fend off attacks than efforts to understand or communicate.

On the other hand, when receivers view their spouses' intent as positive or at least benign, they are more likely to respond warmly to distress expression. Satisfied partners tend to make more generous or forgiving attributions for their spouses' negative behavior than do unsatisfied partners (e.g., Fincham & Bradbury, 1993). In fact partners' responses to their spouses' complaints are influenced more by partners' global feelings toward their spouses than by the spouses' immediate behavior (Alberts, 1988). In good relationships, in which interactions are generally positive and satisfying, spouses can get away with a bit of bad behavior and still get a good response. In bad relationships, spouses may be damned by their partners before they open their mouths. This relates to the idea of relational efficacy that we discussed in terms of avoiding the cross-complaining of the angry couple. When couples have had experiences of resolving conflicts together, they gain confidence that they can do so again. So, they are more likely to view their spouses' distress expression as perhaps unpleasant but ultimately beneficial. They are more likely to see it as communication rather than an attempt to be hurtful, so they are more likely to respond positively.

Receivers' Coping Capacity

The final type of threat-related interpretation that receivers make involves asking themselves, "Can I deal with this?" Even if all the other threat-related interpretations are positive, receivers might still respond negatively if they perceive their spouses' distress expression as something that exceeds their capacity to cope. It might just seem like more than they can handle.

The couples in our anecdotes expressed emotions that were not only negative but also extremely intense and long-lasting. This necessarily makes them more threatening to receivers than minor, transient difficulties. In the distressed–caregiver couple, Claire was helpful and solicitous when Dan first hurt his back, but his continued distress, with no sign of improvement, wore her down. In the bereaved couple, the intensity of Brenda's grief was unbearable for Bob, especially given his own feelings of loss. In the angry couple, the intensity of the hostility expressed by each partner precipitated even more hostile responses from the other partner.

Circumstances or efforts to make distress expression seem more manageable make positive responses from receivers more likely. We noted that being able to moderate the intensity of conflicts is an important skill for resolving difficulties and avoiding negative escalation cycles. Similarly, the strategies of embedding emotionally "hot" discussions in a context of "cool" activities and expressing positive as well as negative emotions are likely to prompt greater cooperation and less avoidance from receivers than unrelenting distress expression.

CONCLUSION

Expressions of distress in intimate relationships are shaped by the reciprocal influence of partners' emotional behavior: One person's emotional expression evokes a corresponding response from the partner, which in turn influences the first person's emotional behavior. This reciprocal influence can move in a positive direction, toward greater intimacy and improved well-being, or in a negative direction, toward rejection, animosity, and greater distress. The consequences of distress expression depend on how receivers interpret it. Receivers draw on verbal and nonverbal aspects of their partners' emotional behavior to infer the degree of threat that the distress expression entails for them. The more threatening receivers find the distress expression, the less likely they are to respond positively.

The view of distress expression that we have presented in this chapter carries a number of implications for clinical practice. First, it means that therapists need to identify interpersonal patterns involving distress expression, such as those illustrated by the couples in our anecdotes. Helping clients to identify these maladaptive patterns, and to understand how both partners contribute to the development and maintenance of these patterns, can be an important step in modifying them. Often, having just one partner, either partner, *not* respond negatively is enough to change the direction of a maladaptive interpersonal cycle.

Second, our discussion underscores the importance of a longitudinal view in examining distress expression. Patterns can take time to emerge, and short-term results don't necessarily match long-term consequences. Sometimes it is helpful for unhappy couples to realize that their relationship wasn't always this way, which suggests that it can change for the better.

Third, and most important, our discussion suggests that therapists need to understand (and perhaps modify) not only clients' emotional behavior but also the construed meaning of that behavior. It is the subjective meaning that receivers infer from their partners' expression of distress that guides receivers' responses and fuels maladaptive cognitive-interpersonal cycles. Strategies or contexts that make distress expression seem less threatening to receivers can elicit more positive responses.

PART IV

Treatment Implications

8

Expression and Nonexpression in Psychotherapy: Facilitating Emotional Understanding and Behavioral Change

INTRODUCTION

Therapist and Client Views of Emotional Expression

Most clinicians believe that the expression of emotion is critically important in psychotherapy. They view it as a sign that therapy is going well. They rate sessions in which clients cry or express difficult feelings as deep and powerful (Stiles, 1984). Every orientation has at least some techniques that draw upon and encourage expression. For example, cognitive-behavioral therapists focus on expression as a means of identifying "hot cognitions," which are emotion-laden beliefs (Goldfried, 1982; Safran & Greenberg, 1982; Safran & Segal, 1990). They also emphasize communication training as a means of teaching clients to effectively articulate their feelings to others. Psychodynamic therapists discuss the importance of catharsis and the importance of working through emotional experience (Eagle, 1984; Freud, 1914/1963). Expression is probably most central for experiential therapists, who see it as a means of symbolizing emotional experience and drawing upon that experience as a guide to adaptive coping (Daldrup, Beutler, Engle, & Greenberg, 1988; Bohart, 1993; Bohart & Tollman, 1998; Goldfried, 1982; L. S. Greenberg et al., 1993; L. S. Greenberg, Watson, & Lietaer, 1998, C. Rogers, 1965).

In contrast, clients are often considerably less enthusiastic than therapists about emotional expression (Rennie, 1993; J. C. Watson & Rennie, 1994). They describe expression as difficult (Stiles, 1984). They often resist

205

and try to avoid therapists' attempts to elicit emotional expression in session. Sometimes clients fear that they will be overwhelmed by their feelings if they express them. Other times, clients expect that expressing their feelings will be futile or will elicit rejection from the therapist or significant others.

Clinical research points to both the benefits and the risks of expression. On the one hand, expression in a therapeutic context can lead clients to enhanced self-understanding and greater self-acceptance (Mergenthaler, 1996; Roemer & Borkovec, 1994). It can also be a bridge toward new ways of acting and communicating in day-to-day life. On the other hand, not all forms of expression are helpful (Nix, Watson, Pyszczynski, & Greenberg, 1995). As we described in earlier chapters, when expression involves an impulsive spilling over of poorly processed emotional responses, it can interfere with coping efforts and can drive other people away. Expression that is indiscriminate, prolonged, and extremely intense tends to elicit interpersonal rejection. Expression that involves a rehearsal of entrenched feelings tends to compound distress rather than foster emotional insight. Brief bursts of expression that entail a surface compliance with therapist demands are also unlikely to enhance well-being.

Characteristics of Adaptive Emotional Expression

How do we distinguish between adaptive and maladaptive forms of expression? In terms of outcome, expression is adaptive when it (1) leads to resolution and new understanding rather than rehearsal of negative feelings and/or (2) communicates feelings to others in a desired way. Emotional expression is not an end in itself, but it can be a means of facilitating adaptive coping and enhancing well-being.

In terms of process, a key characteristic of adaptive expression is that it reflects a balance between reason and emotion (L. S. Greenberg et al., 1993; J. C. Watson & Greenberg, 1996a). People have two different ways of processing information: experiential or rational (Bohart, 1993; Elliott & Greenberg, 1993; S. Epstein, 1994; Gendlin, 1974, 1981; L. S. Greenberg et al., 1993; Zajonc, 1980). The *experiential processing system* is global and holistic. It draws upon affect and imagery. It processes information quickly, in an integrative way, but once activated, its impressions are slow to change. In contrast, the *rational processing system* is analytic, dominated by logic and fact. It processes information more slowly, in a more differentiated way, but its conclusions can change quickly. Both rational and experiential processing of information are important for well-being: Relying solely on rational processing means that one is cut off from a rich source of information about oneself and the impact of the environment, whereas relying solely on experiential processing entails being driven blindly by diffuse affective responses. An integration between thinking and experiencing is both a sign and a result of adaptive emotional expression.

The process model of emotional expression that we described in Chapter 1 lays out the steps involved in the processing of emotional experience, resulting in an integration of rational and experiential knowledge. Successive steps in the model involve increasing cognitive differentiation of affective experience. This cognitive elaboration is guided by felt experience and also transforms that experience. People first become aware that they feel something, then they label what they feel, then they go on to determine the meaning of those feelings for themselves and others. Problems involving emotional behavior can arise when this process is either thwarted or circumvented.

It is important for clinicians to be able to recognize when to heighten clients' awareness of their feelings and when to facilitate reflection. Attending to the content of what clients' say provides an indication of their expressive stance toward their experience. Expressive stance (Rice, Watson, & Greenberg, 1993) refers to the focus of clients' attention and the activity in which they are engaged during the session. It describes, for example, whether they are actively engaged and exploring their experience or are being more distant and analytical.

When clients are engaged in productive exploration and expression of emotion, they are inwardly focused on their thoughts and feelings, actively experiencing their feelings in the session, and intensely engaged in examining and evaluating their experience to create new meaning. When clients are in touch with their feelings in this way, their voices are soft, hesitant with ragged pauses and emphasis in unexpected places. Their language is often poignant and vivid, creating a sense of immediacy and aliveness.

In contrast, less productive processing and expression are characterized by more distant and disengaged descriptions and analysis of experience and feelings. At these times, clients often have an outward focus, describing the events and people in their lives in a rehearsed and lifeless manner (Rice et al., 1993; J. C. Watson & Greenberg, 1996a). Clients may talk about what is happening in their lives but pay little attention to its impact on them and their own inner responses. They may talk in a well-modulated, rhythmic tone, as if they were presenting a well-rehearsed speech or chatting to a friend. They are not in touch with their feelings but seem distant from them and appear to be talking about them rather than experiencing or expressing them in the moment.

In this chapter, we present general guidelines for therapists concerning how to facilitate clients' adaptive emotional expression. Our model of expression and nonexpression provides a framework for understanding in what way clients are stuck in the processing of their emotional experience. Different problems related to emotional behavior require different therapeutic approaches. Our purpose in this chapter is *not* to provide an exhaustive list of all possible clinical strategies related to emotional expression. Rather, we discuss general goals for addressing different problems involving emotional behavior and provide examples of some therapeutic techniques that can be helpful in achieving these goals. First we describe therapeutic strategies for problems involving *nonexpression*, then we consider ways of addressing problems involving *expression*.

ADDRESSING PROBLEMS INVOLVING NONEXPRESSION

Problems involving nonexpression occur when people do not process their emotional experience (Mongrain & Zuroff, 1994; Roemer & Borkovec, 1994). Different forms of nonexpression vary in terms of the degree to which people have processed their experience before stifling it. Below, we describe instances of nonexpression stemming from difficulties in accepting, understanding, or perceiving emotional experience and offer some clinical strategies for dealing with these problems. Each of these forms of nonexpression refers to a disruption at a different step in our process model of emotional expression. We start by examining the most surface level disruption and then describe increasingly more pervasive forms of blocking.

Negative Attitudes toward Emotion

One type of nonexpression stems from difficulties accepting one's feelings because of negative attitudes toward emotion. Clients sometimes deliberately refrain from expressing because they judge their feelings to be dangerous, wrong, or shameful. This is frequently an issue at the beginning of therapy. Clients may be reluctant to focus on their feelings and be fearful of the consequences of doing so.

Psychotherapy process research shows the importance of having clients and therapists agree on the goals and means of therapy (Hovarth & Greenberg, 1994), so it may be necessary to address clients' negative attitudes toward emotion before launching into any techniques aimed at increasing emotional expression. Therapists need to be very careful not to ride roughshod over clients' expression-related beliefs, especially when they do not match therapists' own beliefs (J. C. Watson & Greenberg, 1994, 1995). Clients' negative attitudes toward emotion may be deeply rooted in their sense of identity and based on powerful experiences or highly meaningful family or cultural values. Simply dismissing these beliefs or forcing clients to act in a way that is contrary to their values may impede the development of a good working alliance and is unlikely to lead to a positive outcome in therapy.

When nonexpression stems from negative attitudes toward emotion, therapists can help clients to articulate their personal goals and values concerning emotional behavior (see Chapter 4). Making these beliefs explicit gives clients the opportunity to reexamine and perhaps revise them. There are two main ways of doing this: two-chair dialogues and Socratic questioning.

Two-Chair Dialogues

One way of helping clients to articulate and reconsider their negative attitudes toward emotion is through the gestalt two-chair technique (L. S. Greenberg et al., 1993; Perls, 1969, 1973; Robins & Hayes, 1993). In the following example, the therapist uses the two-chair technique to help the client negotiate a compromise between the part of herself that wants to express her feelings and the part that doesn't. The client was not ready to commit to the work of therapy until she dealt with her negative attitudes toward emotion.

> Natasha was a bright, articulate graduate student who had returned to school after the collapse of her marriage. She was quite depressed and uncertain about her career path. At first, Natasha was very open and responsive to a variety of therapeutic techniques aimed at helping her access her feelings. Then, it was as if the spring ran dry. She suddenly stopped talking about her feelings in any immediate way. She put limits on what topics could be discussed in therapy. For instance, she insisted that she did not want to discuss anything about her childhood, since this had been done in an earlier therapy experience and did not seem helpful.
>
> Soon, it became clear to both Natasha and her therapist that she was not making any progress. As she began to explore the meaning of this lack of progress with her therapist, Natasha acknowledged that she found it difficult and anxiety-provoking to be in therapy.
>
> Her therapist encouraged her to engage in a two-chair dialogue between the part of herself that wanted to be in therapy and the part of herself that was scared. Through this dialogue, Natasha was able to articulate her fear that therapy would somehow change her irrevocably, so that, instead of remaining the competent, analytical person she prized, she would become an irrational creature driven by her emotions. In the course of the dialogue, Natasha was able to negotiate between the two sides of herself to come up with a compromise view of what she wanted to accomplish in therapy. She decided that she wanted to be able to honestly acknowledge her feelings without being blindly ruled by them. She recognized that both her analytic side and her feeling side were vital parts of herself and that they could work together. Natasha was subsequently able to resolve some of the more pressing issues contributing to her depression.

Socratic Questioning

Another way of addressing nonexpression stemming from negative attitudes toward emotion is through the Socratic questioning used by cognitive therapists (Beck, 1983; Person & Miranda, 1991). For instance, therapists might ask clients questions such as "What would it mean to you if you let yourself express your feelings?", "What do you fear might happen?", "How likely is this outcome?", "Is there anything you could do to make it less likely that this outcome will occur?" Socratic questioning does *not* involve trying to convince clients of the wrongness of their beliefs. Instead, the therapist's questions are aimed at helping clients to understand their expression-related beliefs and to figure out the basis of these beliefs and the consequences of adhering or not adhering to them (see Chapter 4). Explicating their beliefs in this way may prompt clients to realize that these beliefs, while once adaptive, are no longer relevant to their current circumstances. Alternatively, instead of forbidding themselves any kind of expression, clients may discover a way of expressing their feelings that is consistent with their values. For instance, they may decide to express their feelings in some situations but not others, or they may realize that it is easier for them to write about their feelings before talking about them.

After using Socratic questioning to fully articulate clients' beliefs, cognitive-behavioral therapists sometimes help clients to devise experiments to test the validity of some of the assumptions underlying their negative attitudes toward emotion. These experiments are done in a spirit of collaborative empiricism (Beck, 1983), as therapists and clients discover together, "What would happen if . . . ?" These experiments may take place in the context of the therapeutic relationship, or they may involve interactions with people outside of therapy. For example, a client who is reluctant to discuss his sexual feelings because he believes they are "sick and twisted" and would make other people see him as disgusting may decide to confide "a little bit" of these feelings to his therapist. When his therapist responds with acceptance, rather than disgust, this client has a new piece of information that contradicts his previous assumptions. This may prompt him to revise his view of his feelings and himself by becoming more self-accepting and to continue testing his assumptions by expressing more of his feelings. Similarly, a client who believes that expressing any anger toward her husband will destroy her marriage and cause her husband to abandon her may decide to assert herself with him concerning a minor irritation. If this interaction goes well, or even if it simply doesn't produce the disastrous consequences she expected, this client may begin to revise her expression-related beliefs in a way that gives her the confidence to talk to her husband about her feelings concerning more important issues.

Skill Deficits in Emotional Processing

Nonexpression can also stem from difficulties understanding one's feelings because of limited emotional processing skills. Clients' adaptive emotional expression is sometimes impeded because they lack the skills required to label and interpret their feelings. They may realize they feel "bad" but be unable to elaborate on exactly what they feel or why or to understand what these particular feelings mean to them.

Two Skills in Emotional Processing

According to experiential therapists, two key skills are involved in processing emotional experience: symbolization and reflexive self-examination (Gendlin, 1981; L. S. Greenberg et al., 1993; Mahoney, 1993, 1995; Neimeyer, 1993a; Rosen, 1996; Rogers, 1965; J. C. Watson & Greenberg, 1996a). *Symbolization* involves labeling inner subjective states by expressing them in words. It allows clients to translate their inchoate, bodily felt sense into highly differentiated and meaningful feelings. As we described in Chapter 3, symbolization both represents and creates feelings. In the process of representing their experience, clients come to understand it in ways not possible before they put their feelings into words (Lane & Schwartz, 1987; J. C. Watson & Greenberg, 1996a; J. C. Watson & Rennie, 1994). For instance, whether a client characterizes her inner experience as feeling "lost" or feeling "abandoned" carries very different implications for how she perceives herself and her environment.

The second skill involved in emotional processing is *reflexive self-examination.* This involves interpreting emotional experience by thinking through the personal implications of one's symbolized experience. Clients consider their experience in the context of past, present, and future circumstances and spell out how these feelings are related to their goals, values, needs, and desires. For instance, the client who realizes she feels "lost" could consider in what way she is lost, how long she has felt lost, what it would take for her to no longer feel lost. . . . Similarly, the client who feels "abandoned" might need to explore the roots of this feeling. She might consider what this feeling means about her perceptions of herself and others and what patterns of interaction in her current relationships contribute to this feeling. Through reflexive self-examination, clients can draw upon their feelings in order to gain new perceptions of or new responses to themselves, other people, or stressful situations.

Both emotional processing skills, symbolization and reflexive self-examination, involve an integration of the rational and experiential knowledge systems, in that they draw upon and make sense of emotional experience. Both are important for well-being. One cannot understand one's feelings unless they are clearly symbolized. However, psychotherapy process research shows that expression and symbolization of emotion are helpful only if they lead to some kind of resolution (Klein, Mathieu-Coughlan, & Kiesler, 1986; J. C. Watson, Goldman, & Greenberg, 1996). Reflexive self-examination allows clients to productively draw upon their feelings as a guide to self-understanding and adaptive coping.

An important outgrowth of symbolization and reflexive self-examination is that these skills can help clients not only to understand their feelings but also to determine how they wish to act in particular situations. As they process their emotional experience, clients become aware of their emotion-related action tendencies (e.g., wanting to run away from a fearful situation, wanting to fight back in an anger-arousing situation). Sometimes clients decide that these action tendencies are appropriate and necessary coping responses. In this case, emotional processing provides the impetus to visualize and carry through desired coping strategies. Other times, as they consider their emotion-related action tendencies in light of their personal goals and values, clients may decide that these spontaneous action tendencies would not be productive responses in their particular situation. In this case, emotional processing may help clients to choose an alternative course of action that will yield more satisfying consequences or to change their emotional experience by altering the way they construe their situation.

Two techniques that can be helpful in enhancing clients' emotional processing skills are empathic reflection and systematic evocative unfolding. We describe each of these below.

Empathic Reflections

A key way of helping clients to cultivate their emotional processing skills is through empathic reflections (Bohart & Greenberg, 1997; Burns & Nolen-Hoeksema, 1992; L. S. Greenberg & Elliott, 1997; C. Rogers, 1951, 1965; J. C. Watson, Goldman, & Vanaerschot, 1998; J. C. Watson, in press). Empathic reflections are therapist statements that attempt to distill the essence of what clients are saying and to give form to the unstated feelings or perceptions that lie immediately below the surface of clients' remarks. Empathic reflections are not simply parrot-like repetitions of clients' words. Rather, they are sophisticated attempts to uncover buried thoughts and feelings. They are conjectures concerning the subtexts of clients' inner lives.

Accurate empathic reflections ring true to clients in a deeply felt way and provide clients with access to new views and understanding of their inner experience. Clients have an inner barometer that informs them of the rightness or wrongness with which certain symbols characterize their experience. Once they discover an adequate symbol that "fits" their feelings, clients often experience a sense of relief. This frees them to explore the impact and meaning of their feelings.

In the example below, the therapist uses empathic responses in the context of a focusing exercise[1] (Gendlin, 1981; Leijssen, 1990). Focusing involves asking clients to attend to their inner experience, as it occurs in the moment, and to symbolize their experience in words or pictures. Therapists then use empathic statements, metaphors, or direct questions to help clients articulate their inner reactions.

Steve is a 25-year-old client who feels depressed. He has lost interest in his work and is experiencing difficulties in his relationship with his girlfriend. Three years ago, his brother died of cancer, and 2 years before that, his father had a fatal heart attack. In therapy, Steve reports that he has difficulty talking about his feelings because they seem vague and confusing.

THERAPIST: I wonder if we could try a focusing exercise. Close your eyes and try to tune in to what is happening inside. I want you to attend to your inner experience, can you do that?

STEVE: I will try.

THERAPIST: What are you aware of now?

STEVE: There is this empty space almost . . . I don't know, just a hole . . .

THERAPIST: Stay with that! Can you try to give it words or tell me what the hole is about?

STEVE: I feel so alone, so numb. It is as if there is no one there. Every thing is so bleak, and I can't get the energy together to do anything about it.

THERAPIST: It almost sounds as if you feel like the lone survivor of some catastrophe. I have an image of you sitting among the ruins, shocked and despairing.

STEVE: Yes, that is exactly how I feel. I feel as if I have been through so much since my father died, and then my brother's death a few years ago just laid waste to what I was trying to build.

In this dialogue, the therapist's remarks are tentative attempts to represent the client's inner experience. The remarks carry an implicit request for the client to check whether this symbolization matches his felt experience. The therapist uses vivid imagery to help Steve focus on and clarify his feelings, and Steve resonates with this imagery—it feels right to him.

A particularly potent form of empathic responding is evocative empathic responses (Rice, 1974). These are statements in which the therapist uses colorful, imagistic, and concrete language to try to bring the clients' experience alive in the session. As the following example shows, evocative empathy leads clients to open up emotionally, bringing forth new therapeutic material.

Maureen is living away from her husband while pursuing her graduate studies. In the dialogue below, Maureen talks about her annoyance following a visit by her brother on one of her weekends home. Her therapist's empathic reflections help her to become aware of her previously unacknowledged fears that her marriage will not survive this separation.

MAUREEN: I can't understand why I feel so upset and irritated by my brother's presence.

THERAPIST: Mm-hmm.

MAUREEN: It's like he is stealing something from me that I really value, something that needs to be really protected and nurtured. It's probably the time of day that I get the most out of my relationship . . . It's like there is this fragile core but it seems so vulnerable to outside influence.

THERAPIST: So somehow this time you have with your husband seems very precious . . . vital. I don't know. Am I right in getting the sense that somehow the relationship seems threatened to you, that somehow it may not survive? Without this glue or time together it may fall apart?

MAUREEN: Yeah. Yeah, I mean it's the only time . . . I guess that captures it. I haven't admitted it to myself but I'm really, really worried that the relationship won't withstand my being away. (*now quietly sobbing*) That's the only time we have to keep it going.

Two important points should be emphasized about this dialogue: First, the therapist's empathic reflections prompt a marked shift in Maureen's emotional understanding. She moves from an intellectual, almost legalistic focus on her brother's transgression to a vivid comprehension of her unrecognized fears. Second, the therapist's empathic reflections are offered in a tentative way. Therapists can make conjectures, but clients are the final authority on their own inner experience. Only clients can tell whether therapists' empathic reflections accurately elucidate their feelings. In this case, Maureen's tears and her direct statements attest to the validity of the therapist's reflections.

Systematic Evocative Unfolding

Another technique that can enhance clients' emotional processing skills is systematic evocative unfolding (Rice & Saperia, 1984). This technique is particularly useful when clients report being puzzled by their emotional reactions. It involves asking clients to vividly describe the scene or situation in which they experienced the feelings so as to evoke their emotional responses during the therapy session. Describing their experience in this way helps clients to identify the triggers to their reactions and gives them the opportunity to label and interpret their feelings. The therapist encourages clients to bring an emotional scene alive, using concrete, image-laden, and evocative language. Clients are asked "to play a mental movie of the scene" in order to conjure up a sufficiently vivid memory so that clients can reexperience and thereby reexamine their feelings.

The following dialogue illustrates how this might be done. Susan is a competent, independent college student who unexpectedly experienced a panic attack during a thunderstorm. Her therapist asks her to recall that evening.

SUSAN: I was alone at home, quietly reading. I think I was preparing for an exam and had taken a break.

THERAPIST: So, there you were alone at home. Do you recall which room you were in?

SUSAN: Uh-huh. I had gone into the kitchen to get a drink and I think it was as I reached up to take a glass out of the cupboard that I heard the first thunder roll. I recall being startled and then remembering to check the windows . . . So, I went into the bedroom and living room to see if any needed fastening. Then I went back to my bedroom and lay down with the book I was reading.

THERAPIST: OK, so there you are, lying on the bed, and it's growing dark and threatening outside. You can hear the storm building, and . . . I'm not sure how you are feeling at that point.

SUSAN: OK, I was kind of looking forward to an evening alone. My mom was out and I wanted to relax. But after I picked up my book, I began to become aware of the storm. The lightning was cracking and the thunder was very loud. I began to feel a little anxious . . .

THERAPIST: So, somehow the loudness of it all began to disturb you?

SUSAN: No, it wasn't that so much as I began to be aware of a door banging. That sound really got me going . . . Something about it was so disturbing, I began to feel scared.

THERAPIST: So there was just something about the banging that somehow left you . . . what? Vulnerable?

SUSAN: I guess so. I never really thought of that, but that reminds me of last year when I was visiting a friend out west, I got caught up in a storm on Vancouver Island. I remember feeling so vulnerable that whole time, because I had no way of reaching my family.

Susan then goes on to examine how vulnerable she feels in her current family situation. Her mother is an alcoholic and very reliant on Susan for support. Susan had begun to feel weighed down by her mother's concerns and dependence, but she did not know how to initiate any changes in this relationship. In this dialogue, she begins to process her feelings of anxiety and vulnerability as a precursor to being able to separate emotionally from her mother. She moves from a sense of being taken over by an alien sense of incomprehensible panic to a more targeted and personal understanding of her fears concerning separation. Susan's incomprehensible panic did not suggest any viable coping responses for her. This panic seemed to come out of nowhere. After articulating a more specific understanding of her feelings, Susan was able to deal directly with the issues that troubled her.

Motivated Lack of Awareness of Emotional Responses

The most difficult type of nonexpression to address clinically involves problems in perceiving one's feelings due to motivated lack of awareness of emotional responses. With the other two forms of nonexpression that we discussed, clients are aware of their feelings but have difficulty accepting or understanding them. In this case, clients are not consciously aware of their feelings, because these feelings are so profoundly threatening to them. Although all interventions require a good therapeutic alliance, a strong alliance is critically important when dealing with problems involving a motivated lack of awareness of emotional responses. Clients need to feel safe in order to stop hiding from their threatening feelings. Once clients have articulated their blocked feelings, they have the opportunity to revise their perceptions of these feelings. They may come to see their feelings as painful but bearable, and therefore have less need to avoid them (see Chapter 2).

Numerous therapeutic techniques can be used to help clients become aware of their feelings. We describe two of them: recognizing signs of emotional blocking and drawing attention to clients' nonverbal signs of emotion.

Recognizing Signs of Emotional Blocking

One way of helping clients to become aware of the unacknowledged feelings is to help them to recognize their signs of emotional blocking (see Chapter 3). For instance, clients might quickly bypass talking about very emotional material to focus on less threatening topics, or they might suddenly "freeze up" while discussing certain feelings. Rhythmic, "chatty" speech, which makes clients sound like newscasters reporting well-rehearsed material, can also be a sign of emotional blocking (Rice, Koke, Greenberg, & Wagstaff, 1979).

Therapists need to be very gentle when approaching clients' signs of emotional blocking. Observations of possible blocking behaviors should be made in the context of a question rather than a criticism. Therapists can point out the behavior and inquire about what is happening for clients at that moment. Sometimes, when the blocked feelings are especially threatening, having a therapist point out the blocking behavior is extremely anxiety-provoking for clients. In these cases, it is imperative that therapists *not* push clients to express their blocked feelings. Instead, therapists should help clients to simply acknowledge the block and perhaps explore what this block is like for them and what it means to them.

A 50-year-old client named Maisy frequently blocked her feelings from awareness by talking rapidly, almost cheerfully, about many different topics. She barely paused for breath, and her therapist had difficulty following the rapid topic changes. Her therapist commented about this, noting that although Maisy was not moving in her seat, her therapist experienced her as constantly in motion. This remark prompted Maisy to describe her emotional block as a brick wall, sealing off dangerous feelings, that she constantly needed to fortify. She said that she knew there was something large behind the wall that could consume her, but she didn't know what it was, and she didn't want to look at it. Her therapist empathized with her terror at these unknown feelings and her desperate need to keep the wall in place. She offered some reassurance, saying that when and if Maisy decided she wanted to look at these feelings, the therapist would help. She also suggested that these feelings might seem less frightening in the light of day than they did hidden behind that wall. However, the therapist emphasized that it was up to Maisy to decide what she wanted to address in therapy and whether she was ready to deal with these feelings.

For many sessions, Maisy skirted around these feelings, although she was able to acknowledge the emotional block when it came up and even to talk about some of the ways that she kept her dangerous feelings walled off. Then one day, instead of changing the topic when she came across her emotional block, Maisy paused and then slowly recounted how, over 30 years ago, after a series of devastating personal losses, including the death of her child, and abandonment by her husband, she had "gone into shock" and been institutionalized in a state mental hospital. She described being locked in a room by herself for a long period of time. She said she wasn't sure how she got out of this institution, but she thought that her brother might have had something to do with her eventual release. Although she had had no relapses in the intervening decades, Maisy lived in fear that her "secret craziness" would one day reemerge and she would again be institutionalized. In all these years, she had spoken to no one about her experiences or her fears, and she had done her best not to think about it herself. She equated any feelings of helplessness or sadness with her "secret craziness" and said it was easier for her to feel nothing.

In this example, because the therapist helped the client to recognize her emotional blocking without pushing her to go beyond it, the client was eventually able to begin dealing with some of her unacknowledged feelings. In other cases, having therapists point out the blocking behavior prompts clients to look more carefully inward to draw out their experience. The next example describes a client who learned to see his emotional blocking as a cue to focus on and become aware of his emotional experience.

Mica was a 27-year-old client who found it difficult to stay with his subjective experience during therapy sessions. When emotional topics came up, he described "going blank." Once, while recalling a violent argument between his parents that took place when he was a child, he suddenly stopped talking and stared at the wall. When his therapist asked what was going on for him at that moment, Mica replied that he had gone blank and didn't know what he wanted to say. His therapist asked him to stay with what was happening for him. Mica observed that he was fascinated by a particular painting that hung on the wall and was curious about its content. When his therapist asked what he had been feeling just prior to becoming entranced by the painting, Mica acknowledged that he had begun to feel anxious while talking about his parents' argument. He realized that he often turned to intellectual pursuits to calm himself. After recognizing this emotional blocking, he was able to move past it, to begin to acknowledge the feelings that his parents' conflict elicited in him. For this client, an important therapeutic goal was to help him become aware of his feelings rather than tuning them out.

Drawing Attention to Clients' Nonverbal Signs of Emotion

Another way of helping clients become aware of their emotional responses is to draw their attention to their nonverbal signs of emotion. Because of expressive leakage, once affective responses are elicited, some signs of that response tend to "leak" out, even without conscious awareness or intent (see Chapters 1 and 3). This is particularly the case with strong emotional reactions. Helping clients notice their nonverbal signs of emotion can prompt them to become aware of previously unacknowledged feelings. For instance, therapists might comment on a client's furrowed brow, tapping fingers, clenched fist, or swinging foot. The therapist can ask clients to exaggerate the relevant expressive sign and to give words to that behavior, so that clients can begin to have a sense of their inner experience (Polster & Polster, 1973; Yontef, 1991, 1995; Yontef & Simkin, 1989).

Physiological signs of arousal can be drawn upon in a similar way to enhance emotional awareness. For instance, while talking about highly emotional material, one client insisted that he felt "fine." However, his chest, neck, and face had turned bright red. His therapist pointed out that he was flushed and commented, "Your words say you are feeling fine, but your body seems to be saying something different." On this and subsequent occasions, the client was able to use his flushing as a sign that he was experiencing "something" emotional and to try to perceive and articulate what those feelings were. Other clients might use different physiological cues such as sweaty palms, tense shoulders, a dry mouth, or a racing heart as signs of unacknowledged feelings.

Clients' vocal quality can also provide clues concerning unacknowledged feelings:

Moira, a manager in her mid-30s, often felt disempowered at work. She complained that her colleagues did not take her seriously, and she despaired of ever being promoted. In therapy, she had difficulty attending to her own inner experience, but she was able to describe the events in her life in great detail. Her therapist's attempts to have her turn her attention inward and articulate her feelings were unsuccessful. Other than a general dissatisfaction with how others treated her, Moira was not able to discern any of her feelings.

One day, Moira's therapist remarked on the fact that Moira sometimes spoke in a high-pitched, girlish voice. The therapist urged Moira to exaggerate the girlish quality of her voice for a few moments, so that she would be more aware of it. After doing so, Moira made a connection between this girlish voice and her desire, as a child, to appease her brutal father by appearing weak, fragile, and nonthreatening.

After this session, Moira began to pay more attention to how she spoke when she was at work. She realized that she often used a girlish voice around her male colleagues and that this voice was a sign that she felt frightened. With the help of her therapist, Moira was able to articulate her fear that if she did not placate men and let them feel superior to her, they would retaliate and hurt her somehow. Moira also observed that her girlish voice sounded flaky and inept. She realized that her previously unacknowledged fears were causing her to undermine herself at work, by squashing her strength and initiative. With this new understanding of her feelings and their meaning and implications, Moira was able to cope more directly with her fears and to adopt a more confident and competent stance at work.

Summary

In this section, we described clinical approaches to three different forms of nonexpression, involving difficulties in accepting one's feelings due to negative attitudes toward emotion, difficulties in understanding one's feelings due to limited emotional processing skills, and difficulties in perceiving one's emotional experience due to motivated lack of awareness of emotional responses. In all three of these cases, the general therapeutic approach involves helping clients to recognize and give voice to their experiential knowledge system, which had been stifled by their rational knowledge system. The goal is to help clients achieve an integration of their experiential and rational systems. The specific techniques we described for each form of nonexpression differ because each form entails a different level of disruption in the process of emotional expression.

For conceptual clarity, we discussed these three forms of nonexpression separately. However, they can co-occur. For instance, people who maintain a conscious negative attitude toward emotion may have had little practice processing their emotional experience and therefore be less skilled at doing so. Over time, negative attitudes and limited processing skills may crystallize into motivated lack of awareness of emotional experience, as clients come to see feelings that they don't like and don't understand as unbearably threatening to acknowledge (Weinberger, 1990). This means that a particular client may benefit from multiple interventions aimed at multiple levels of nonexpression.

ADDRESSING PROBLEMS INVOLVING EXPRESSION

As we mentioned at the beginning of this chapter, as well as in previous chapters, clinical difficulties can arise not only from nonexpression but also from maladaptive forms of expression. Maladaptive forms of expression occur when the experiential system swamps the cognitive system, so that steps in the process of emotional expression are circumvented. Problems involving expression often create interpersonal difficulties. For adaptive functioning, clients not only have to know what they feel, they also have to know how to communicate their feelings to others in a way that accomplishes their interpersonal goals.

In this section, we describe two types of problems involving expression—flooded expression and ambiguous expression—and offer some suggestions concerning how they might be addressed therapeutically.

Flooded Expression

Flooded expression occurs when clients have such intense levels of emotional experience and arousal that their feelings seem to burst out of them with little control and minimal cognitive processing (see Chapter 2). At high levels of emotional arousal, people can't think straight (D. G. Gilbert, 1991; Gottman, 1993b). They are so swamped by their feelings that they can't organize their thoughts, can't communicate clearly, can't process new information, and can't consider another person's point of view. Their behavior tends to be impulsive and extreme.

The primary therapeutic task for clients with difficulties involving flooded expression is to contain their feelings sufficiently so that they can engage in rational processing aimed at differentiating and evaluating their feelings and emotional behavior. Just as being completely cut off from one's feelings impairs functioning, the opposite extreme of being completely dominated by one's feelings is also maladaptive. Therapists need to help these clients achieve an optimal psychological distance from their emotional experience so that they can draw upon these feelings without being driven blindly by them (Rice et al., 1979; Scheff, 1979).

For some clients, flooded expression causes intrapersonal difficulties. They may feel frightened by what they perceive as their uncontrollable waves of expression and may see these as a sign that something is wrong with them (Thoits, 1985). An experiential technique that can be useful in these circumstances involves providing the client with a persona to act as an alter ego (Hudgins, 1998). For example, a bereaved client who is distressed by his unpredictable bouts of intense sobbing might find it useful to visualize an alter ego in the form of a strong and benevolent self. This alter ego can offer the client support and encouragement and provide some psychological distance from the bereavement-related feelings and events that the client is grappling with in therapy. Grounding techniques (Briere, 1989; McCann & Pearlman, 1990), which focus clients' attention on concrete details in the here and now, can also be useful when clients feel overwhelmed by their feelings (see Chapter 10).

For other clients, flooded expression causes primarily interpersonal problems. For example, a client who flies into uncontrolled rages may find that his work performance suffers because his colleagues don't want to interact with him, and his marriage suffers because his wife feels abused by his scathing tirades that erupt following even the most minor frustrations. In this case, a two-pronged approach involving arousal regulation and communication skills training may be helpful.

Arousal regulation skills enable clients to lessen the intensity of their emotional responses so that they are capable of cognitive processing and inhibiting maladaptive expression. Specific techniques to foster arousal regulation include relaxation training, devising cognitive self-statements aimed at deescalating emotional responses, and implementing self-soothing techniques (e.g., Bandura, 1977; Borkovec & Costello, 1993; Deffenbacher, 1994; Goldfried, De Canteceo, & Weinberg, 1974; J. C. Watson et al., 1998; Zeiss, Lewinsohn, & Muñoz, 1979; Zillmann, 1993). For example, a therapist might help a client to recognize the early signs that he is starting to become enraged and to use these signs as a cue to begin deep breathing exercises or to think about calming statements that, in his own words, encourage him to control his rage (e.g., "It's not worth getting worked up over this," "It's my choice whether I let this get to me," "My rages hurt me more than other people," or "I kept my head last week. I can do it again today"). Another important arousal regulation technique is active listening. Concentrating on understanding what another person is saying helps people to step out of their own emotional frame of reference and reduces physiological arousal (D. G. Gilbert, 1991).

In communication skills training, therapists help clients to learn to express their feelings in assertive rather than aggressive ways. They teach clients to talk about their feelings in the context of specific incidents rather than global judgments and to acknowledge responsibility for their own feelings rather than blaming their feelings on other people. The general goal is to help clients express their feelings in a way that is more likely to be heard and responded to positively by others, rather than evoking hostile or defensive reactions.

Cognitive-behavioral therapists emphasize that arousal regulation and effective communication are skills that are acquired through practice. It is not enough for clients to have a general idea of what they ought to do to manage flooded expression, they need to actually try implementing these skills often enough that they feel comfortable using them. These two sets of skills complement each other: Arousal regulation skills are necessary for using communication skills. If clients can't control the intensity of their emotional responses then they won't want to or won't be able to express their feelings to others in adaptive ways (Gottman, 1993b; Jacobson & Holtzworth-Monroe, 1986). Conversely, unless clients can communicate their feelings effectively, they will not be able to resolve interpersonal difficulties, and their arousal regulation abilities will be taxed excessively.

Ambiguous Expression

In addition to flooded expression, another type of maladaptive expression involves ambiguous expression. Ambiguous expression can take a variety of forms, such as too subtle expression, mixed signals, expression that the sender is not aware of, or expression that creates an unintended impression (Noller, 1984). The key characteristic of all of these instances of ambiguous expression is that the client is not able to convey the desired emotional message to others. Often, anxiety and poor social skills are at the root of ambiguous expression. These clients are so preoccupied with their own emotional responses that they are not able to anticipate or accurately perceive how others respond to their emotional communication.

One way of approaching problems involving ambiguous expression is to help clients to understand their feelings more clearly, using the techniques we described earlier when we talked about enhancing emotional processing skills. When clients can accurately label and interpret their feelings, they are better able to communicate these feelings clearly to others and less likely to have poorly understood feelings leak out in socially detrimental ways.

Another approach to ambiguous expression focuses more directly on the interpersonal impact of expression by (1) providing clients with feedback concerning how their expressive behavior is coming across to others, (2) comparing these observations to clients' intended emotional message, and (3) providing clients with practice in expressing themselves clearly. Sometimes clients' friends or family members are available to come in for therapy and provide clients with feedback regarding the impact of their ambiguous expression. For instance, in marital therapy, partners can reflect clients' expressions ("What I hear you saying is . . . ") or communicate about how clients' emotional behavior makes them feel ("When you say that, I feel . . . "). When significant others are not available to come in for therapy, the therapist can be a source of feedback about clients' interpersonal impact. Having clients role-play another person's part as well as their own can also be a means of helping them understand the impact of their expression on others. Moreover, in-session role play can be helpful in providing clients with practice in expressing their feelings clearly.

Andrew was a young man in his mid-20s who was distressed by his inability to develop a romantic relationship with a woman. He feared that there was something fundamentally wrong with him because he had never had anything approaching a serious relationship with a woman. He said he didn't know what this personal flaw might be, but he thought that women were able to intuitively sense it and therefore got scared off by him. Andrew was very bright in a scientific way, but he seemed bewildered by social interactions. He was highly motivated to find out what was "wrong" with him.

Andrew's therapist asked him to observe and remember specific examples of what happened when he tried approaching women. The next session, Andrew returned with copious notes describing several instances of him approaching women in blow-by-blow detail. In each of these examples, Andrew had expressed interest in the women by making sarcastic comments.

Andrew's therapist asked him to role-play a scenario of how he wished a first interaction with a woman would proceed. She asked Andrew to play both his own part and the woman's part. Playing himself, Andrew seemed extremely nervous but attempted to cover this nervousness with caustic remarks that he intended to be amusing, but that the therapist suspected might intimidate or annoy the young women he hoped to impress. He was at a complete loss trying to imagine how the woman might respond.

Andrew's therapist suggested that he might be shooting himself in the foot by trying too hard to come across as witty in a first encounter. She asked him to try the role play again, expressing his interest in the imaginary woman merely by being pleasant. This time, the dialogue proceeded more easily. Andrew made some polite comments as himself and was able to enact similarly polite responses as the woman. When the therapist asked how he felt during this role play, Andrew said that as the woman he felt mildly positive, and as himself he felt pleased that the interaction was going more smoothly but frustrated about not knowing when or how the interaction was going to "get off small talk and get serious."

Subsequent work with Andrew involved more role play and in vivo practice expressing his interest in women in positive ways. This enabled Andrew to become more relaxed and comfortable in these interactions. It helped him to focus on enjoying a woman's company in the moment and paying attention to what she said and how she felt rather than trying to be an instant "success" at "getting" a woman.

Summary

To summarize, the two examples we discussed of maladaptive expression involve instances in which the experiential system swamps the cognitive system, so that clients' expression involves an unintended leakage of poorly understood feelings. Therapeutic strategies for maladaptive expression involve efforts to help clients contain their emotional experience and cognitively process it, considering the meaning of these feelings for themselves and the impact of their expression on others.

CONCLUSION

In this chapter, we presented an overview of therapeutic approaches related to emotional behavior. We argued that adaptive expression involves an integration of cognitive and experiential information-processing systems. Positive outcomes of adaptive expression include self-understanding, self-acceptance, and effective communication with others. We described a number of different problems involving nonexpression and expression that occur when the process of emotional expression is blocked or circumvented, and we outlined clinical strategies for fostering adaptive expression.

Psychotherapy provides a unique and valuable context for fostering adaptive expression. Therapists' accepting, containing stance can lessen clients' fears of being overwhelmed by expression or eliciting rejection. Therapists can support and extend clients' abilities to understand their emotional experience by helping clients to articulate their feelings. Therapists can draw on observations of clients' subtle expressive cues to enhance clients' awareness of their emotional responses. Through modeling and in-session practice, therapists can help clients learn new and more effective ways of communicating their feelings. They can also provide feedback to clients, in a supportive way, concerning possible reactions of others to clients' use of particular forms or styles of emotional expression.

In the next four chapters, we describe how these general therapeutic strategies related to emotional behavior can be used in the context of particular clinical difficulties. Specifically, we look at the role of emotional behavior in depression, trauma, marital distress, and health-related problems. These clinical difficulties encompass problems involving nonexpression, problems involving expression, and vacillation between the two.

NOTE

1. The therapeutic dialogues in Chapters 8–10 have been modified for clarity, confidentiality, and readability.

9

Beyond Sadness:
Therapeutic Approaches
to Emotional Constriction
in Depression

INTRODUCTION

Rosa knocks on her roommate's bedroom door. "Deborah, can I come in?" she calls.

"It's unlocked," Deborah answers listlessly.

Rosa opens the door and tentatively pokes her head in. The room smells stuffy. The blinds are half drawn. The bed is unmade. There are piles of clothes on the floor. Deborah is sprawled sideways in an easy chair. Although it is early evening, she is dressed in her bathrobe and her hair is unbrushed. There are some magazines on her lap, but she is not reading them. She is staring out the window. "A bunch of us are going out for pizza. Do you want to come?" Rosa offers.

"No thanks," Deborah answers without turning around.

Rosa looks concerned. Hesitantly, she asks, "How are you doing?"

"OK," she replies with a deep sigh.

"You can't just sit here all the time, Deb. It would do you good to get out."

"I know," Deborah replies. "I just don't feel like it."

Looking worried and frustrated, Rosa stares at her roommate's profile for a moment then turns to leave. "Well, if you change your mind, we'll be at Gino's." Deborah doesn't answer.

In this vignette, Deborah is clearly depressed. Her listlessness, unkempt appearance, and messy room suggest that even minor chores are beyond her coping abilities right now. What can we say about Deborah's emotional behavior? On the one hand, she is very expressive of her misery. Her sighs, her lethargy, her lack of eye contact, and her short utterances are all behaviors that communicate her dysphoria. On the other hand, Deborah's expression is very passive and poorly differentiated. We know she is feeling miserable, but we have no idea whether her misery involves feeling disillusioned, or rejected, or inadequate, or helpless, or any number of other possibilities. She shows absolutely no sign of any positive feelings, such as curiosity or enthusiasm.

Interpersonally, Deborah's emotional expression keeps her isolated. Deborah is unable to respond to her roommate's invitation or to communicate her needs. Rosa seems concerned but also unsure of how to respond to Deborah and somewhat frustrated that her efforts to be helpful have no effect.

In this chapter, we focus on the role of emotional behavior in depression and how it can be addressed therapeutically. We then look at clinical strategies concerning expression and depression. These strategies help depressed clients move beyond passive and diffuse expressions of sadness toward more focused, positive, and emotional behavior that reflects their sense of urgency. Specifically, we describe therapeutic ways of processing depressed feelings, cultivating agentic feelings, and modifying maladaptive interpersonal patterns of expression.

PROCESSING DEPRESSED FEELINGS

Signs of sadness and despair pervade the emotional communication of depressed people (Segrin, 1998). They speak slowly and softly. Their faces are not animated. Their posture and gestures seem listless and uninvolved with their social context, and the content of their speech is usually negative. Depressed people are preoccupied with their distress, but their descriptions of both their inner experience and external events tend to be global and fuzzy (L. S. Greenberg, Watson, & Goldman, 1998). It is as if they are in a fog of depressive pain, that makes it difficult for them to clearly perceive either their own emotional responses or the environmental circumstances surrounding their responses. Deborah's passive sighs and mutters are a sign of her depressed feelings, not a way of working through them. She is mired in a chronic haze of dysphoria.

One key function of emotional expression in the treatment of depressed clients is to facilitate processing of depressed feelings. In virtually every therapeutic orientation, the first step in treating depressed clients involves allowing them to express their feelings in an environment where they can feel safe and accepted. This expression is essential for establishing a therapeutic alliance. Depressed clients need to know that their therapist has heard and understood their feelings in an empathic way in order to develop a sense of trust in the therapeutic relationship (Barrett-Lennard, 1997; Bohart & Greenberg, 1997; Linehan, 1997). Having the receptive ear of their therapist is especially important given that expression of depressed feelings tends to elicit rejection in everyday life (Segrin, 1998). For some depressed clients, just being able to confide their feelings and have those feelings validated can bring a sense of relief.

However, therapeutic expression of depressed feelings is very different from the kind of passive, perseverative expression that depressed people show in their day-to-day interactions. Therapists can help clients to be more focused as they describe their emotional reactions, so that clients can label their responses more accurately and perceive the impact of events more clearly. The general goal in having clients talk about their depressed feelings is to give them an opportunity to symbolize and differentiate their emotional experience. Therapists need to encourage depressed clients to express their feelings in active and specific ways, in order to process that experience and draw upon it as a guide for self-understanding and adaptive coping.

By representing their depressed feelings in words, clients come to know and perceive their emotional experience in new ways. Attending to clients' idiosyncratic language as they describe their feelings can help draw out the meaning or implications of those feelings. For instance, clients might report feeling "raw," "wounded," or "beaten down." As we described in Chapter 3, putting feelings into words fosters emotional insight by labeling those feelings, structuring them, and actively constructing their meaning (Lane & Schwartz, 1987; Meichenbaum, 1990; Pennebaker, 1993b; J. C. Watson & Greenberg, 1996a; J. C. Watson & Rennie, 1994). Giving form to their depressed feelings in this way can enable clients to perceive these feelings as less overwhelming. Their depressed feelings become objectified, scaled down, and less diffuse, and therefore seem more manageable (Watson & Rennie, 1994).

Three expression-related techniques that can be useful for processing depressed feelings are systematic evocative unfolding, metaphor, and identification of critical self-statements (Arnkoff & Glass, 1992; Beck et al., 1979; L. S. Greenberg et al., 1993, 1998; Hollon, Shelton, & Loosen, 1991; Mahoney, 1993; Rice & Saperia, 1984; Safran & Segal, 1990). These techniques, which we describe below, are means of accessing depressed feelings in focused ways that allow clients to clarify their emotional responses and anchor their feelings to specific events, times, or perceptions.

Systematic Evocative Unfolding

Systematic evocative unfolding (Rice, 1974; Rice & Saperia, 1984) involves asking clients to describe certain events in detail, while the therapist helps them to track their emotional responses at the time. In order to make the events more vivid and to help clients access their inner subjective state, therapists can use colorful, imagistic language to highlight aspects of clients' experiences. This helps clients to get a clearer sense of their emotional reactions in the moment and the impact of various events.

For example, Miriam, a 35-year-old woman who had recently had a child, sought treatment because she was depressed. She mentioned it was often tense at home, but she did not understand why she felt so despondent. Her therapist asked her to tell her what was going on in her life.

MIRIAM: Nothing much, basically I am at home with Joshua. I usually go for a walk with him in the afternoon, and then I try to get things done around the house. Yesterday was more difficult though and Joe was irritable.

THERAPIST: Can you tell me more about this? It would help if you could almost play me a movie of the scene so that I can get a good feel for it.

MIRIAM: It was when he got home from work, the baby had had a difficult day. He had been crying most of the afternoon, so I had not had a chance to get supper ready. Then when Joe got home he was irritable.

THERAPIST: OK. So, it had been a difficult day for you. I am not sure . . . You were cooped up, alone with Joshua who was squalling and hard to comfort? I guess you must have felt pretty wrung out . . . exhausted by the end of the day?

MIRIAM: Yes! I was exhausted because he had been up during the night, too. I feel as if I am in a fog these days. I am getting so little sleep.

THERAPIST: So, there you are, sleep-deprived, lost in a fog, waiting impatiently for Joe to come home to give you some relief. Then he arrives. What happens?

MIRIAM: Well, I guess I was hoping he would take Joshua for a while and let me have a nap. But he seemed grumpy, so I didn't want to trouble him.

THERAPIST: So there was no relief, no escape for you after he got home. How did you know he was grumpy? What did he do? Did he talk gruffly to you, snap at you, or was there some other indication that he was feeling miserable?

MIRIAM: Oh, I don't know . . . I guess his brow was furrowed and when I said "Hi" he didn't reply. He just walked off into the family room . . .

THERAPIST: What was that like for you? There you are impatiently waiting for some relief, and when Joe arrives he is silent and gruff.

MIRIAM: It made me feel tense . . . I just shrink up inside . . . I so wanted to ask him for help . . . I guess it makes me feel very alone.

In this example, the therapist helps the client process the events of her life more slowly. The therapist uses concrete language and tries to get a vivid sense of what occurred between Miriam and her husband. As they continue to explore her interaction, Miriam observes that she often suppresses her feelings when Joe appears grumpy. She realizes how alone and vulnerable she feels in the marriage. As they process her feelings, Miriam begins to get a better sense of her own needs and a better understanding of what was contributing to her depression.

Highlighting the specific situational context of clients' feelings can help clients to feel more in control of their emotional responses. Depressed clients often have difficulty identifying the antecedents of their emotional experience. This makes them feel like victims of their moods. Therapists can help depressed clients to articulate their feelings while recognizing the situational context of those feelings. This enables clients to see links between their depressive moods and external circumstances, to clarify their needs and desires, and to effectively target problem-solving efforts. For instance, instead of having a diffuse sense of general misery, exploring their situationally specific emotional responses might lead clients to realize that they felt pressured by a spouse under these circumstances or disappointed by a friend in that situation. This more specific understanding of their emotional responses enables clients to spell out the personal significance of these events and to explore alternative ways of coping with these situations. In Miriam's case, recognizing that she felt alone, exhausted, and unsupported prompted her to get outside help and ask her mother to relieve her for a few hours during the week, so she could nap.

Metaphor

In addition to systematic evocative unfolding, therapists can use metaphors to help clients process their depressed feelings. Metaphors heighten clients' access to their inner experience and emphasize the subjective, temporally specific nature of their distress (Angus & Rennie, 1988; Carlsen, 1996; J. C. Watson & Greenberg, 1996a). For instance, a therapist might reflect a client's despair by saying, "It seems that the world is a bleak, cold place to be right now." This response not only clarifies and communicates empathy for the client's current experience, it also implicitly suggests that this is only one view of the world and that this view might change in the future.

Identification of Critical Self-Statements

A final expression-related technique for processing depressed feeling involves identification or critical self-statements. As clients express their feelings in clear and specific ways, they may be able to access core cognitions or critical introjects underlying these feelings (Beck, 1983; L. S. Greenberg et al., 1993). These are negative self-statements that incapacitate clients and compound their feelings of depression. Examples of these kinds of self-statements might be "I mustn't express my own feelings or needs or I will hurt other people" or "No one would like me if they really knew me." Usually such thoughts operate automatically, outside of conscious awareness, but when clients are vividly in touch with their feelings, they may be able to articulate these thoughts. Articulating such thoughts is a necessary step in order to recognize the impact of these thoughts and to modify them. Process–experiential therapists usually focus on helping clients to negotiate a compromise between the critical side of themselves—the one that wants to silence and restrict them—and the experiential side; the one that gives voice to clients' needs and wants (see later discussion on assertiveness). Cognitive-behavioral therapists help clients to modify their negative self-statements by encouraging clients to come up with counterarguments to these critical and restrictive beliefs and to seek out experiences that contradict these negative beliefs.

So far, we have talked about the role of emotional expression in processing depressed feelings. We have suggested that helping clients to actively express their depressed feelings in a clear, differentiated manner, tying these feelings to specific situations, times, and underlying beliefs, can enhance clients' self-understanding and coping abilities. However, this is not the only way in which emotional expression can be useful in the treatment of depression.

CULTIVATING POSITIVE AND AGENTIC FEELINGS

Depressed clients are cut off from the full range of their emotional experience. They are unaware of anything but the pain of their depression. Deborah, in the anecdote at the beginning of this chapter, is silently drowning in misery. She shows no signs of interest in going out with friends, reading her magazines, or even taking care of herself.

Thus, in addition to processing depressed feelings, another important task in working with depressed clients is to increase the range of their emotional responses by cultivating positive and agentic feelings (P. Gilbert, 1991). Specific expression-related strategies that can be used to access agentic feelings include empty-chair work, two-chair work, attending to positive feelings, and scheduling and discussing pleasant events.

Empty-Chair Work

Experiential therapists often use empty-chair work to expand depressed clients' emotional repertoire (L. S. Greenberg et al., 1993). This technique involves having clients imagine that an important person in their lives is present in the therapy session and then talking to that person and for that person. Empty-chair work is a very effective means of helping clients to get in touch with their feelings and reactions to others because it allows clients to visualize and represent the other person in a vivid and concrete way. Sometimes it is not the words that people use that convey their attitudes but rather their nonverbal behaviors. For example, it may be the toss of the head or the movement of the wrist that conveys the other person's contempt, thereby triggering the client's feelings of resentment. Furthermore, playing the role of the other person can help clients to decenter from their own immediate experience, widening their view of reality and expanding their emotional range (L. S. Greenberg & Watson, 1998; R. L. Greenberg, 1993; Nix et al., 1995; Sommers, 1981; J. C. Watson, 1997).

Empty-chair work can help foster feelings of self-acceptance. Consider the following example:

> Doug was a depressed client whose feelings of worthlessness were linked to his perceptions that his mother neglected him when he was a child and did not want to bother with him. His therapist encouraged him to imagine his mother in an empty chair. In vividly presenting his mother's account, Doug realized that she was exhausted from caring for six children under dire financial straits with no help from her husband or her extended family. She always worried that they would not have enough to eat. After expressing his sadness at not having felt his mother's love, Doug imagined his mother replying that she loved him dearly and just wished she could have provided more for them.

Even if Doug's representation of his mother is not completely accurate, imagining a nurturing response to his distress can act as an antidote to his view of himself as worthless. It can create positive feelings of acceptance or compassion for himself.

Empty-chair work can also be a means of accessing angry feelings. What we are talking about here is not the diffuse hostility that depressed people often express in their close relationships (Florin, Nostadt, Reck, Franzen, & Jenkins, 1992; Segrin, 1998), but rather a more targeted and empowering feeling that clients can drawn upon to counter the passivity of depression. For instance, abused clients might use empty-chair work to express their anger at the abuser. They might assert that they did not deserve to be treated in so uncaring a fashion (Elliott et al., 1996; L. S. Greenberg & Paivio, 1998). They can hold the abuser accountable for the abuse, thereby diminishing their own sense of responsibility as the recipient of abuse. Because the abuser is not actually present, clients can script the encounter the way they want, fostering a sense of control and agency.

In the following example Bill, a 25-year-old engineer, came to therapy because he was feeling depressed. He told the therapist that he hadn't spoken to his mother or brother for almost a year. He also revealed that his father had left the family and severed all contact with them when Bill was 11. The therapist observed that Bill expressed a lot of sadness and resentment at his father, so she suggested an empty-chair exercise.

THERAPIST: I wonder if you can imagine your father in this chair. What does he look like? Is he tall? Heavy?

BILL: He was a big man, slightly overweight. He had a beard . . . brown hair and blue eyes.

THERAPIST: What is the expression on his face? Is he smiling or does he look stern?

BILL: He is frowning . . . uhmm . . . his expression is sort of contemptuous.

THERAPIST: So he looks contemptuously at you. Can you tell him how you feel at his leaving? Can you tell him how that made you feel?

BILL: This is hard . . . I feel so nervous imagining him there not caring . . . I don't know what to say.

THERAPIST: What about "You let us down, Dad . . . "?

BILL: Yeah! You did. It was hard for me when you left. You just didn't seem to care what became of us . . . Mom, Nick, and I. Mom had to struggle to make ends meet . . . She was always tired. I used to worry so much about her. You were so selfish, and even when you were around you always used to criticize Nick and me, and you would play us against each other. I guess that is why we don't get along now.

During this dialogue, Bill was able to express his long-buried feelings to his dad. He recalled how he had always been terrified of him as a boy. As he expressed his anger and disappointment to his dad, he noted that his dad seemed to shrink. Instead of the bully he recalled from childhood, Bill saw his dad as a weak, selfish person. He resolved to get in touch with his mother and brother and to repair the breaks in their relationships.

Two-Chair Work to Resolve Depressive Splits

Another expression-related technique for cultivating positive and agentic feelings is two-chair work aimed at resolving depressive splits. Clients who are depressed often talk about the conflict between wanting to do things and feeling too tired or unable to get started. It can be helpful to engage clients in a dialogue between the part of themselves that feels discouraged and hopeless and the part that would like to get moving and start participating in life again. In this dialogue, it is especially important to access the feelings of the side of the self that is fighting the depression. Clients often describe this counterdepression side of themselves as feeling very vulnerable and at risk. For example, in speaking for this side, clients often say things like "I feel as if I am dying, that I am just going to fade away." They may enact the counterdepression side pleading with the depressed side to start living again and to become more engaged with life. Initially, the depressed side may not be able to respond except with exhaustion and tiredness. Moreover, the depressed side is often fed up with being exhorted and pushed to accomplish things. However, as it listens to the pain expressed by the other side, usually the two sides can begin to negotiate a compromise that acknowledges the depressed side's need to rest while beginning to allow the other side to meet some goals. The goal of this intervention is to access more life-affirming parts of the client and to promote more self-nurturing behaviors.

Attending to Positive Feelings

Expression can also be a means of helping clients to attend to positive feelings. From a mood-regulation perspective (Gross & Muñoz, 1995; Kirsch et al., 1990; Zeiss et al., 1979), therapists might encourage clients to become aware of variability in their depressed feelings, paying particular attention to times and circumstances in which they feel "less bad." Fleshing out these "less bad" feelings by talking about them not only expands depressed clients' emotional repertoire, it can also enhance positive perceptions of self-efficacy and provide important information to guide adaptive coping efforts.

> Dalia was a 49-year-old depressed client who felt crushed by the constant demands of her grown children. Her three daughters called her daily, asking her to fix their dilemmas. They asked her to turn in forms they had forgotten about, to pick up one of her grandchildren because they had left it too late to arrange a car pool, to drive them to a job interview because they had lent their car to someone else. Dalia found it extremely difficult to say "No" to her daughters' demands. She despaired that they would ever change, but she felt trapped in her role of rescuer because she couldn't bear to have the consequences of her daughters' irresponsibility affect her grandchildren. One day, Dalia inadvertently missed a frantic phone call from one of her daughters because she was attending a church function. Dalia heard the message on her answering machine when she got home. By then, there was nothing she could do to help her daughter. In describing her feelings about this incident, Dalia noted that she felt guilty and worried after listening to the message, but she also felt relieved, and even . . . gleeful. She smiled shyly as she admitted this, saying she felt like she had gotten away with something, because if she had been home to receive the call, she would have rushed to the rescue as usual.
> Accessing these positive feelings and elaborating on what they meant to her was a turning point for Dalia. She still had a lot of work

to do in negotiating her relationships with her daughters and finding her own sense of identity outside her role of rescuer. However, she was able to draw upon her exploration of these positive feelings to clarify her therapeutic goals and to motivate herself to make changes in the way she viewed herself and the way she interacted with her daughters.

Scheduling and Discussing Pleasant Events

Behavioral therapists often encourage clients to schedule pleasant events (Hollon & Jacobsen, 1985; Hollon & Beck, 1979; Lewinsohn, 1974; Zeiss et al., 1979), and then talk about their feelings surrounding these events, as a means of cultivating positive emotional responses. This needs to be done with some delicacy. Unless there is a strong therapeutic alliance, unless clients sense that the therapist truly accepts and understands their depressed feelings at a meaningful level, pleasant-events scheduling can come across in a way that is as invalidating as the well-meaning but unempathic efforts of significant others to cheer up depressed people. In order not to compound depressed clients' sense of powerlessness, it is essential that clients, rather than the therapist, take the lead in coming up with and scheduling pleasant events.

In introducing the idea of pleasant events scheduling, it may be helpful to first get clients to talk about whether they have noticed any behaviors or events that make them feel *worse* (e.g., staying in bed all day, spending time with a critical and unsupportive relative). This can be a means of broaching the idea that what clients do can impact on how they feel. Often depressed clients insist that there is nothing that they enjoy doing. In this case, the therapist can encourage them to think of things that they used to enjoy doing or things that they could do which at least won't make them feel worse (e.g., promising themselves that they will get dressed every morning or take a short walk every afternoon, even if they don't feel like it).

Talking about the pleasant events afterward and encouraging clients to describe any positive (or less bad) feelings these events elicited is an important part of this intervention. Research shows that talking about positive feelings can be a means of rehearsing, prolonging, and intensifying them (Langston, 1994). Again, though, it is important that clients take the lead in these discussions. The therapist's stance should be one of helping clients to discover variability in their emotional responses and to gain a sense of emotional self-efficacy, rather than pressuring clients to feel a certain way and thereby devaluing their actual emotional experience.

In this section we discussed the therapeutic use of expression as a means of cultivating positive and agentic feelings. We described how expression can be a means of helping clients to expand the range of their emotional response by becoming aware of nondepressed feelings and spelling out the personal meaning of these feelings. Clients can draw upon these feelings as a guide to effective coping and as a resource for countering the passivity of depression.

So far, in this chapter our discussion of therapeutic strategies concerning expression and depression has focused on using in-session expression to cope with individuals' difficulties in processing depressed feelings and accessing nondepressed feelings. However, as we describe below, depressed people often have problems in their interpersonal relationships. This suggests that it is not enough to foster adaptive individual expression within a therapeutic session. Therapists also need to address how depressed clients express their feelings with the people in their daily lives and how these others respond.

MODIFYING MALADAPTIVE INTERPERSONAL PATTERNS OF EXPRESSION

Depressed people are often involved in unsatisfying relationships characterized by maladaptive patterns of emotional expression involving both the depressed person and the other person (Alloy, Fedderly, Kennedy-Moore, & Cohan, 1998; Coyne, 1976b, 1990; see also Hinchliffe, Hooper, & Roberts, 1978; Hokanson & Rupert, 1991; Keltner & Kring, 1998; Klerman, Weissman, Rounsaville, & Chevron, 1984; Muran & Safran, 1993; Segrin, 1998; Segrin & Abramson, 1994; S. J. Siegel & Alloy, 1990; Chapter 7). A large body of research documents depressed people's difficulties in emotional communication. Because their despair consumes their attention, depressed people find it difficult to connect with others. Their emotional behavior is often unresponsive to and disengaged from their interaction with partners. As we saw in the anecdote about Deborah and Rosa at the beginning of this chapter, depressed people's passive and diffuse expressions of misery can leave other people feeling at a loss as to how to respond. Moreover, depressed people tend to behave in globally hostile ways in their close relationships, which can push others away without ever addressing the depressed person's true concerns.

A similarly large body of research shows that others often respond to depressed people's expression of distress in less than optimal ways. Other people's efforts to "cheer up" a depressed person may communicate to the depressed person that his or her feelings are invalid or inappropriate (Coates & Peterson, 1982; Coates & Wortman, 1980). Furthermore, other people often express overt criticism or rejection of the depressed person (Hooley & Teasdale, 1989). All of these responses from others tend to compound depressed people's distress,

The final therapeutic function of expression that we discuss in this chapter involves modifying maladaptive interpersonal patterns of expression between depressed individuals and their significant others. Ideally, significant others are available to come into therapy, so that both or all parties' contributions to maladaptive interpersonal patterns of expression can be addressed directly. A treatment outcome study by O'Leary and Beach (1990; see also Beach, Sandeen, & O'Leary, 1990) showed that, overall, marital therapy emphasizing communication skills (e.g., active listening, "I statements") is as effective as individual therapy in treating depressed women. Interventions designed to alter the communication pattern called "expressed emotion," or "EE," may also be helpful, given that both depressed people and their significant others tend to show this corrosive type of interaction involving criticism, hostility, and emotional overinvolvement (Florin et al., 1992; Hooley & Teasdale, 1989; Vaughn & Leff, 1976a, 1976b).

Even when significant others cannot or will not come in for therapy, it is still possible to change maladaptive interpersonal patterns of expression by helping depressed clients to change the way that they relate to others. Sometimes just having the support of a therapist can positively alter depressed people's close relationships by alleviating some of the strain on these relationships: A therapist's acceptance and understanding can help depressed clients to feel that they have another relationship in which they can express their negative feelings, so that they feel less need to do so in their daily lives and therefore become less demanding of their significant others. At the same time, because a professional is involved, significant others may feel less pressured to "fix" the depressed person, and they may find their depressed partner's less frequent or less intense expressions of distress more tolerable. Beyond these general benefits of therapeutic emotional support, maladaptive interpersonal patterns of expression can also be addressed directly in individual therapy with depressed clients. This involves helping them to express their feelings assertively, to counter depressive passivity and diffuse hostility, and, using expression to cultivate empathy, to counter depressive self-focus and interpersonal disengagement.

Enhancing Assertiveness

Helping depressed clients to clearly, specifically, and assertively express their feelings to others can improve their interpersonal relationships. If depressed people can express their feelings and needs clearly and directly, they are less likely to resort to maladaptive forms of expression and more likely to elicit the kinds of responses they want and need from others. Two techniques for enhancing assertiveness are two-chair work to address self-criticism and assertiveness training.

Two-Chair Work to Address Self-Criticism

Process–experiential therapists sometimes use two-chair work to enhance assertive emotional expression. With this technique, clients act out a dialogue between the critical aspect of themselves—the one that restricts their feelings and behavior—and the more spontaneous, experiential part of themselves—the one that is in touch with their basic needs and desires. Alternatively, clients can act out a dialogue between themselves and a critical other person. In two-chair dialogues, clients do not challenge the validity of critical statements with reason or evidence. Instead, they respond emotionally to the harshness or unfairness of the criticisms, expressing the pain and life-affirming feelings provoked by these criticisms. Once the experiencing side asserts itself by telling the critical side about the impact of the criticisms, the critical side is usually able to respond sympathetically. The critical side may then be able to express the feelings of fear or concern that underlie the criticism.

The goal of two-chair dialogues is to reach a compromise between the two sides. For instance, clients might come to realize that there are ways for them to achieve the expressive objectives of their spontaneous side without threatening the need for self-protection represented by their critical side. Or, they may decide that the standards of their critical side can be applied more flexibly, in some situations but not others. Two-chair dialogues give clients an opportunity to express their feelings in a powerful way, so that they come to view their needs as important and worthy of attention. Once they have voiced their feelings and confronted their critical, restrictive inner voices, depressed clients feel more empowered. They are more aware of aspects of their experience that they had previously silenced, and therefore they may be less likely to squelch expression of these feelings in their daily interactions with others.

Deirdre was a 27-year-old, recently divorced woman who came to therapy because she felt depressed. She had a long history of subjugating her needs for the sake of others. Growing up, as the eldest of three children, she was responsible for looking after her younger siblings and generally taking care of the home during her mother's frequent bouts of illness. While she was married, somehow her needs always took second place to her husband's demanding job and numerous hobbies. Deirdre had difficulty expressing her wishes directly to her husband. However, she often found herself snapping at him for no obvious reason, fuming in silent resentment, or sulking in resignation when her desires were ignored or overlooked by her husband. Many times Deirdre didn't even realize what her wishes were in a particular situation until it was too late to do anything about them. Then she felt foolish for not speaking up but also guilty for having "selfish" desires. When her marriage ended despite (or because of?) her constant self-sacrifice, Deirdre was determined to make a new beginning for herself. Through two-chair dialogues between the critical and spontaneous sides of herself, Deirdre learned to tune into her own needs, begin to respect her own limits, and not always put other people's needs first.

Assertiveness Training

Whereas the experiential two-chair technique fosters assertiveness by helping clients to acknowledge their feelings and give themselves permission to express them, cognitive-behavioral techniques enhance assertiveness by providing direct training and practice in how to get one's feelings across to others effectively (Becker & Heimberg, 1985). For instance, therapists might explain to depressed clients the difference between assertive, unassertive, and aggressive communication, providing examples of each. They might provide clients with phrases to use in order to express their feelings assertively—phrases that are specific, nonblaming, and emphasize clients' ownership of their own feelings (e.g., "When you do X, I feel Y," rather than "You make me Z"). Role playing, in which the therapist acts the part of the significant other and clients practice expressing their feelings assertively, can help clients gain confidence before they try out these skills in their daily lives. In some cases, depressed clients may decide to proceed directly from these exercises to asserting themselves with significant others. In other cases, clients may prefer to work up to important encounters with significant others by first practicing expressing their feelings assertively under less important and less threatening circumstances (e.g., asserting themselves with telephone solicitors, asserting themselves with an acquaintance).

All of these assertiveness-enhancing techniques aim to provide depressed clients with alternatives to their usual expressive passivity and diffuse hostility. Clients are encouraged to recognize their specific feelings and to take responsibility for clearly communicating these feelings to their significant others. Obviously, there is no guarantee that others will respond positively to depressed clients' assertive expressions of emotion. Therapists should discuss directly with clients the possibility of unsupportive responses from others. However, assertive expressions are more likely to elicit desired responses from others than either passive withdrawal, muddled moaning, or indiscriminate snarling. Even if others respond negatively, having the ability to communicate their feelings assertively can be important for depressed clients' self-esteem. This ability is empowering. It means that depressed clients can choose to articulate their feelings to others rather than sitting as passive victims of their moods.

Cultivating Empathy

In addition to enhancing assertiveness, another therapeutic use of expression that can address the interpersonal difficulties of depressed clients involves using expression to cultivate empathy (Barrett-Lennard, 1997; S. M. Johnson & Greenberg, 1994b). Empathy enables depressed clients to step out of their preoccupation with their own distress and relate warmly and effectively to others.

In family or marital therapy, empathy can be cultivated by having clients reflect back their partners' thoughts and feelings (e.g., "What I hear you saying is that you feel . . . "). Partners can then acknowledge that their emotional message has come across accurately, clarify misunderstandings, or elaborate on their message until they feel fully understood. Then partners switch speaking and reflecting roles.

If the significant other is not available for therapy, the empty-chair technique can be a useful way of helping depressed clients to step out of their own framework and vividly understand the other person's perspective and feelings. With this technique, clients visualize and act out the other person's verbal and nonverbal expressions of emotion thereby gaining a concrete and highly personal view of what the other person might be feeling. For instance, in playing the role of a rejecting spouse, a depressed client might discover that this rejection stems from the spouse's feelings of helplessness and inadequacy at being unable to help the depressed client. This new understanding could lead the depressed client to feel and express more compassion toward the spouse. It could also change how the depressed person responds to the spouse's negative comments. Seeing these comments as a sign of the spouse's feelings of insecurity, the depressed person might feel less hurt by these remarks and might be less likely to withdraw completely or obsessively seek reassurance at the first sign of rejection.

CONCLUSION

Depressed people are highly expressive in some ways but nonexpressive in other ways. They show many signs of general misery, but they tend to be unresponsive to those around them. They feel enveloped in a fog of despair, but they are unable to articulate their feelings with any specificity or to tie these feelings to particular thoughts or events. They may communicate a diffuse hostility, but they are unable to access positive or agentic feelings.

In therapy, helping clients to express their feelings in a clear and differentiated manner can be a means of enabling them to process their depressed feelings and to expand the range of their emotional responses so that they can draw upon their emotional experience to guide adaptive coping efforts. The general goal is to help depressed clients move beyond diffuse expressions of paralyzing sadness and despair, toward greater self-understanding and self-efficacy. Because depressed people often have difficulties in their relationships, addressing interpersonal patterns of emotional expression is also important. Expression can be a means of enhancing assertiveness and cultivating empathy.

10

Flooding or Blunting: Vacillating Expression and Nonexpression in Bereavement and Trauma

EMOTIONAL BEHAVIOR FOLLOWING TRAUMATIC EXPERIENCES

There is a famous story about Psammetichus, King of Egypt, who is beaten and taken prisoner by the King of Persia. Psammetichus remains outwardly impassive about his own dire circumstances. He also shows no reaction when he sees that his daughter has been enslaved and forced to haul water. However, upon seeing that one of his servants has been captured, he weeps and wails and beats his head in sorrow. When his captor, the King of Persia, asks about his reactions, Psammetichus explains, "It is because only the latter grief can signify itself by tears, whereas the former goes way beyond means of expressing itself" (story told by Montaigne, 1580/1965, cited in Frijda et al., 1992). This story illustrates the extremes of both expression and nonexpression that can occur following traumatic experiences. Psammetichus feels unable to express his grief over his own or his daughter's tragedy. He is frozen in emotional silence during his capture and beating and upon viewing the maltreatment of his beloved daughter. Yet, his grief over his servant's conditions bursts forth in dramatic expression.

The emotional behavior of trauma survivors is often characterized by emotional blunting, emotional flooding, or vacillation between these two extremes (Courtois, 1988; Herman, 1992; Foy, 1992; Litz, 1992; van der Kolk, 1987; Horowitz, 1985). In terms of the model that we described in Chapter 1, these extremes involve either disruption or circumvention of

240

steps in the process of emotional expression, so that clients do not adequately recognize, label, interpret, or accept their trauma-related feelings.

At one extreme, the emotional blunting of trauma survivors can entail disruptions at several different levels in the process of expression. For instance, a war veteran who feels that no one could possibly understand his feelings or that other people would be horrified at what he had seen and done might deliberately suppress his feelings because he perceives that he lacks a social context for expression. A rape survivor who blames herself for somehow causing the rape might deliberately refrain from expressing because she considers her feelings of helplessness to be unacceptable. A recently widowed man might not express because he lacks the skills to articulate his profound and confusing feelings. Finally, a survivor of childhood sexual abuse might not express his feelings because they evoke such intense distress and are too painful to acknowledge consciously.

How completely trauma survivors block their emotional expression is likely to depend on characteristics of the trauma—for example, whether or not the trauma was expected, how long it lasted, whether other people were involved, as well as characteristics of the individual—for example, age, coping resources, past experience with loss, social support, or expression-related beliefs. When in an emotionally blunted state, survivors are cut off from their affective responses and therefore cannot adequately process or "work through" their trauma-related feelings (Horowitz, 1986; Zahava, Mikulincer, & Arad, 1991).

At the other extreme, the emotional flooding of trauma survivors involves expressive leakage of minimally processed affective experience. Because trauma-related feelings are intense, they tend to leak out in ways that trauma survivors experience as unintended, unpredictable, or incomprehensible. Trauma survivors might burst into tears in the middle of a happy social event. They might find themselves shaking with terror upon hearing an ostensibly innocuous sound. They might fly into a rage at what they consider a minor provocation. When survivors are emotionally flooded, they experience their feelings as intrusive and out of control. They are unable to modulate, organize, or process their emotional experience or expression (Horowitz, 1986).

Some researchers suggest that individuals with limited social, personal, and physical supports and those whose early experiences have left them physiologically and psychologically ill-prepared for coping are especially prone to experience symptoms of posttraumatic stress following events of extreme threat, loss, or assault (Elliott et al., 1996; Herman, 1988; Horowitz, 1986; van der Kolk, 1987; McCann & Pearlman, 1990). van der Kolk (1987) notes that this may be particularly true for children who suffer disrupted attachment histories. These people may have difficulty modulating their affective reactions and early abuse may leave them in states of chronic hyperarousal, which can lead to their having more intense emotional reactions to events than other people. People suffering from complicated mourning or symptoms of posttraumatic stress may try to avoid the feelings of grief and pain that ensue after a traumatic event because these are experienced as too overwhelming and devastating to be confronted. Effortful avoidance of trauma-related feelings may eventually inhibit longer term adaptation and adjustment (see Chapter 2).

Trauma-related distress can typically last a surprisingly long time. Wortman and her colleagues have conducted longitudinal studies of several different populations who have experienced irrevocable traumatic losses (see reviews by Wortman & Silver, 1987, 1989, 1990; Wortman, Silver, & Kessler, 1992). These losses involved sudden, permanent paralysis due to spinal cord injury, loss of a child due to sudden infant death syndrome (SIDS), loss of a child or a spouse due to a motor vehicle accident caused by someone else's negligence, or widowhood. Data from these studies show that resolution of grief reactions can take much longer than people might expect, and it doesn't necessarily involve finding meaning in the event. For instance, in the motor vehicle study, 72% of respondents were unable to find meaning in their loss, even after 4 to 7 years. Wortman, Kessler, Bolger, and House (1991) found that widowed men and women took about 10 years before they approached control subjects' levels of life satisfaction and about 20 years before they achieved levels of depression comparable to controls. Enduring distress following major losses may be normative rather than indicative of pathological grieving.

However, a lack of expression of trauma-related distress is sometimes a sign of especially good coping. Amazingly, the majority of people who experience severe traumatic events such as combat, nuclear accidents, and disasters do *not* develop chronic symptoms of posttraumatic stress disorder (M. A. Greenberg, 1995). Furthermore, a substantial minority of people do *not* experience or express significant distress even shortly after traumatic losses. Perhaps because they have coped effectively with previous losses or because they have a religious or philosophical orientation that allows them to incorporate traumatic events into their world view, some people are less affected by traumatic experiences than others (Wortman, Sheedy, Gluhoski, & Kessler, 1992). For instance, in a study of SIDS, 30% of parents showed no signs of depression only 1 month following the loss (Wortman & Silver, 1987). Minimal distress early on is *not* generally associated with delayed or prolonged grief. Instead, initial reactions are highly predictive of later reactions. People who express little distress initially continue to show little distress at subsequent assessments (Bonanno, Keltner, Holen, & Horowitz, 1995; Wortman, Sheedy, Gluhoski, & Kessler, 1992).

These empirical findings concerning the emotional responses of trauma survivors have important clinical implications. First, they suggest that therapists should not assume that clients "ought" to be over their trauma-related distress within a certain time frame or that clients "must" express distress to resolve trauma-related feelings. There is an enormous amount of variability in how different people respond to traumatic events. Forcing clients to grieve in a particular way is disrespectful and probably harmful (Wortman & Silver, 1987, 1990). Second, these findings suggest that the mere presence or absence of distress expression is not indicative of how well clients are coping with traumatic experiences. Distress expression can be a sign that clients are working through their trauma-related feelings or that they are experiencing devastating emotional flooding. Nonexpression can be a sign that trauma survivors are coping particularly well or that they are in a paralyzed state of emotional blunting. The emotional behavior of trauma survivors needs to be understood in the context of their overall functioning and in qualitative rather than quantitative terms. Whether or not clients express their feelings is less important than how they express their feelings and how they perceive their emotional behavior.

In order to rebalance the constriction and intrusion of affect clinicians need to encourage and facilitate clients' adaptive expression of affect in therapy (Briere, 1989; Courtois, 1988; Elliott et al., 1996; McCann & Pearlman, 1990; Winn, 1994). To this end one of the primary goals of therapy is to have people begin to reenact and narrate the traumatic situation so as to process their original affective response in a situation of diminished threat and where their levels of arousal can be carefully modulated. By helping clients to process both their affective responses to and memories of traumatic situations clinicians can help clients regain balance of their emotions and address symptoms of constriction and intrusion.

In this chapter, we describe therapeutic techniques related to emotional expression that can help trauma survivors process their emotional experience. As in previous chapters, our emphasis is on helping clients to achieve an integration of cognitive and experiential processing. We consider three broad categories of clinical strategies involving (1) laying the groundwork for expression, (2) facilitating adaptive forms of emotional expression, and (3) using emotional expression to achieve resolution.

LAYING THE GROUNDWORK FOR EXPRESSION

The first step in fostering adaptive emotional expression in clients who have experienced traumatic events often involves laying the groundwork for expression. In all cases, it is imperative that therapists provide trauma survivors with a respectful and compassionate environment in which they can process their trauma-related feelings. In some cases, it may be necessary for clients to resolve their ambivalence concerning expression or to cope with self-criticism that limits their expression before they can effectively process their feelings. Addressing these issues helps clients to give themselves permission to acknowledge, express, and understand their feelings.

Resolving Ambivalence about Expression

At the beginning of therapy, clients are often reluctant or fearful to talk about their trauma-related feelings (see Chapter 3). Ambivalence over expression can also emerge later in therapy, when clients encounter new emotionally laden material. Sometimes clients indicate their ambivalence about expression indirectly. For instance, they might report suddenly going blank when a therapist asks about their feelings, or they might seem tense or reluctant to engage in interventions involving expression. Alternatively they may continually correct their therapist's understanding as a way of staying in their heads and not accessing their underlying feelings. Other times, clients are very explicit about their ambivalence and question the efficacy or usefulness of specific techniques. For instance, clients might ask, "What is the point of discussing my feelings if it only makes me feel worse?"

When clients show signs of ambivalence concerning expression, it is important for therapists to be carefully attuned and empathic to their clients' concerns. Therapists should help clients to articulate their concerns, and they should genuinely acknowledge clients' fears or difficulties.

Sometimes clients' ambivalence over expression stems from a mismatch in their own and their therapists' understanding of the goals and means of therapy (J. C. Watson & Greenberg, 1994; 1998). For instance, clients may see their therapeutic goal in terms of wanting to "feel better," and they may be puzzled by their therapists' encouragement to examine painful feelings. In this case, it may be helpful for therapists to explain the rationale behind the specific therapeutic intervention that prompted clients' ambivalence. Therapists can summarize their understanding of clients' goals in therapy and describe how this intervention could help clients realize their objectives.

It is difficult to make progress if clients and therapists disagree concerning the goals of therapy, so therapists need to check that their formulation of clients' difficulties is congruent with clients' views of their problems. If there is disagreement concerning therapeutic goals, therapists need to talk about this with clients, to gather more information, and to negotiate with clients in order to tailor their formulation to more closely match clients' conceptualizations of their problems. Finding the fit between clients' views of their problems and therapists' theoretical and technical expertise can be challenging, but it is essential for the development of a good working alliance.

Other times, ambivalence over expression is a function of conflicting goals within clients themselves. Part of them may want to express their feelings, but another part may be reluctant to do so. In this case, therapists can help clients to negotiate a compromise between their conflicting goals (see Chapter 4). Tricia is an example of a client who needed to address her ambivalence concerning expression before she was able to work effectively with her feelings.

> Tricia was a young woman in her 30s who had sustained severe facial and bodily injuries as a result of a car accident in which she was a passenger. She came in for therapy when she began showing signs of depression and having problems at work, such as missing appointments with clients and failing to meet deadlines.
>
> At the start of therapy, Tricia was sure that she had put the accident behind her. She was tired of talking about it and felt that she had cried herself out. She was also sure that other people were tired of hearing her talk about the accident. Everyone was encouraging her to move on with her life. However, Tricia still found herself overcome by fear at the sight of certain cars or pictures of automobile accidents. Every night, she had nightmares that left her soaking with sweat, but when she awoke, she couldn't recall the content of these nightmares. Tricia also noticed that she had become more socially withdrawn since the accident, and she was having difficulties in her relationship with her fiancé. She found herself feeling irritable and distant from him.

In terms of our model, Tricia is deliberately refraining from expression because of her own dislike of her feelings as well as her perceptions of other people's lack of acceptance of these feelings. However, her fears, her nightmares, her work problems, and her relationship difficulties all suggest that she has not adequately processed her feelings concerning the accident.

When Tricia's therapist asked her to talk about her feelings concerning the accident, Tricia initially balked. She said she was afraid that she would be overcome by panic, the way she was when she woke up from her nightmares. In the following dialogue, Tricia's therapist uses the experiential technique of two-chair work to help Tricia resolve the split between her desire to deal with her feelings and her reluctance to face them. (For descriptive purposes, we have labeled the nonexpression chair "Side N" and the expression chair "Side E.")

THERAPIST: Can you separate out the two parts of yourself, the part that wants to express the feelings about the accident and the losses that have ensued and the other part that says, "Don't! It's too painful and overwhelming"? Let's put them in different chairs. Which side are you most in touch with now?

TRICIA [Side N]: The part that says, "Don't! It's not worth it."

THERAPIST: OK. Let's start there. What does that side say?

TRICIA [Side N]: Don't feel. It is just too painful. What's the point, anyway. It is not going to improve things.

THERAPIST: So, this side is scared of the pain. It feels pointless. What does the other side respond?

TRICIA [Side E]: I know it will be painful, but it has to be done. We can't carry on like this. You just have to face up to it.

THERAPIST: So, this side says, "Grin and bear it." How do you feel when she says that?

TRICIA [Side N]: I feel that she does not understand. She is so cavalier. She has no idea how difficult it is.

THERAPIST: How do you feel about her lack of concern?

TRICIA [Side N]: It scares me. I feel I can't trust her—that we might just be swept away.

THERAPIST: What do you need from her?

TRICIA [Side N]: I need her to be careful. I need her to see how difficult this is for me and to go slow, stop pushing.

THERAPIST: So, you need her to slow down and take care of you.

TRICIA [Side N]: Yes.

THERAPIST: How do you respond to this side's request that you stop pushing and slow down?

TRICIA [Side E]: I can try, but I need to know she will do this. She will need to tell me when we are going too fast. I will try to listen better. I know it is going to be hard, but it is the only way that we are going to be able to move on with our lives.

In this dialogue, Tricia manages to negotiate a more comfortable pace for dealing with her trauma-related feelings. Permitting herself to control the pace with which she expresses her feelings gives Tricia a sense of strength and safety that helps her manage her intense affective reactions and resolve her ambivalence about expression.

Addressing Self-Criticisms and Strengthening Self

In addition to resolving ambivalence about expression, another issue that can be important in laying the groundwork for therapeutic expression involves addressing clients' self-criticisms. Trauma survivors are often preoccupied with blaming themselves for what happened or wishing they could somehow undo what happened. They may ruminate about "If only I had done this . . . " or "If only I hadn't done that. . . . " This kind of self-criticism can cause trauma survivors to inhibit their emotional expression.

For instance, a rape survivor who blames herself for causing the rape because of how she dressed or how she acted is also, in effect, telling herself that she has no right to express pain or to feel sorry for herself.

It is important that therapists do not dismiss self-blame as unrealistic or silly, even though from an outsider's perspective it may be clear that the client is blameless and a victim of uncontrollable circumstances. To clients, these concerns feel very compelling. The expressions of self-blame and wishes to undo the event can be viewed as important first steps in helping clients develop stronger and in some cases new assumptive frameworks about themselves and the world that will enable them to confront the traumatic event more easily. Instead of discounting these concerns, therapists can help clients to redirect their attempts to control their emotional experience from unhealthy self-criticism, which inhibits what they are allowed to feel and express, toward healthy self-assertion, which enables them to express their feelings in life-affirming ways. This assertion of self is important in strengthening the person to engage in the work of reconstructing the event and permitting the self to express emotion. In clients who have suffered from sexual assault it is particularly important to help them develop a stronger sense of self because often these clients have introjected social values that shame them and hold them culpable for the assault either by virtue of their position, dress, or demeanor. By helping clients to access their critical introjects, and how they feel in response to the accusations, particularly how oppressive and life denying they are, therapists can help clients get in touch with their own needs and more life-affirming attitudes. Once these attitudes have been activated clients are in a position to reject their critical introjects and can begin to develop more accepting, nurturing, and soothing ways of being toward themselves. As the following example illustrates, one way of doing this is by helping clients to confront their inner critic.

> Tanya was a 19-year-old woman who was raped while on a date. She had participated in a group for sexual assault survivors. In the group, members had explored issues concerning their sense of culpability and their unfair treatment by authorities. Tanya felt compassion toward the other members of the group. She was able to support them and clearly see that they were not responsible for the events that befell them. However, she still castigated herself and felt that she was somehow to blame for allowing the rape to occur.

Tanya's self-criticism prevented her from acknowledging or expressing her feelings of loss and vulnerability. In the dialogue below, Tanya's therapist uses the two-chair technique to help Tanya confront her inner critic and begin to develop a more accepting, nurturing, and soothing way of being toward herself.

THERAPIST: So, you are able to support Odette and reassure her that she was not to blame for what happened, but somehow it is different for you?

TANYA: Yes. I know that the others had to do what they did to save their lives and to protect themselves and were not to blame, but I don't believe that with me. I still feel I should have done something differently. My mom and aunts have told me that only a woman who deserves it gets raped. So, somehow I feel as if I did something to make him attack me.

THERAPIST: So, somehow it's your fault?

TANYA: That's what everyone believes, isn't it?

THERAPIST: This seems important to work with. Let's set up a two-chair exercise. Can I ask you to put your mom and aunts in this chair. What do they say to you?

TANYA [as mother]: You should have stopped it. You know that this only happens to bad girls.

THERAPIST: Come over here. How does it feel when she says you should have stopped it, and that somehow you are to blame for being bad?

TANYA [as self]: She's right. I should have stopped it. I just . . . I just did not know what to do. He was so big. . . . He totally overpowered me.

THERAPIST: Come be your mother again. What else does she say?

TANYA [as mother]: You must have done something to bring it on. I have always told you that your skirts are too tight. It's you fault. You can't blame anybody else but yourself.

THERAPIST: Come over here. What happens when you hear your mom say it was the way you were dressed and does not respond to your being overpowered.

TANYA [as self]: I feel demolished, silenced.

THERAPIST: Tell her what it is like to be silenced.

TANYA [as self]: Mom, I feel like you do not want to listen to me. I feel like my pain does not even count with you, that it does not matter that I felt so frightened and helpless when he threatened me. He pinned me down. I could not move.

THERAPIST: What do you need from her?

TANYA [as self]: (crying) I need you to hear me, Mom. I need you to see how bruised and hurt I am. I didn't want this to happen. I used to be happy; now I feel spoiled, dirty. I need to know that you still love me. It's not fair that you are taking his side against me.

THERAPIST: How does you mother respond?

TANYA [as mother]: It is so hard for me to see you like this. It hurts me to see you bruised. I wish it could have been different. I did not want this to ever happen to you. That is why I kept nagging you about your clothes, warning you about men. I am sorry you are hurting. I wish I could make it better.

In confronting her self-criticism (voiced through the image of her mother), Tanya helps to lay the groundwork for the expression and processing of her trauma-related feelings. As she argues for fairness and acknowledgment of her pain, she begins to shift responsibility for the rape from herself to the perpetrator. She begins to assert herself and to express her affective responses in a circumscribed way. She gains a stronger and more compassionate sense of self that will enable her to express her painful feelings about the rape without being totally overwhelmed.

In this section, we have described ways of helping clients to prepare themselves for engaging in effective emotional expression. We talked about addressing blocks to expression in the form of ambivalence over expression or self-criticism. We now turn to a discussion of therapeutic techniques for facilitating adaptive forms of emotional expression.

FACILITATING ADAPTIVE FORMS OF EMOTIONAL EXPRESSION

Clinical strategies for facilitating adaptive expression in trauma survivors have two aims: (1) helping clients access their feelings to counter affective blunting, and (2) helping clients to pace their expression to counter affective flooding. In combination, these strategies enable clients to find a middle ground between being completely cut off from their feelings and being utterly overwhelmed by them. These strategies allow clients to express their feelings in a context of safety and adaptive self-control, so that they can begin to process their trauma-related experience.

Accessing Feelings

Most therapists, regardless of orientation, believe that an important way of helping trauma survivors to access and process their feelings is to have them recount the traumatic event in detail. A number of interventions have been developed to assist clients to access their memories and feelings about traumatic events. Cognitive-behavioral therapists use systematic desensitization. They may begin by having clients talk about more peripheral events and tolerable feelings and work up to talking about more painful feelings and events, or they may simply encourage clients to describe the traumatic event as it occurred. Clients can narrate the events to the therapist during the therapy hour, or they can narrate the events into a tape recorder that they can then play back a number of times during the day (Foa et al., 1989; Foa, Rothbaum, Riggs, & Murdock, 1991; Foy, 1992). As clients stay with their feelings, they come to see these feelings as tolerable, rather than unbearable.

Similarly, experiential therapists use a technique called *systematic evocative unfolding,* in which the therapist helps clients to build concrete, visual, and kinesthetic representations of traumatic events. Clients describe details of what they saw, heard, felt, thought, and did at the time of the trauma, as if they were creating a movie of the event. As clients reconstruct the event, the therapist asks about their feelings at the time of the trauma and in the present context, so that clients can acknowledge, articulate, and understand these feelings. Describing traumatic experiences can elicit intense feelings, such as terror, self-loathing, or helplessness. It is important to take time to fully explore and process these feelings as they occur, rather than pushing on with the reconstruction of the event.

In the dialogue below, Tricia, the client we described earlier who had been injured in a car accident, and her therapist use systematic evocative unfolding to reconstruct the events of that day and access the related feelings.

THERAPIST: Can you begin with what you remember that day? What sort of day had it been?

TRICIA: It was warm, muggy, and overcast. Then, it began to rain soft, drizzly rain. My fiancé and I had been invited to a pool party later in the afternoon.

THERAPIST: So, fill me in. What had the morning been like?

TRICIA: I hung around in the morning, doing things around the house. I remember thinking that the weather was so icky that perhaps we should cancel.

THERAPIST: OK. So, the day was somewhat wet and dismal and it sounds like part of you was reluctant to go out.

TRICIA: Yeah! But then Frank came over and insisted it would be fun, so I gave in.

THERAPIST: So then what? You both got ready to leave?

TRICIA: Yeah, we went out to the car. I sat in the back with Olivia and the guys sat up front. Otto was driving.

THERAPIST: So, how were you feeling at this point? Still reluctant or more looking forward to the day?

TRICIA: I was starting to get more into the spirit of it. They were both laughing and kidding around. But there was still a part of me that thought I would be better off at home, working on a proposal for a client.

THERAPIST: OK. So, you are going along somewhat reluctantly and then what happens?

TRICIA: We decided to pick up some snacks on the way . . . some beer. When we got back in the car, Olivia asked if she could ride up front. I remembered that I forgot to lock my door.

THERAPIST: You sound upset as you recall not locking your door.

TRICIA: Yes, if only I had locked the door or even . . . If I had stayed home, it wouldn't have happened. I would have been safe and then, because I didn't lock the door well, that caused most of my injuries. I feel angry with myself. I don't remember much after that. I think the last thing I remember was speaking to Ken . . .

At this point, the therapist decided to forgo reconstructing the event and changed to two-chair work to address Tricia's self-blame. During the two-chair work, Tricia was able to stand up to the critical part of herself that held her responsible for what happened. She asserted that this blame was unfair and that she had no way of knowing that she was in any danger. However, she did acknowledge that she needed to listen to herself more and not allow herself to be overridden so easily by the needs and demands of others.

Over the next few sessions, Tricia and her therapist continued to work at reconstructing the accident. Tricia described what it was like riding in the car, what she was feeling, and what she saw and heard after stopping at the store. At first, Tricia could remember nothing immediately prior to the accident except the tinkling of shattered metal and glass. However, by building the details of the scene and drawing from others' accounts of the accident, she slowly reconstructed a clearer sense of what had happened. She remembered hearing her friend gasp and recalled the motion of the car swerving before she blacked out. After the accident, doctors told Tricia that she had been thrown from the car and had hit a barrier at the side of the road.

By re-creating the scene and putting it together piece by piece, Tricia came to fear it less. She eventually concluded that there was nothing more to be recalled about the accident. Tricia realized that her nightmares and other symptoms were the result of not having adequately processed her feelings concerning the accident. As she recounted the details of the accident and its aftermath, Tricia was able to get in touch with her feelings of sadness and loss. She was able to mourn the loss of some of her physical capacities and the person she would never again be.

By the end of therapy, Tricia no longer had nightmares and she seemed less anxious. She was able to be a passenger in a car with less stress, and she no longer felt the need to avoid seeing pictures of accidents in movies or on television. Tricia no longer blamed herself for her injuries, but she did resolve to trust her gut more and try to stay more in tune with her own needs and wishes in the future. She also made some changes in her career plans as part of coming to terms with her physical limitations.

Pacing Expression

In addition to helping clients access their trauma-related feelings, another important aspect of facilitating clients' expression of painful feelings and memories is to help them to pace their expression, so that it takes place in tolerable doses. As the story about King Psammetichus at the beginning of this chapter illustrated, traumatic events often leave clients feeling at the mercy of unpredictable and uncontrollable bouts of intense emotional expression. Providing clients with strategies that allow them to express their feelings in a more voluntary and controlled fashion can enhance their sense of mastery. The ability to examine their feelings in a context of present safety makes it possible for clients to process their feelings effectively.

It is important for the therapist to help clients set their own pace with respect to how fast they will go in exploring trauma-related feelings in therapy. Therapists should check in with clients when they seem particularly emotional to make sure that the pace feels comfortable to them. Sometimes clients show that they need to slow down by failing to remember certain details, as Tricia did at the end of dialogue above. Clients may also want to devise signals to inform the therapist when they want to slow down the pace of expression because they are beginning to feel overwhelmed by their feelings. Such signals might involve raising a hand or turning away.

When clients indicate that they are starting to feel out of control, it is important to respect their need to slow down the pace of expression. It may be necessary to forgo further exploration of feelings until the next session and instead to focus on helping clients feel less overwhelmed.

Relaxation or grounding techniques can be useful for intercepting unbearable feelings (Briere, 1989; McCann & Pearlman, 1990). For instance, the therapist might ask clients to put their feet on the ground and become aware of the floor, or to look at the therapist and concentrate on what they are seeing in the here and now. These techniques allow clients to take a break from their immersion in their trauma-related feelings and memories, refocusing on the present, so that they can modulate their emotional responses.

Sometimes modifications to expression-related therapeutic techniques can provide clients with a sense of safety and control. For example, before engaging in experiential chair work, clients may wish to increase the distance between chairs or to turn a chair so it faces away from them. Other clients might wish to use art or writing to express their feelings before they talk about these feelings (Pennebaker, 1993b). Clients may also want to gradually work up to talking about their most painful feelings. L. S. Greenberg and Paivio (1997) suggest that it is important not to have clients express vulnerable, sad feelings to a perpetrator, these should rather be expressed to the therapist who can then respond empathically and provide a soothing, caring response that the client can internalize.

To summarize, in this section we described techniques for facilitating adaptive emotional expression. These techniques involve helping clients to access their feelings while pacing their expression so that it occurs in manageable doses. The goal is to find a middle ground between emotional blunting and emotional flooding, so that clients can effectively process their feelings.

In working with trauma survivors, it is essential to bear in mind that emotional expression rarely proceeds in an orderly fashion. Clients may express a little, then retreat from their feelings, then express a little more, then need to return to laying the groundwork for expression. Therapists need to be sensitive to these fluctuations and to let clients take the lead in determining how much they can handle and how fast. Forcing clients to express their feelings before they are ready to do so can lead to emotional flooding and can compound clients' sense of victimization. On the other hand, helping trauma survivors achieve a sense of mastery in their ability to articulate and manage their feelings can help counter the sense of vulnerability and lack of control that traumatic events often evoke.

USING EXPRESSION TO ACHIEVE RESOLUTION

As we have maintained throughout this book, emotional expression is not an end in itself, but it can be a means to an end. What is important therapeutically is not only that trauma survivors express their feelings, but that they are able to use their emotional expression to reach some sort of resolution. Achieving this resolution generally involves helping clients to think through the meaning and implications of the feelings they have accessed, and thereby to acquire new perspectives on themselves, others, and the world (Elliott et al., 1996; M. A. Greenberg, 1995). These new perspectives provide clients with a sense of mastery that enables them to let go of the past and focus on taking care of themselves in the present and planning for the future.

Accessing and Revising Core Beliefs

Janoff-Bulman (1992) suggests that people have three core assumptions: First, the world is a benevolent place, where other people are trustworthy and misfortune is rare; second, life events are meaningful, such that outcomes are determined by people's own behavior, and people get what they deserve or at least no more than their fair share of difficulties; and third, the self is worthy and relatively invulnerable to negative events because of personal decency, sound judgment, or good luck. Traumatic events can shatter any or all of these assumptions, resulting in terrifying ambiguity that leaves survivors feeling deeply distraught and paralyzed. According to Janoff-Bulman, the coping task facing survivors is to either reinterpret the traumatic experience in ways that are more compatible with these core assumptions or to revise these assumptions to accommodate the trauma.

In the process of expressing their feelings, trauma survivors may be able to access their core beliefs and gain new understanding that allows them to preserve or even enhance their sense of self-worth, their connection with others, and their ability to cope in the world. Because core beliefs tend to be emotion-laden, they are often only available to conscious awareness when clients are actively immersed in their feelings. Therapists can encourage clients to spell out the personal meaning and implications of their feelings as a means of articulating their core beliefs.

The techniques we described in the previous section on facilitating adaptive emotional expression can provide a starting point for drawing from expression to achieve resolution. As clients express their feelings in a context of safety, they may gain new perspectives on themselves and their feelings, which the therapist can help them articulate. For instance, they may come to see their feelings as bearable rather than unbearable (see Chapter 2). They may begin to view themselves as capable of managing their intense feelings rather than as helpless victims of emotional hijacking (Goleman, 1995). Janoff-Bulman (1992) emphasizes that supportive responses by other people to trauma survivors' expressions of distress can be very important in helping survivors restore their self-esteem, trust in others, and hope for the future.

Expressing and processing their feelings may prompt trauma survivors to experience a moment of striking affective insight (Kuiken et al., 1987; see Chapter 3) that enables them to understand their suffering as meaningful somehow. They may see their suffering as imparting some important lesson or unexpected benefit (Elliott et al., 1996; Janoff-Bulman, 1992). For instance, spelling out the implications of their trauma-related feelings may help survivors to realize with sudden clarity and certainty what truly matters to them in life (e.g., "I almost died without telling my wife how much I love her"). They may also gain a new appreciation for their own courage, dignity, or resilience in response to the trauma (e.g., "This experience let me see what I'm capable of when I'm pushed to my limits"). Alternatively, trauma survivors may perceive that their suffering was worthwhile because it helped others or brought them closer to people they care about (e.g., "My father's death was a tragedy, but it brought me closer to my brother"). Such efforts to create meaning out of experience are central to constructivist psychotherapies (Neimeyer, 1993; Rosen & Kuehlwein, 1996).

In addition to the techniques we have already mentioned, two other therapeutic strategies that can be helpful in drawing from expression to achieve resolution are empty-chair work and psychodrama.

Empty-Chair Work

Empty-chair work This can foster resolution by enabling clients to express their feelings to another person in a way that they previously couldn't. It can provide clients with a new perspective on the other person.

> Tim was a 21-year-old man who, as a child, had been emotionally and physically abused by his father. He sought therapy because he felt like he had no direction in his life. He was also socially isolated and had difficulty trusting other people.
>
> Tim characterized his father as a mean, powerful, and domineering man. He recalled feeling helpless and manipulated by his father when he was a child.
>
> Tim's therapist asked him to imagine his father sitting in an empty chair. She encouraged Tim to tell his father how difficult it had been to live under his reign of terror. Tim expressed feelings of helplessness and frustration as he acted out a confrontation with his father. He accused his father of having destroyed the family. He became more assertive as he expressed his anger and contempt for his father's actions. Tim also began to express his sadness at being cut off from his brothers. In his effort to break away from his father's abuse, Tim had also lost touch with his three younger brothers.
>
> Subsequently, in an interview about this therapy session, Tim reported that as he expressed his feelings during this exercise, his image of his father began to change. Instead of seeing him as unassailably powerful, he began to see his father as small and weak. This represented a turning point for Tim. As a result of his new perspective on his father, Tim was better able to assert himself and to hold his father accountable for the disintegration of his family. He also decided to reconnect with his brothers.

The example above shows that the importance of empty-chair work is not only that it provides an opportunity to express previously inhibited feelings, but also that it is a means of drawing upon expression to construct new perceptions of the self and others. By imagining asserting himself with his father, Tim comes to see his father as less indomitable. He also comes to see himself as empowered. Instead of perceiving his only options as hiding from or being victimized by his father, Tim begins to see that he is capable of taking care of himself. He begins to let go of his preoccupation with his past traumas and to focus on acting to fulfill his life-affirming needs and wants in the present and future.

Psychodrama

Psychodrama is another therapeutic technique for drawing from expression to achieve resolution of traumatic experiences. Psychodrama in effect gives clients the opportunity to enact and undo events in their imagination so that they can once again feel more masterful and able to go on with their lives (Winn, 1994; Hudgins, 1998). As clients have the opportunity to narrate and enact the original situation new information can emerge. Reenactments can be made less overwhelming as other group members can play protective roles for clients during the traumatic incident. In later reenactments clients may be encouraged to engage in those behaviors that were inhibited or suppressed in the original situation as a result of fear and threat.

For instance, Tanya, the date rape survivor, might want to portray herself yelling and fleeing her attacker in her reenactment. Alternatively, Tim, the childhood abuse survivor, might want to enact a scene of someone intervening to protect him from his father. This someone could be another adult, such as his mother or his teacher, or it could be his adult self acting to defend his childhood self. By making the traumatic event less overwhelming, clients can create a stronger sense of self and feel better able to move on with their lives.

CONCLUSION

In this chapter we noted that the emotional behavior of trauma survivors often vacillates between emotional flooding and emotional blunting. Sometimes survivors feel hijacked by what they perceive as unpredictable and uncontrollable bursts of expression. Other times they feel numb and disconnected from their emotional responses. Therapeutically, the goal in working with trauma survivors is to enable them to find a middle ground between these two extremes. They need to be able to express their trauma-related feelings without being overwhelmed by them, so that they can process and resolve these feelings.

We described three broad categories of clinical strategies for working with trauma survivors. The first category pertains to laying the groundwork for expression. This involves helping clients to give themselves permission to access their feelings. The second category involves facilitating adaptive expression by helping clients to access their feelings and pace their expression. The third category involves helping clients to draw from their expression to create new perceptions of themselves, others, and the world.

As the clinical examples we described in this chapter suggest, clients may need to move back and forth between these three categories of expression-related interventions. For instance, they may suddenly encounter a block while expressing their feelings and need to return to use strategies aimed at laying the groundwork for expression. Similarly, after gaining new perceptions from their emotional expression, they may become aware of other feelings in need of expression. In combination, these three categories of expression-related clinical interventions can help clients to resolve their trauma-related feelings and move on with their lives.

11

Emotional Expression
in Marital Therapy

INTRODUCTION

Cathy and William had been married less than 6 months, but already their relationship was beginning to show signs of strain. This was evident in an exchange that occurred around a decision about whether or not to purchase a piece of furniture. The couple was struggling financially. They were living in a basement apartment with borrowed odds and ends. Cathy was eager to turn their apartment into a comfortable home, despite their makeshift belongings. She wanted their small space to be tidy, but this was difficult because they had very limited drawer space. Cathy told William that she wished they could purchase a chest of drawers. William ignored Cathy's request.

Not wanting to provoke William, Cathy did not pursue the matter for a while. However, she felt hurt and disappointed by what she saw as William's uncaring response. Why couldn't they even talk about the purchase? Didn't he care about her wishes? Didn't he care about their home? A few days later, she tried again to broach the topic. She spoke about the need for space for their clothes and repeated her wish that they could purchase a set of drawers. William said "No" and withdrew to the television.

So began an escalating cycle of Cathy complaining and criticizing the lack of space in their small apartment with increasing insistence, while William became more rigid and withdrawn. Whenever Cathy raised the issue of purchasing a piece of furniture, William responded with angry defensiveness. He swore and said he refused to discuss the matter, and Cathy ended up in tears.

From William's perspective, Cathy's unrelenting complaints about their lack of furniture felt like a personal attack on him. Didn't Cathy appreciate how hard he was working and how carefully he was managing their money? Why was she focusing on a silly dresser when they were not even sure they could pay the rent? Why couldn't she help and support him instead of finding fault all the time? He began to feel more and more inadequate and distressed that he was unable to please his young wife.

One day, in desperation, William snarled at Cathy, "If you're so unhappy with our life together, why don't you leave?!" Cathy felt shocked and deeply hurt by this remark. She could not understand why William would suggest a solution as radical as leaving. She had no intention at that point of moving out—she was trying to build a life not tear it down. William's continued refusal to even try to understand her concerns left Cathy feeling helpless, cut off, and trapped.

The pattern of complaint and criticism coupled by withdrawal and defensiveness became endemic to Cathy and William's relationship. Twelve years later, they divorced.

The reader with greater wisdom and experience may see this as a trivial argument between two immature young people. However, Cathy and William's interactions illustrate three key problems involving emotional behavior that are related to marital dissatisfaction and dissolution: First, Cathy and William express their negative emotions in destructive ways. Rather than leading to greater understanding or conflict resolution, their emotional expression exacerbates their problems and leaves both partners feeling worse.

Second, underlying Cathy and William's difficulties is the incongruity between their emotional expression and their emotional experience. Neither partner is able to clearly communicate his or her feelings. Cathy feels helpless, hurt, and unloved, but what she communicates to William is dissatisfaction with him and with their living circumstances. William feels attacked and unappreciated, but what he communicates to Cathy is disinterest and rejection.

Third, Cathy and William are trapped in a pattern of rigid expressive roles. Cathy is always criticizing; William is always withdrawing. Each partner's emotional behavior pulls for the other partner's opposing behavior. The result is a power struggle and a stalemate. With each interaction, Cathy and William's expressive roles become more and more entrenched. Neither partner is able to step out of his or her habitual role to understand the other person's perspective or to reach a compromise.

In this chapter, we describe therapeutic approaches to problems involving emotional behavior in the context of marital relationships. Specifically, we describe ways of helping couples to minimize destructive expression of negative emotion, to address incongruity between emotional expression and emotional experience, and to modify rigid expressive roles.

Many of the techniques we describe are also relevant for individual therapy. However, marital therapy provides a unique opportunity for understanding and modifying the interpersonal context of emotional expression. Partners reciprocally influence each other through their emotional behavior. Each person's expression or nonexpression can elicit emotional responses in the other, determine the other person's opportunity for expression, and provide consequences for the other person's emotional behavior. Marital therapists can work with how and what couples express, as well as how partners interpret each other's emotional behavior, in order to help couples communicate their feelings effectively.

MINIMIZING DESTRUCTIVE EXPRESSION OF NEGATIVE EMOTION

We have emphasized throughout this book that emotional expression is not necessarily beneficial. As the interaction between Cathy and William illustrates, some forms of emotional expression can be harmful to individuals and to relationships, particularly critical and intrusive behaviors (N. Epstein & Baucom, 1988; Gottman, 1993b, 1994; Kuipers, 1979; Strachan, Leff, Goldstein, Doane, & Burtt, 1986). Similarly, longitudinal and observational studies of interactions of married couples by Gottman (1994) noted that criticism, contempt, defensiveness, and withdrawal are particularly corrosive emotional behaviors that are deleterious to marital satisfaction and stability.

An important goal in marital therapy is to minimize destructive forms of expression of negative emotion. Broadly speaking, therapeutic techniques aimed at modifying destructive forms of negative emotional expression focus on deintensifying emotional responses and/or teaching communication skills. The goal is not to forbid clients to experience or express negative feelings, but rather to enable clients to express these feelings to their partner in ways that promote understanding and conflict resolution. In terms of the process model of emotional expression described in Chapter 1, this involves minimizing expressive leakage of poorly processed emotional experience and fostering greater cognitive processing of experience and more adaptive forms of emotional expression.

Deintensifying Extreme Emotional Responses

When people are in the throes of experiencing very intense emotions, their behavior tends to be extreme and impulsive. Spouses are likely to lash out at each other with hurtful remarks. They are unable to organize their thoughts, communicate clearly, or consider their partner's point of view. Thus a key strategy for minimizing destructive expression of negative emotion is to help clients to deintensify extreme emotional responses, so that they can think about and adaptively act upon their feelings rather than being driven blindly by them. Therapeutic techniques for deintensifying extreme emotional responses include communicating empathy, reducing physiological arousal, and engaging cognitive processing.

Communicating Empathy

The most basic and essential means by which therapists can help clients to deintensify their extreme emotional responses is by communicating empathically with their clients. Therapists need to show that they have heard and understood what their clients are experiencing. Perceiving that finally someone hears and understands their feelings can reduce clients' frustration and even provide them with some sense of relief (S. M. Johnson & Greenberg, 1994b; Wile, 1994).

Communicating empathy in the context of marital therapy can be tricky for therapists. Typically both spouses consciously or unconsciously try to get the therapist to take their side. Each spouse has a spoken or unspoken desire to have the therapist, as an objective outsider, declare that his or her feelings are the most "right" or "justified."

Therapists need to communicate empathy for both partners so that each person feels heard, validated, and supported in the relationship. As therapists join with each member of a couple they have to take care not to alienate the partner. Therapists should try to use descriptive rather than evaluative language in reflecting clients' feelings, and they should try to validate each spouse's experience without attributing blame to the other (Guerney, 1994; L. S. Greenberg & Johnson, 1988; S. M. Johnson & Greenberg, 1994b). Connecting with both partners is essential for creating a positive working alliance in marital therapy. By refusing to take sides and communicating empathy for both partners, therapists can help create a collaborative rather than a combative atmosphere between spouses, thereby deintensifying clients' extreme emotional responses and laying the groundwork for further therapeutic progress.

Reducing Physiological Arousal

Another technique for deintensifying extreme emotional responses involves teaching clients to recognize and reduce their physiological arousal. With this technique, clients learn to become more aware of their internal responses as they are occurring during interactions, so that they can short-circuit the escalation of negative affect. For instance, a husband might notice that, for him, the early signs that he is becoming angry include a racing heart and feelings of tension in the back of his neck. Once he has identified these early signs of anger, he can use them as cues to initiate various coping strategies so that his feelings of anger don't escalate into blind rage. He might use muscle relaxation or deep breathing exercises to regulate his emotional thermostat to within moderate ranges, or he might tell his wife that he needs to take a break from their discussion and agree to resume the discussion when he is feeling calmer.

Engaging Cognitive Processing

A third technique for deintensifying extreme emotional responses involves helping clients to engage their cognitive processing so that they can get some psychological distance from their feelings and thereby allow themselves the opportunity to cool down (Bowen 1978; Epstein & Baucom, 1988; Goldfried et al., 1974). There are several variations on this technique, but all of them involve helping clients to step out of their immediate emotional experience.

For instance, Bowen (1966, 1978; see also Papero, 1995) in his systemic approach to marital and family therapy, deliberately alters clients' narrow focus of attention from the marital unit to the wider family system. Each spouse is required to focus on his or her own family of origin and try to identify patterns of functioning and interaction that characterize the wider system. Each spouse is also encouraged to seek out and meet with members of his or her extended families to assist them in building his or her understanding.

This approach seems to serve two very important functions in marital therapy: First, it activates people's rational, analytical, or cognitive systems as they begin to think about their own families of origin, which has the effect of cooling their emotional responses and reorients their focus of attention. Second, it diffuses emotional attention to the wider family system and provides the opportunity for partners to have emotional needs and concerns met by people other than their spouses. This can take a lot of emotional pressure off the family or marital unit and can help to reduce anxiety.

Encouraging Active Listening. Encouraging spouses to actively listen to and reflect each other's thoughts and feelings is another way of helping clients to step out of their own immediate experience, engage their cognitive processing, and therefore deintensify their extreme emotional responses (e.g., Margolin & Fernandez, 1985). Often distressed spouses are so caught up with experiencing and expressing their own intense feelings that they do not listen to their partner. Therapists can ask spouses to take turns talking in session, designating one partner as the speaker and the other as the listener. While the speaker expresses his or her feelings, the listener's job is just to pay attention to and try to understand what the speaker is saying, without evaluating it or worrying about how he or she wants to respond. The listener does not have to agree with what the speaker is saying, just understand it. At appropriate intervals, the therapist asks the listener to repeat back to the speaker what he or she heard the speaker say. If necessary, the speaker can then clarify or elaborate on his or her meaning. When the speaker is satisfied that the listener has heard and understood what he or she is saying, the spouses switch roles, so that the listener is now the speaker, and vice versa.

This intervention slows down each respondent's reactions. It gives more time and space to think about the other person's perspective, rather than being flooded by one's own experience. It also encourages clients to express their feelings more carefully and deliberately rather than impulsively. Knowing that they have the listening spouse's full attention, speaking spouses can concentrate on helping the listener to understand their feelings, rather than lashing out desperately.

Identifying Core Beliefs. Still another way of engaging cognitive processing as a means of deintensifying extreme emotional responses involves having clients identify and articulate the core beliefs underlying their emotional responses (Baucom, Epstein, & Rankin, 1995; Gurman & Jacobsen, 1995). For example, with careful questioning by her therapist, Cathy might realize that her distress over William's withdrawal stems from her unspoken belief that "if he really loved me he would agree to buy the chest of drawers."

Once she articulates her underlying beliefs, Cathy can explicitly examine these beliefs and perhaps modify them. Cathy's therapist might encourage her to consider whether William does in fact expresses his love for her in ways that do not involve purchasing furniture, and whether there might be reasons other than a lack of love behind William's reluctance to buy furniture. These considerations might prompt Cathy to realize that, although she very much wants a chest of drawers, purchasing furniture is not necessarily the only or even the best indicator of William's love. With less absolute beliefs about how their relationship "must" be, Cathy is likely to be less distressed by William's behavior, better able to understand his point of view, and more willing to reach a compromise.

So far, we have described techniques for deintensifying extreme emotional responses as a means of minimizing destructive expression of negative emotion. Couples need to be able to regulate the intensity of their emotional responses so that they can inhibit impulsive and maladaptive bursts of expression. However, usually this is not enough. In order to minimize destructive expression of negative emotions, couples also need to know how to express their negative feelings in constructive ways. In the next section, we talk about ways of teaching clients emotional communication skills.

Teaching Emotional Communication Skills

Emotional communication skills can be taught indirectly or directly. Therapists' empathic reflections of clients' feelings are a means of indirectly modeling constructive forms of emotional expression that clients can internalize and use with each other. Therapists' reflections can convey several important messages that foster adaptive emotional expression.

First, therapists' reflections underscore the importance of feelings. As couples describe their difficulties, often in factual terms, therapists listen for and reflect feelings, thereby indicating that clients' feelings are valuable and worthy of attention. For instance, Cathy, from the anecdote at the beginning of this chapter, might go on at length about the details of their lack of drawer space, but by reading between the lines or noticing Cathy's tone of voice, her therapist might reflect Cathy's feelings of helplessness, or loneliness, or her wish for a sense of home.

Second, therapists' reflections are nonblaming. They place ownership of feelings clearly with the person feeling, rather than seeing them as thrust upon people by others. William might complain, "Cathy is such a nag! She pisses me off!" but his therapist is likely to reflect his feelings by saying, "You feel angry when Cathy asks you about buying furniture." When spouses verbally attack each other, therapist reflections can rephrase what each partner is saying and feeling in less accusatory terms, making it easier for the other partner to understand and accept. Christensen, Jacobson, and Babcock (1995) note that the expression of pain plus accusations of blame lead to marital discord, whereas the expression of painful feelings without blame can lead to acceptance and greater understanding between spouses.

Third, therapists' reflections are specific. They attempt to clearly symbolize and differentiate clients' feelings and to connect them to specific events. Clients might say that they feel "bad," but therapists' reflections encourage them to articulate how they feel bad and under what circumstances.

Adaptive forms of emotional expression can also be taught directly, through communication training (Christensen et al., 1995; Jacobson & Margolin, 1979; Margolin & Fernandez, 1985). This involves explicitly providing clients with specific guidelines for expressing their feelings and encouraging clients to practice using these guidelines until they feel comfortable with them. Examples of such guidelines include:

1. *Remarking on a positive aspect of the partner's behavior prior to making a complaint.* For example, before discussing her desire to buy furniture, Cathy might tell William, "I really appreciate how hard you are working to provide for us." Having his efforts acknowledged might make William more willing to listen to her complaint.

2. *Using "I" statements.* William might explain to Cathy, "I feel inadequate. You seem so unhappy. I worry that I'm not doing a good enough job as your husband, but I feel like I'm trying as hard as I possibly can." These comments clearly describe William's feelings and perceptions, which may or may not match Cathy's. Such statements underscore the subjective

nature of experience. They give Cathy a chance to understand William's feelings, without necessarily having to agree with them.

3. *Connecting negative feelings to specific behaviors rather than global traits.* Cathy might tell William, "When you withdraw, I end up feeling very isolated and confused and frustrated." When the speaker focuses on a specific behavior, the listener is more likely to see it as a manageable problem and be willing to discuss it. In contrast, global criticisms and character assassinations, such as, "You are an uncaring lout," are more likely to prompt defensiveness or counterattack than cooperation.

4. *Acknowledging one's own contribution to the problem.* Cathy might say, "I know I've been bringing up buying furniture a lot, and I realize my timing is terrible, since we're so strapped for money. I just want you to know how important this is to me." When one partner is able admit his or her role in creating the problem, it makes it easier for the other spouse to listen to that partner's concerns and perhaps to reciprocate by similarly acknowledging some responsibility for the couple's difficulties. This makes the problem's solution a collaborative endeavor and one in which neither spouse has to assume total responsibility.

Summary

To summarize, a first step in marital therapy often involves helping clients to minimize destructive expression of negative emotion. Destructive forms of emotional expression wound partners and interfere with mutual understanding and problem solving. Therapists can help couples to minimize destructive expression of negative emotions by helping them to deintensify their emotional responses, so that they are less likely to lash out with impulsive outbursts, and/or by teaching them emotional communication skills, so that they are capable of expressing their negative feelings in constructive ways.

The therapeutic techniques we have described so far in this chapter address *how* couples express their feelings. However, at least as important as how people express is *what* they express. Couples can be very adept at regulating the intensity of their emotional responses and can have exquisite communication skills, but unless they are talking about the issues that truly matter to them, they are unlikely to resolve their differences.

If therapists only attend to how couples express their feelings, they may be standing so close to clients' remarks that the wider picture of what couples want or need to express is obscured (Christensen et al., 1995; S. M. Johnson & Greenberg, 1994b, 1995; Ruckdeschel & Hazan, 1994; Wile, 1995). For instance, a wife might be quite articulate in expressing her displeasure about her husband's extensive activities outside the house and his heavy involvement with his career. However, underlying her complaints may be her fear that her husband is no longer interested in her. One approach to this scenario is to have the couple use their communication skills to renegotiate the time he spends outside the home. However, if this negotiation does not address the wife's underlying concerns, it is unlikely to be helpful in any lasting way. Another approach to this scenario is to help the wife to acknowledge and communicate her underlying fear. This gives the couple the opportunity to talk about the wife's basic concerns. Her husband may be able to reassure her of his love, and perhaps together they can come up with solutions that allow her to feel more important. This may involve more expression of affection, more time spent together, or some other way that would symbolize for the wife that her husband cares about her. Some of the solutions might not entail the husband changing his routine at all.

In the next section, we describe therapeutic strategies for addressing incongruity between emotional expression and experience. These strategies address what spouses express to each other, with the goal of helping them to articulate their most central feelings and concerns.

ADDRESSING INCONGRUITY BETWEEN EXPRESSION AND EXPERIENCE

One of the key reasons that Cathy and William were unable to resolve their difficulties is that neither of them was able to communicate his or her most important feelings. As the model presented in Chapter 1 illustrates, incongruity between expression and experience can arise for various reasons. Clients may have difficulties perceiving, understanding, or accepting their feelings, or they may perceive their social environment as disallowing expression. Different forms of nonexpression require different therapeutic approaches (see Chapter 8).

When incongruity between expression and experience stems from difficulties in perceiving or understanding feelings, therapeutic techniques aimed at heightening clients' access to their internal affective states and helping them to symbolize their experience may be useful. For instance, therapists can help clients to become aware of their nonverbal expressive behavior by asking clients to exaggerate fleeting facial expressions or repeat certain actions of their hands and feet and then put these expressions into words (L. S. Greenberg & Johnson, 1988; S. M. Johnson & Greenberg, 1994b; Pierce, 1994; Wile, 1995). Therapists can also reflect clients' feelings using vivid language and metaphor to capture each partner's experience in the moment.

When incongruity between expression and experience stems from clients' difficulties in accepting their own feelings, therapists need to create a context of safety so that clients feel able to acknowledge their feelings. Wile (1994) suggests that one reason partners may not be able to be congruent in expressing their affective experience is that they may be ashamed of certain feelings and may not be able to represent these accurately to themselves let alone their partner. For example, William expresses anger at Cathy's demands because he cannot face his own fear of being an inadequate husband and a poor provider. If therapists detect shame, then they have to be especially careful to empathize with their clients and help them articulate their own disowned feelings. Therapists' acceptance of and responsive attunement to clients' shameful feelings can help clients give themselves permission to acknowledge and communicate these feelings to their partner.

When incongruity between expression and experience stems from clients' fears concerning their partner's reactions, therapists can help clients to acknowledge their fears and bring them into awareness so that they can be tested and disconfirmed. Sometimes clients' fears regarding expression are based on their partner's actual rejecting or unresponsive behavior in previous interactions. In this case, therapists need to work with the partner using the techniques we described earlier in this chapter in the section on minimizing destructive expressions of negative emotion, in order to help the partner respond empathically. Other times, clients' expression-related fears stem from their attachment history. Perhaps in their family of origin emotional expression was ridiculed or punished. In this case, therapists can help clients to distinguish between their past and their present context and to test the current validity of their previous assumptions about the consequences of expression. For instance, based on his past experience, William might fear that expressing vulnerable feelings to Cathy will lead her to see him as a wimp. However, if, with his therapist's help, William musters his courage to tell Cathy about his feelings of inadequacy, and Cathy responds by expressing love and concern for him, William not only connects with Cathy at an emotionally meaningful level, he also gains new information that contradicts his old fears. The experience of having expression-related fears disconfirmed in the session creates positive interactions between spouses that facilitates trust and increases the likelihood of this happening in the future.

Addressing incongruity between expression and experience is central to emotionally focused marital therapy, developed by L. S. Greenberg and Johnson (1988). Using this approach, therapists help clients to access and communicate their previously unacknowledged feelings of vulnerability, fear, or resentment. Therapists then redefine or reframe clients' problems in terms of these newly accessed feelings. By identifying and accepting these feelings, clients gain new information about what is significant for them. By expressing their basic needs and wants to their partner, clients can achieve new understanding of their difficulties, generate new solutions, and establish new patterns of interaction with each other.

The therapeutic strategies we have described so far are focused primarily on individuals, in that they address each spouse's expression of his or her own feelings. However, it is also important to consider how partners' emotional behavior fits together in an interpersonal pattern. In the next section, we look at ways of modifying couples' rigid expressive roles.

MODIFYING RIGID EXPRESSIVE ROLES

In the anecdote about Cathy and William, both partners are locked into rigid expressive roles. Each partner's emotional behavior pulls for an opposing behavior from the other partner, resulting in a maladaptive interpersonal cycle. The more Cathy criticizes, the more William withdraws; the more William withdraws, the more Cathy criticizes. As we described in Chapter 7, maladaptive interpersonal cycles can take a number of different forms (e.g., the mutually hostile pattern, the miscarried helping pattern, the demand–withdraw pattern), but the key features of these cycles are that they are entrenched and that they compound participants' distress. Rigid expressive roles often result in power struggles or power imbalances within relationships. Partners are so focused on protecting or defending themselves or counterattacking that they are unable to understand each other or to resolve their difficulties.

Therapeutic strategies aimed at modifying rigid expressive roles help spouses to step out of their entrenched and unproductive ways of relating to each other. Below we describe techniques pertaining to three general strategies for modifying rigid expressive roles. These general strategies involve (1) shifting the focus beyond the immediate dyadic interaction, (2) reinterpreting partners' emotional behavior, and (3) expressing novel, role-inconsistent feelings.

Shifting the Focus beyond the Immediate Dyadic Interaction

One general strategy for modifying rigid expressive roles involves helping clients to shift the focus of their attention beyond their immediate dyadic interaction. There are several specific techniques for accomplishing this.

Recognizing Interpersonal Patterns

One technique for shifting clients' focus involves helping clients to recognize interpersonal patterns in their emotional behavior. Therapists can encourage spouses to step back and observe their interactions rather than automatically responding in habitual ways. This allows spouses to understand the reciprocal nature of their emotional behavior and their mutual responsibility in creating maladaptive interpersonal cycles. Instead of concentrating on protecting themselves from "the awful things he/she does," spouses can begin to focus on "the terrible traps we dig for our-selves." Recognizing maladaptive interpersonal patterns of emotional com-munication is often a necessary first step in changing these patterns.

Externalizing the Problem

Another technique for shifting clients' focus beyond their immediate dyadic interaction is to use the empty-chair technique to externalize their problem (Koerner & Jacobson, 1994). Instead of locating the problem within one of the partners, spouses visualize it as a separate entity apart from the couple. The goal here is to identify a common problem that partners can unite against. In Cathy and William's case, the therapist might ask them to imag-ine their financial difficulties sitting in an empty chair and then invite each spouse to talk to and about these difficulties. By conceptualizing their prob-lems as separate from themselves, couples can gain some emotional dis-tance from their distress and can join together to share their problems instead of struggling against each other.

Fostering Self-Care

A third strategy for shifting clients' focus beyond their immediate dyadic interactions is to foster self-care. Therapists can encourage partners to nourish themselves and meet their needs in as many different ways as possi-ble rather than relying on their partner to take care of them. When spouses expect each other to meet all of their needs, it can put tremendous strain on the relationship (Koerner & Jacobson, 1994). On the other hand, cultivat-ing autonomy and independence by helping each member of the couple to identify his or her needs and think of ways of meeting these outside the re-lationship can provide some breathing space so that spouses become less in-vested in maintaining their rigid expressive roles with each other. For example, a wife who feels neglected because of the long hours her husband works might decide to develop interests and friendships in the community as a means of meeting some of her social needs. This may lead her to be less demanding of her husband. Her husband, in turn, may become more will-ing to pay attention to her because he no longer feels coerced by her de-mands.

Reinterpreting Partners' Emotional Behavior

In addition to shifting couples' focus beyond their immediate dyadic inter-actions, another general strategy for modifying rigid expressive roles in-volves reinterpreting partners' emotional behavior.

Therapists can reframe partners' expression or nonexpression by ex-plaining it in an empathic way or pointing out the positive features of certain behaviors (Beach & Fincham, 1994; L. S. Greenberg & Johnson, 1988; Koerner & Jacobson, 1994; Margolin & Fernandez, 1985). Therapists might also urge spouses to generate alternative, kinder explanations for their partner's behavior. For example, William might come to see Cathy's requests for a dresser as an expression of her desire to be a good wife to him and to create a home for them rather than as a personal attack on him. Cathy might come to see William's withdrawal as a sign that he feels threatened or overwhelmed, rather than as an indication that he doesn't care about her. Reinterpreting partners' emotional behavior in a more benign light can help spouses experience greater tolerance and acceptance of each other. It also encourages compassionate rather than adversarial responses, allowing spouses to modify their rigid expressive roles.

Expressing Novel, Role-Inconsistent Feelings

A third general strategy for helping couples to modify their rigid expressive roles involves encouraging them to express novel, role-inconsistent feelings. Expressing role-inconsistent feelings provides an opportunity for partners to experiment with different roles and ways of being with each other. This allows them to develop new views of themselves and each other and to create new interactional patterns. Expressing role-inconsistent feelings usually involves accessing and communicating positive or vulnerable feelings.

Expressing Positive Feelings

When spouses' interactions are dominated by direct or indirect expressions of hostility, evoking role-inconsistent expressions of positive feelings can help them to modify their rigid expressive roles. One way of doing this is to have couples remember and talk about what they liked about each other before their difficulties began or what attracted them to each other initially. By recalling positive memories, partners' moods can be changed so that they are able to be more responsive and forgiving toward each other. By expressing positive feelings, such as love and empathy, partners act in affirming and validating ways toward each other. This helps them to reconnect with each other, fosters a sense of intimacy, and offers a vivid contrast to their usual adversarial patterns of interaction.

Expressing Vulnerable Feelings

When spouses' interactions are dominated by a power struggle or a power imbalance, evoking role-inconsistent expressions of vulnerable feelings can be a means of helping them to break out of their rigid expressive roles. By revealing their vulnerable feelings to each other, spouses can promote understanding, elicit compassion and care, and create a sense of trust. For instance, a husband whose angry, blaming expressions usually elicit counterattacks from his wife might find that telling her instead about his feelings of fear or insecurity gives his wife a chance to respond in a supportive way. His wife's warm response may then prompt the husband to be more willing to express other vulnerable feelings, more confident that she will respond compassionately the next time, and less likely to resort to his usual angry tirades. The wife may also be more willing to reciprocate by expressing some of her vulnerable feelings.

However, expressing vulnerable feelings to each other is risky for unhappy spouses. What if they bare their souls and their partners rip them apart? In this case, the partner that is exposed may feel betrayed and cling even more tightly to his or her rigid expressive role (L. S. Greenberg & Johnson, 1988; S. M. Johnson & Greenberg, 1994b; Koerner & Jacobson, 1994).

Prior to initiating the expression of vulnerable feelings by one of the partners, it is important for therapists to assess whether the other will be able to respond with compassion and care. In predicting partners' likely response to the expression of vulnerable feelings, therapists can consider several different clues:

1. How much positive affect is there between spouses? Are they able to recall and reevoke positive memories of what they like and enjoy about each other? Do they laugh together in the session? Do they report having good times together outside the session?
2. How willing are spouses to see each other's behavior in a benign light? Are they able to respond to their therapists' attempts to reframe their problems in terms of a common enemy or a mutually created pattern of interaction? Are they willing to accept an explanation of their partner's emotional behavior in terms of positive intentions or understandable concerns?
3. How good are their emotional communication skills?
4. How committed are they to each other—for example, is one or both spouses seriously contemplating separation or have they voiced a strong commitment to each other in spite of their difficulties?

If these clues look promising, therapists can be reasonably confident that partners will respond positively to the expression of vulnerable feelings. If these clues do not look promising, it is probably best to lay further groundwork before encouraging spouses to express vulnerable feelings. Therapists may also want to suggest individual therapy for each spouse so that partners can address some of their individual needs and concerns prior to coming together to renegotiate their relationship and develop new patterns of interaction.

Summary

We described three general strategies for modifying couples' rigid expressive roles: shifting the focus beyond the immediate dyadic interaction, re-interpreting partners' emotional behavior, and expressing novel, role-inconsistent feelings. All three of these strategies attempt to help spouses to step out of their automatic and maladaptive patterns of interaction. By developing a more benign view of each other's emotional behavior and communicating to each other in new ways, couples can move beyond their entrenched power struggles toward greater understanding and problem resolution.

CONCLUSION

In this chapter we looked at ways of addressing problematic emotional behavior through marital therapy. We described therapeutic techniques for helping couples to minimize destructive expression of negative emotion, to address incongruity between emotional expression and emotional experience, and to modify rigid expressive roles.

For conceptual clarity, we presented these three problems separately, but, as the story at the beginning of this chapter suggests, these problems often feed off of each other in a dynamic fashion. When spouses express their feelings in destructive ways, they limit each other's expression, fostering incongruity between expression and experience, and trapping each other in rigid expressive roles. When partner's interactions are dominated by rigid expressive roles, they are cut off from expressing positive or vulnerable feelings, resulting in incongruity between expression and experience, and they are more likely to resort to destructive forms of expression of negative emotion.

Therapists need to use their judgment in deciding which problem involving emotional behavior they will focus on first. With highly combative couples, it is often important to help them turn down the emotional thermostat and develop skills for regulating the expression of negative emotions before addressing other issues. Alternatively, in cases where incongruity between expression and experience prevents couples from focusing on their most central concerns, this issue may take top priority. In the case of long-standing, highly entrenched difficulties, therapists may be aware that rigid expressive roles seem to be the most inimical factor in having the couple deal with difficulties in their relationship, and the therapist may address this issue first. Before attempting any interventions, therapists need to make sure that they have fostered an empathic connection with each partner and that both partners feel safe in the therapeutic encounter. Therapists need to be able to supply a supportive and caring environment so that couples can address their problematic emotional behaviors.

12

Expression-Related Interventions in Health Psychology

INTRODUCTION

Henry sighed. He had drunk enough that his thoughts were becoming hazy. A sense of numbness was beginning to set in. He glanced around the bar, seeing familiar faces, but nobody he particularly wanted to talk to. He took a last drag on his cigarette, stubbed it out, then stared dully at the dregs of the beer he was holding. He noticed that his hands still had some unhealed cuts from the fight he got into last weekend. He'd been drinking, and some loud-mouthed young punk had gotten on his nerves. Luckily, this time, he hadn't been arrested.

Henry supposed he had always talked with his fists. As a kid, he was often suspended from school for fighting. His family was poorer than most of the other families in the neighborhood, because neither of his parents was able to hold down a steady job. Henry hated the fact that everybody in their small town knew about his family's problems. He was always ready to lash out at anyone he thought looked down on him.

Henry shifted uncomfortably in his chair. He guessed he ought to call it a night and head home, but it wasn't like there was anything or anyone waiting for him there. He supported himself, more or less, by doing occasional, small-scale construction work, so his place wasn't much to look at. He'd been married, briefly, when he was in his early 20s, but his wife walked out on him after only 6 months. He never hit his wife, but he did break things when he got mad, and once he punched a hole in the wall. His wife had hated his temper. Henry didn't even try to talk her out of leaving. He concluded he just wasn't the "married happily ever after" type. He hadn't bothered to date anyone seriously since then.

Henry felt a growing ache in his chest. He had been having these

273

pains a lot lately. He supposed he ought to see a doctor, but he didn't have the money, and he figured they were all quacks anyway. Henry lit another cigarette and motioned for the bartender to give him another beer.

Could helping Henry to express his feelings in adaptive ways enhance his psychological well-being? Undoubtedly. Would it make him physically healthier? Possibly.

Our description of Henry (which is based on H. S. Friedman, 1992, pp. 5–6) suggests many possible avenues for expression-related interventions that could lessen Henry's distress, enhance his coping efforts, and perhaps improve his health. For example, teaching Henry to minimize and control his rages might decrease the rage-related hormone surges that place a strain on his heart. Providing him with the opportunity and the skills necessary for appropriate emotional expression might lessen his distress, guide active coping efforts, and help him to cultivate positive social relationships. Gaining better understanding of his problems and learning more adaptive coping options by talking over his feelings with a therapist could also make it less likely that Henry will resort to drinking as a way of drowning his sorrows and his angina.

A number of recent reviews describe mechanisms by which emotions might influence physical health (e.g., Adler & Matthews, 1994; Cohen & Rodriguez, 1995; Gross, 1989; Leventhal & Patrick-Miller, 1993; Robinson & Pennebaker, 1991; Smith, 1992; J. S. Tucker & Friedman, 1996). These reviews point to laboratory findings of short-term changes in the immune and/or endocrine systems associated with emotional experience and emotional expression. They suggest that, over time, such reactions could have a medically significant impact on physical health (e.g., see discussions by Davison & Petrie, 1997; Levenson, 1994). These reviews also point to the impact of emotional responses on patients' symptom perception and health-related behaviors (e.g., compliance with medical treatment regimens).

Drawing from this theoretical and empirical work linking emotions and health, psychologists have developed interventions for virtually every medical condition (see examples in Baum, Newman, Weinman, West, & McManus, 1997). Many of these interventions explicitly or implicitly address emotional expression. They are based on the assumption that being able to express their feelings in adaptive ways makes it possible for patients (1) to minimize the psychological and physiological toll of intense or enduring distress and (2) to rely less on unhealthy ways of managing distress (e.g., fighting, smoking, drinking, and avoiding medical care). The goals of these interventions are to help patients to cope with the stress of their illness, to enhance their psychological well-being, and perhaps even to improve the course of their disease.

In this chapter, we describe some representative examples of expression-related interventions that are commonly used with medical patients. Specifically, we discuss the role of expression in enhancing self-awareness and effective problem solving among psychosomatic patients and in fostering social support among cancer patients. We also consider therapeutic ways of modifying maladaptive patterns of anger expression among cardiac patients. Although we include some discussion of theoretical and empirical rationales, our emphasis is on describing a variety of clinical techniques. But first, we want to mention some cautions that therapists need to bear in mind when using expression-related interventions with medical patients.

SOME CAUTIONS CONCERNING THE USE OF EXPRESSION-RELATED INTERVENTIONS WITH MEDICALLY ILL PATIENTS

Peggy Orenstein, a 35-year-old woman with breast cancer, recently published some excerpts from her diary concerning how she coped with finding out about her diagnosis. One passage in particular highlights the danger of overstating and oversimplifying the links between psychological and physical well-being:

> Over lunch today, an old friend asked me in all seriousness whether I thought I had a "cancer personality." What would that be? Someone who holds anger in, she said. She's been on antidepressants for over a year, and *I* have the cancer personality?
>
> Maybe deep down the reason it bothers me so much when people say I should change my diet or get rid of stress is that I am afraid I did do something wrong. . . .
>
> It doesn't help that there is a distinct undercurrent of accusation in many of the books supposedly promoting "healing." I can't believe what I've found skimming best sellers in the health sections of bookstores. Bernie Siegel writes, "There are no incurable diseases, only incurable people." Louise Hay claims that cancer returns when a person doesn't make the necessary "mental changes" to cure it. Those are tidy ideas, placing the onus of the illness on the ill and letting the healthy off the hook.
>
> Still, I doubt I gave myself cancer because I'm reluctant to tell one of my best friends she's an idiot. (Orenstein, 1997, p. 32)

Interpreting the empirical literature concerning emotional behavior and health is not easy. Inconsistencies among empirical findings and practical difficulties involved in spelling out the connections between immediate psychological events and long-term physical outcomes mean that *no* link has been unequivocally established.

Experts disagree concerning precisely what sort of emotional responses are toxic, because asking this question in different ways yields different answers. Some investigators argue that distress in general is problematic. For instance, H. S. Friedman and Booth-Kewley (1987a) combined the results of over 100 studies looking at personality and illness. They did not find evidence for links between specific emotions and specific diseases, but they did find that chronically experiencing negative feelings such as anxiety, sadness, and hostility made it twice as likely that people would suffer from a variety of physical problems, including asthma, headaches, ulcers, and heart disease. Other investigators insist that experiencing and expressing different emotions has different health consequences. For instance, drawing from laboratory observations, Leventhal and Patrick-Miller (1993) note that different emotions are associated with different patterns of psychophysiological response, which argues for the importance of considering specific emotion–disease links. Still other investigators suggest that it is not so much what people feel but how they handle those feelings that determines the health consequences of emotional responses. Based on experimental studies in which participants are instructed to express or inhibit their feelings, Traue (1989) argues that expression of particular emotions is linked to specific physiological changes, whereas inhibition of expression results in a generalized physiological stress response.

Clinicians need to be cautious about inferring treatment implications from general patterns of relationship between expression or nonexpression and physical health. Even when specific, robust associations are found between emotional behavior and illness, it doesn't necessarily imply that changing emotional behavior will alter illness outcomes. The links between expression and health are not necessarily simple or direct. For instance, H. S. Friedman and his colleagues (1993) analyzed longitudinal data and found links between a number of emotion-related personality traits in childhood and later mortality. One of their findings was that the trait of cheerfulness was associated with increased mortality. Obviously, this does *not* mean that clinicians should try to stamp out cheerfulness so that clients will live longer. In this case, J. S. Tucker and Friedman (1996) speculate that the link between cheerfulness and mortality is likely to be mediated by a constellation of health-related behaviors, such as smoking and drinking, and psychosocial variables, such as life stressors and coping strategies.

Moreover, even when expression-related interventions help medical patients, they may not work for the reasons originally hypothesized. For instance, a number of theorists have suggested that cancer patients who participate in support groups might have enhanced immune function. Fawzy et al. (1993) conducted an intervention study with cancer patients in which, as predicted, they found theoretically positive changes in immune parameters associated with treatment. The intervention also enhanced survival. However, the observed immune changes were not related to cancer mortality. Similarly, many theorists have suggested that anger-management programs might help cardiac patients to minimize the excessive cardiovascular reactivity that puts a strain on their heart. However, although many studies have demonstrated the health benefits of such programs, Johnston (1992) concludes that, at present, there is no convincing, direct evidence that Type A reduction interventions (which focus on anger and hostility reduction) work by modifying cardiovascular reactivity.

The confusion that remains concerning theoretical and empirical links between emotional behavior and physical health suggests three important caveats that therapists should bear in mind when using psychological interventions with medically ill patients: First, these interventions are definitely *not* a substitute for appropriate medical care. Second, many medical patients don't want psychological treatment (e.g., Meyer & Mark, 1995; Pennebaker, 1990). Refusal plus dropout rates are often as high as 50% (see review by B. L. Andersen, 1992); thus these should not be considered universal treatments. Third, when medical patients do agree to psychological treatment, it is critically important that therapists communicate a rationale for treatment that neither blames patients for their illness nor suggests that patients' ailments are "all in their heads."

Medical patients' concerns about the implications of psychological treatment should be addressed in the first session. For instance, patients might wonder, "Does this mean my doctor doesn't believe I'm really sick?" or "Does this mean I'm crazy as well as sick?" or even "Is it my fault that I'm sick?" They might benefit from some reassurance that the therapist believes that their symptoms are real, that they aren't crazy, and that illness arises because of multiple factors including biological vulnerabilities and environmental triggers and it certainly isn't anyone's fault. Clients might be asked, in a nonthreatening way, whether they have noticed any connections between their mental and physical health. Are their symptoms more bothersome when they are distressed? Do their symptoms make them feel anxious or irritable? Are they less apt to follow medical directives when they feel sad or overwhelmed? Client observations such as these may provide an inroad to discussing emotion–health connections in a personal sense, while acknowledging that these connections are not fully understood in a general sense. In discussing the goals of treatment, therapists should emphasize managing distress rather than curing or preventing illness. Alleviating distress is important for psychological well-being, and it might even enhance physical well-being, but there is certainly no guarantee of this.

With these caveats in mind, we now turn to specific examples of how expression-related interventions might be used with particular medical populations.

ENHANCING SELF-AWARENESS AND EFFECTIVE PROBLEM SOLVING AMONG PSYCHOSOMATIC PATIENTS

Psychosomatic illnesses are those disorders, such as ulcers, colitis, asthma, or rheumatoid arthritis, in which psychological processes often play a major etiological role. One theory suggests that psychosomatic patients sometimes suffer from alexithymia, which involves an inability to describe one's feelings in words (Sifneos, 1973; Taylor et al., 1991; see Chapter 3). Some investigators even go so far as to argue that alexithymia is a necessary but not sufficient condition for the development of psychosomatic disorders (e.g., Anderson, 1981).

Sachse (1998) explains how alexithymia might result in psychosomatic illness: Because these clients have difficulty understanding their own feelings, they tend to focus on concrete, external facts and avoid introspection. Consequently, Sachse argues, these clients do not know themselves very well. Their coping abilities are compromised because they do not know what they want or what matters to them. Because they have a weak sense of identity, they feel worthless, they suffer from social uncertainty and anxiety, they are unable to assert themselves appropriately by saying "No" to excessive social demands, and they tend to react to stressful situations with avoidance rather than direct action. Presumably this self-alienation and impaired coping means that these individuals have chronically higher levels of sympathetic nervous system responding (cf. J. B. Martin & Pihl, 1986; Rabavilas, 1987; Wehmer et al., 1995). Sachse suggests that this puts a strain on the body, which combined with physical vulnerabilities, ultimately results in illness.

Sifneos (1991), who originally coined the term *alexithymia,* believes that these individuals are poor candidates for psychotherapy because of their diminished capacity for introspection. Instead he recommends medication plus support and reassurance from their general physician. However, other therapists have devised interventions specifically addressing alexithymic traits.

For instance, Sachse (1998) recommends goal-oriented client-centered psychotherapy to address the alexithymic characteristics of clients with psychosomatic disorders. This therapy involves using emotional expression to enhance emotional insight. It focuses on the way that clients process their own experience. Specifically, the therapist helps clients (1) to recognize how they avoid processing their emotional experience, (2) to understand how this avoidant processing interferes with clarifying and resolving their problems, and (3) to learn more constructive processing modes as a guide to effective coping.

A key component of this therapy involves the therapist addressing the various strategies that psychosomatic clients might use to avoid self-reflection. For instance, a common strategy is for clients to answer the therapist's questions about their feelings by saying "I don't know." Sometimes, "I don't know" means "I'm afraid I don't have a good answer." In this case, the therapist merely needs to reassure clients that they aren't expected to have a perfect answer, that, in fact, the task in therapy is to deal with those aspects of experience that are still unclear. The therapist gently urges clients to look for hints or traces of feelings that can provide the basis for further work.

More often, "I don't know" means "I don't want to look at my experience." In this case, clients do not attempt to examine their experience, but instead block the process by immediately responding "I don't know." Sachse suggests that clients' desire to avoid discussion of some aspect indicates that this aspect is highly relevant but has not been clarified or integrated, and therefore needs to be processed. He suggests that the therapist increase pressure to stay with the topic and establish a counternorm assuming that a person always has at least some data concerning his or her experience. For instance, the therapist might say, "I know this is difficult for you, but please continue. People always feel or think something, even if it's diffuse."

If clients continue to insist that they don't know what they are experiencing, Sachse suggests that the therapist shift to "processing the processing work" by directly addressing the avoidance. The therapist might ask, "What makes it so difficult for you to stay with and take a closer look at your feelings?" The therapist might also describe the avoidance process, saying, "I noticed that as soon as I asked you how you felt about that, you immediately responded 'I don't know,' without pausing to see if you might have some glimmer of a feeling. What speaks against trying to clarify your feelings right now?" The general idea is not to criticize clients, but to help them recognize difficulties in the way they process their feelings, so that they can have better access to their feelings as a basis for decision and action.

In Sachse's interventions with psychosomatic patients, clients first address how they process their emotional experience, and then shift to clarifying that experience. In order to be able to draw upon their emotional experience as a guide for effective coping, clients must first perceive their experience as an important source of information, be able to reflect upon their experience, and notice and reduce avoidance strategies. After that, therapeutic work involves using expression to understand experience and clarify motives, goals, and values. The therapist encourages clients to seek out ways to apply their new self-understanding to everyday life. For example, clients might do so by asking for something, saying "No," or seeking out new experiences.

Sachse (1998) states that his intervention was effective in a study involving 87 male and female clients with psychosomatic gastrointestinal diseases. Compared to controls, clients receiving this treatment reported more self-acceptance, less conviction that they are externally controlled, and improved coping. He speculates that the resultant stress reduction is likely to improve gastrointestinal symptoms, but he did not directly assess this.

Swiller (1988) describes a similar therapeutic approach with alexithymic clients, involving both group and individual therapy, which also might be helpful with psychosomatic patients. Group therapy sessions provide the opportunity for emotional expression and interpersonal feedback as well as observational learning. Individual sessions help the client understand and accept his or her feelings. Swiller suggests that this combination of group and individual work maximizes clients' opportunities to learn to effectively express their feelings, while protecting their self-esteem and minimizing unproductive stress.

Using expression to help medical patients to "get in touch" with their feelings so that they can use this information to guide and enhance their coping efforts is a common therapeutic strategy. The ideas of Sachse and others concerning how alexithymic characteristics might compromise health and how these deficits in emotional understanding might be addressed therapeutically are interesting. However, to date, there is very little research on these topics, and what research does exist tends to be fraught with methodological problems such as reliance on self-report as the only outcome measure and assessment of alexithymic characteristics using unreliable and unvalidated measures (see Bagby, Parker, & Taylor, 1994, and Bagby, Taylor, & Parker, 1994, for a well-validated and psychometrically sound measure of alexithymia). Until better outcome studies are available, we believe that clinicians treating patients with psychosomatic illnesses should use these interventions only with great caution, regarding them as intriguing but unproven ideas.

FOSTERING SOCIAL SUPPORT AMONG CANCER PATIENTS

Several investigators have suggested that emotional expression is important in coping with cancer and may even influence the course of the disease (e.g., Greer & Watson, 1985; Gross, 1989; Temoshok, 1987, 1990, 1993). The personality trait called *Type C*, which entails "pathological niceness," emotional suppression, and unassertiveness, may be a risk factor for cancer. Type C individuals are aware of their negative feelings, but deliberately refrain from expressing them, and instead present a facade of pleasantness and compliance.

Unlike the link between alexithymia and psychosomatic illness, the link between Type C and cancer has been established based on methodologically sound research. Although there are some conflicting findings, we believe this reflects the complexity of the relationship rather than any intrinsic unreliability of the findings.

As Buck (1993) points out, Type C personality is neither a necessary nor a sufficient cause of cancer. Chronically being nice doesn't make individual cells grow out of control. Rather, research suggests that for some cancers, under some circumstances, emotional factors may interact with biological mechanisms to influence cancer progression. For instance, many investigators have pointed to the effects of emotional processes on immune functioning as a possible mediating factor in cancer (see review by Cohen & Herbert, 1996). Others have suggested that emotional suppression while under stress may cause increased autonomic and hormonal responding with deleterious effects for cancer patients (Pettingale, 1985).

The evidence showing the importance of emotional processes in cancer suggests that interventions addressing these may be helpful for emotional and even physical health. Psychosocial interventions involving cancer patients have received a great deal of attention in both professional (see reviews by B. L. Andersen, 1992; Helgeson & Cohen, 1996; Meyer & Mark, 1995) and lay literature (e.g., B. Siegel, 1986, 1989). These interventions typically involve groups, which may or may not have a therapist leader, and they focus on the expression of emotions as a means of fostering social support.

The intervention study with the most extraordinary results was conducted by Spiegel and his colleagues (Spiegel, Bloom, Kraemer, & Gottheil, 1989; Spiegel, Bloom, & Yalom, 1981). Women with metastatic breast cancer were randomly assigned to either a control group or a discussion group, while receiving routine oncological care. The discussion group had weekly 90-minute meetings for 1 year led by a psychiatrist or social worker and a therapist who had breast cancer in remission. Members were encouraged to express their feelings about their illness and its affect on their lives, to face and grieve losses, and to discuss ways of improving their interpersonal relationships. They were also taught self-hypnosis for pain management. The emphasis of the group was coping with cancer by "living as fully as possible, improving communication with family members and doctors, facing and mastering fears about death and dying, and controlling pain and other symptoms" (Spiegel et al., 1989, p. 890). At no time were clients led to believe that the intervention would affect the physical progress of their disease. In fact, Spiegel and his colleagues undertook this study with the expectation of countering "the often overstated claims made by those who teach cancer patients that the right mental attitude will help to conquer the disease" (Spiegel et al., 1989, p. 890).

Results showed no differences between the discussion and the control group at 4-month or 8-month assessments, but at 1 year, the discussion group clients reported feeling less depressed, more vigorous, less fatigued, and less confused. At a 10-year follow-up, the discussion group clients were found to have survived an average of 18 months longer than control group clients.

Other studies have shown less promising results. For example, Gellert, Maxwell, and Siegel (1993) conducted a retrospective study of women with breast cancer using survival analysis based on death certificates. They compared participants in a cancer support program to another group of women with similar illness characteristics who did not participate in this program. The program involved weekly 90-minute meetings during which clients received individual counseling, patient peer support, family therapy, and instruction in relaxation, meditation, and positive imagery. The goals of the program were to facilitate acceptance of the disease, build hope, and enhance effective coping. Results showed no differences in survival between the two groups. Paez, Basabe, Valdoseda, Velasco, and Iraurgi (1995) also report disappointing results from unstructured cancer support groups.

In a thought-provoking review, Helgeson and Cohen (1996) note that research on social support and adjustment to cancer shows important contradictions between the results of descriptive and correlational studies versus interventions studies. On the one hand, descriptive studies show that the kind of social support that cancer patients find most helpful is emotional support—having someone listen to their feelings, empathize, and care about them. This type of support is more important to them than informational support (offering advice) or instrumental support (providing concrete assistance). Similarly, correlational studies find that cancer patients' psychological adjustment is more closely linked to their perceptions of emotional support than to other forms of support. On the other hand, psychosocial intervention studies with cancer patients show that short-term interventions aimed at providing informational support through education about the disease and how to cope with it are as effective or more effective than short-term interventions focusing on emotional support through group discussion.

If emotional support is perceived as so important by cancer patients, why have short-term group discussion interventions, intended to provide this kind of support, been relatively unsuccessful? In explaining this contradiction, Helgeson and Cohen (1996) suggest that group discussions have the potential to affect clients either positively or negatively. Ideally, expressing one's feelings in a warm, accepting environment enhances self-esteem and optimism about the future. It enables one to understand, accept, or alter these feelings (cf. L. S. Greenberg & Safran, 1989). However, as we have argued throughout this book, emotional expression does not always yield positive results. The impact of expression depends on what is expressed, to whom, and how. Helgeson and Cohen (1996) describe some possible problems with unstructured peer group discussions among cancer patients. One potential problem is that expressing painful feelings in a group context can sometimes exacerbate distress. Unlike education-based interventions, discussion groups can heighten awareness of distress. Talking about feelings and listening to other group members' expressions of emotion may interfere with attempts to deny feelings or threaten clients' beliefs that they are coping well. Moreover, when groups involve clients with differing cancer sites and differing prognoses, members may have difficulty validating each others' feelings. When group members learn that others in the group do not share their feelings, they may feel even more isolated than before. Also, being around people with worse prognoses may diminish optimism.

Some of these issues can be addressed by having appropriately trained group facilitators. These facilitators can urge members to keep conversations on relevant topics, promote acceptance among group members, normalize and validate feelings, and clarify any misunderstandings that arise.

On the other hand, a number of theorists have argued that even when expression results in short-term increases in distress it can be beneficial in the long run (e.g., Coates & Winston, 1983; Pennebaker et al., 1990). The benefits of acknowledging and dealing directly with painful feelings may take time. It is noteworthy that in Spiegel et al.'s (1989) group discussion intervention, improvements relative to another group of women who received only standard medical care were evident at 1 year, but not before.

Another possible problem with peer discussion groups is that they do not address and may interfere with existing sources of support. Helgeson and Cohen (1996) suggest that emotional support from existing network members is more important for well-being than emotional support from other cancer patients. Compared to relationships with friends and family members, relationships among members of peer discussion groups are usually less intimate, less long-lasting, and even somewhat artificial, because they exist only in the context of the intervention. Furthermore, belonging to a peer discussion group may reinforce participants' identity as a member of a separate, stigmatized group, perhaps interfering with participants' ability to obtain support from friends and family in their everyday environment.

This does not mean that peer support is unhelpful. It can be an important adjunct to existing support networks or even compensate to some extent for faulty or lacking networks. Peer support may be the best option when existing relationships are unhelpful or highly conflicted and are not amenable to change. Peer support can also be useful when caregivers are feeling too overburdened to participate in an intervention. In fact, Helgeson and Cohen (1996) suggest that long-lasting peer support interventions may be effective precisely because they cultivate real friendships among group members, thereby changing "artificial" relationships into "real" ones. Spiegel et al. (1989) noted that in their intervention, group members spontaneously wrote poetry for each other, visited each other in the hospital, and even met in the home of a dying member. This kind of closeness is unlikely to develop after just a few meetings.

Helgeson and Cohen (1996) point out that descriptive and correlational research on the importance of emotional support involves existing network members, whereas intervention research generally involves support provided by new network members. They suggest that interventions focused on enhancing communication in existing relationships may be a more efficient and effective way of meeting patients' needs for emotional support than creating new relationships. These interventions could focus on enhancing patients' and family members' abilities to express their feelings clearly, clarifying misunderstandings resulting from mismatched expressive styles, and dispelling myths such as the one that talking about illness or death is bad for the patient. Along these lines, one study found that communication training for postmastectomy women and their husbands led to less depression and increased sexual satisfaction compared to a no-treatment control group (Jamison, Wellisch, & Pasnau, 1978).

If network members are not available to participate in an intervention, another possible approach is to use therapy to help patients to effectively muster support from existing sources outside of therapy (cf. Cohen et al., 1988). Patients could be encouraged to express their feelings and needs clearly to potential support providers and to distinguish between helpful and unhelpful sources of support. They could also be educated about typical responses to caregiver strain, in order to increase understanding of network members' social communications.

Helgeson and Cohen's (1996) review contrasts interventions focused on providing informational support (with little emphasis on emotional expression) versus those focused on providing emotional support (with a strong emphasis on emotional expression). However, they acknowledge that most interventions combine these two elements to some extent. Even the most didactic interventions are likely to evoke feelings in participants that they will want to express. Even the most feelings-oriented groups are likely to cover some factual information. It may well be that both types of interventions are important. Moreover, cancer patients at different stages of the disease may have different therapeutic needs in terms of information versus emotional support.

B. L. Andersen (1992) suggests that interventions focused on practical information may be especially important early on, whereas interventions involving emotional expression may be especially relevant for more seriously ill patients. Based on her review of the literature, Andersen argues that newly diagnosed patients are best served by a crisis intervention approach, involving an emotionally supportive context to address fears about the disease, coupled with provision of information about the disease and medical treatment plus direct training in cognitive and behavioral coping strategies. She notes that multiple studies have documented the effectiveness of these intervention components at reducing the distress of newly diagnosed cancer patients, whereas group support interventions with no structured content have *not* yielded measurable benefits relative to no-treatment controls.

Whereas low- or moderate-risk cancer patients often show improved psychological adjustment without treatment, high-risk patients who do not receive psychosocial intervention tend to become more distressed. B. L.

Andersen (1992) notes that for these patients existential distress is paramount, as their worst cancer-related fears are realized. Grappling with intolerable symptoms, disability, dependence, and dying make feelings of self-efficacy or control fleeting. For these patients, concerns about death and quality of life are central, and being able to express their feelings concerning these issues in a therapeutic environment may be especially important, particularly when they and/or their loved ones feel unable to do so.

MODIFYING MALADAPTIVE PATTERNS
OF ANGER EXPRESSION AMONG CARDIAC PATIENTS

Hostility is an enduring negative mood state characterized by the expression of irritability and anger (Smith, 1992). Cross-sectional and longitudinal studies suggest that hostility may be the toxic element of Type A behavior, leading to the long-term development of arteriosclerosis and increasing the probability of acute coronary events during stress (see reviews by Smith, 1992; Contrada, Leventhal, & O'Leary, 1990).

Of the three expression—health links that we describe in this chapter, the connection between anger or hostility and cardiovascular disease is by far the best documented by research. Physiological, personality, and epidemiological studies suggest that anger is an important risk factor in the development and exacerbation of cardiovascular diseases (Siegman & Smith, 1994). Many intervention studies have attempted to modify anger responses within the context of Type A behavior treatments (e.g., M. Friedman et al., 1986; Bennet, Wallace, Carroll, & Smith, 1991; Thurman, 1985a, 1985b). These studies have shown marked reductions in anger, Type A behavior, and even myocardial infarction rates (M. Friedman et al., 1986), but few of them have directly assessed the effects of anger reduction. Because our focus in this book is on expression, rather than reviewing these broad treatments, we will examine specific interventions aimed at modifying clients' harmful patterns of anger expression.

Cognitive-Behavioral Approaches to Anger Management

Deffenbacher (1994) provides detailed descriptions of four overlapping phases in cognitive-behavioral interventions aimed at anger management, which we describe below. The goal of these interventions is *not* to eliminate anger, but rather to provide clients with coping strategies so that they are not driven blindly by their anger. Instead of automatically responding to anger-provoking situations with explosive outbursts, clients are encouraged to think about these situations and their own reactions in a nonescalatory way and to express their feelings in a more moderate and effective fashion.

Deffenbacher (1994) points out that many clients with anger-related difficulties initially approach therapy feeling guarded or perhaps coerced into coming. They are likely to balk if they feel the therapist is trying to control them or tell them what to do. So, it is especially important with these clients to pay attention to the therapeutic relationship and to use a collaborative approach. For instance, when between-session homework is used, it should stem directly from the client's observations or concerns, and the client should be responsible for deciding the details concerning the specific form of the homework.

Phase 1: Enhancing Personal Awareness of Anger

The first phase in cognitive-behavioral anger management involves cultivating personal awareness of anger. Many clients have a sense that anger "just happens" to them. The goal at this stage is to enhance self-understanding as clients and the therapist work together to develop a thorough understanding of what triggers clients' anger and how they respond. The therapist asks clients to recount the details of specific anger incidents. As clients describe these incidents, the therapist encourages them to elaborate on their feelings (frustrated? furious? stewing?), their thoughts (What images occur? What phrases do clients say to themselves when they are angry? To what extent do they ruminate?), and their physical responses (clenched jaw? tight stomach?). The therapist also asks about the latency, frequency, duration, and intensity of clients' anger reactions.

Spelling out precisely what clients do when angry and how and why these behaviors change over time is essential for understanding their anger expression styles. For instance, do clients stew silently then explode? Do they explode then withdraw? Do they start expressing irritation and progress to fury? Does their anger in one situation (e.g., work) spill over into other situations (e.g., home)? It is also important to note the consequences of clients' anger responses for health, work, personal relationships, and self-esteem. Do clients feel guilty or depressed about their anger responses? Exploring variations in anger responses across different situations can be especially revealing. Helping clients to articulate why they felt or expressed intense anger in one situation but not another may reveal important information concerning their particular triggers, vulnerabilities, or coping resources. In addition to exploring recent anger incidents, discussing how anger was experienced and expressed in the family of origin can help clients articulate their scripts regarding anger.

Along with this in-session exploration, clients are encouraged to ask themselves questions when anger occurs in their daily lives, such as "What am I responding to?", "Is this what I am really angry about?" or "Is this the way I want to handle this?" Self-monitoring, an assessment strategy in which clients record characteristics of actual anger-related incidents shortly after they occur, can be a helpful means of identifying thoughts or situations that are especially likely to trigger angry feelings in a particular client or for obtaining a clear picture of how that client typically expresses anger.

This careful elaboration of clients' anger responses is essential for guiding subsequent treatment and for monitoring progress in therapy. In some cases, becoming aware of patterns in their anger responses may enable clients to more effectively use their existing coping skills to modify their experience and expression of anger. In other cases, the understanding gained from this exploration lays the groundwork for later interventions by providing clients with a multifaceted view of their anger responses. This exploration is also important for establishing a therapeutic relationship. The therapist's ability to show respect for clients' observations and acceptance of clients' feelings while helping clients examine their anger responses can build therapeutic trust.

Phase 2: Response Disruption and Relaxation

The second phase described by Deffenbacher (1994) involves practicing response disruption and relaxation. A variety of strategies are used to reduce the intensity of anger arousal, such as removing eliciting cues, disrupting escalating cognitive–emotional–physiological cycles, and engaging in alternative activities. Which particular strategies are used depends on the particular nature of clients' anger response as well as clients' preferences as to which strategies seem most comfortable or appealing. One example of such strategies is negotiating a time-out, which involves delaying a response ("I'll get back to you about that later this afternoon") or taking a break when an interaction gets too heated ("I'm feeling so angry now, I'm afraid I'll say things I'll regret. Why don't we talk about this again in half an hour, after I've had a chance to calm down?"). Other examples include calming visualization, progressive muscle relaxation, mental distraction (counting to 10, reciting soothing scripture verses), and palliative self-talk (e.g., "I've dealt with worse than this before"). Specific discussion and practice are important in helping clients to use these strategies smoothly and effectively. For instance, a therapist might help clients to brainstorm in order to come up with a number of different phrases for requesting a time-out and then role-play using these phrases.

Deffenbacher points out that although these strategies are simple, clients need to believe that they are "allowed" to use them. For instance, clients whose anger script dictates that "one should never back down from a fight" will not readily use time-out strategies. They first need to identify and articulate their anger script and explore the personal meaning of that script and the consequences of sticking to it or failing to do so. For these clients, it may be helpful to reframe response disruption techniques in terms of showing strength or control rather than backing down.

Phase 3: Cognitive Restructuring and Humor

The third phase involves using cognitive restructuring and humor to address the form and content of anger-engendering information processing. For example, angry clients often jump to malevolent conclusions concerning other people's intentions, without considering benign explanations for other people's behavior. Also, angry clients often have very rigid rules for living. Their personal preferences or desires are framed in terms of "should," "ought," or "must," and they view violation of these dictates as catastrophic and enraging.

Anger-engendering cognitive processes tend to be automatic and habitual. Interventions addressing these generally aim to increase self-awareness and flexibility in information processing and to help clients to understand that anger does not stem directly from a situation, but rather from clients' interpretation of the situation. Whereas the response interruption strategies discussed above reduce maladaptive anger expression by addressing anger responses, cognitive interventions reduce maladaptive anger expression by addressing the elicitation of angry feelings (see Gross's [1998] distinction between antecedent- and response-focused coping, described in Chapter 2).

Cognitive intervention strategies are *not* always appropriate. Under some circumstances, clients' most adaptive option is to work to create changes in an untenable environment or to remove themselves completely from a toxic environment, rather than to simply perceive the environment differently. The therapist can help clients examine their circumstances, understand their responses, consider their options, and speculate about the likelihood of changing the environment and/or the self. However, ultimately it is up to clients to decide whether they just want to be less distressed by their existing circumstances ("I don't want things to get to me so much") or whether they can no longer tolerate their circumstances. If a client observes that circumstances are not likely to change, that no alternative circumstances are available or desirable, and that other people in their circumstances seem to be experiencing less distress than they are, cognitive interventions seem relevant.

The initial task in cognitive interventions is to help clients identify their automatic anger-related thoughts, usually using techniques such as careful interviewing about specific events, visualization, and self-monitoring. Some cognitive therapists label anger-engendering cognitive processes as irrational and even provide clients with a list of such errors (e.g., Ellis, 1977). However, we believe a more respectful approach is to help clients understand how, because of their particular experiences, they have a tendency to jump to certain conclusions or to make certain assumptions that may or may not be valid in a given situation. Rather than using an extensive prepared list, we prefer to encourage clients to articulate, in their own words, just a few important examples of these assumptions.

Rather than dismissing clients' views as irrational, we emphasize that clients' assumptions made sense under past circumstances, but may not be relevant or helpful under current conditions. Rather than setting the therapist up as the ultimate arbitrator of rationality, we help clients to explore and test the basis and the consequences of their assumptions.

Once identified, automatic anger-related thoughts can be explicitly examined and tested. A therapist may use Socratic questions such as "What's another way of looking at that?", "What evidence is there for that?", or "And that would mean . . . " Clients are encouraged to think of ways of testing their assumptions in their daily life and to articulate new insights as counterresponses to old assumptions. For instance, a client whose old assumption was "Everything *must* go according to plan" might come up with a counterresponse of "It's not worth sweating the small stuff," and then practice identifying small stuff not worth sweating over whenever his or her plans go awry. The therapist could encourage the client to notice the consequences of following the initial assumption versus the counterresponse.

Deffenbacher (1994) notes that humor can sometimes be useful in this phase, both because it is an anger-incompatible affect and because it allows clients to gain cognitive distance and shift perspectives toward a more benign interpretation of provocative situations. However, he cautions that humor should be silly, rather than hostile or sarcastic. Furthermore, it should only be attempted later in therapy when there is a strong therapeutic alliance, because some clients may react to humor by thinking they are being laughed at. An example of humor is claiming that a child is "just doing his or her job" by frustrating parents, rather than blaming misbehavior on the child's malevolent personality. Another example is encouraging clients to visualize, in a concrete way, someone they have labeled as an "ass."

Phase 4: Cognitive and Behavioral Skill Enhancement

The fourth and final phase in Deffenbacher's (1994) description of cognitive-behavioral anger management involves enhancing problem-solving and social skills. In this phase, the client works on enhancing skills for dealing with provocative situations in a constructive way. For instance, clients may work on developing skills related to effective problem solving (including recognizing when to stop trying to solve unsolvable problems), interpersonal communication, assertiveness, employee management, or parenting. Which skills are emphasized depends on clients' particular circumstances and concerns. The work in the previous phases, helping clients to understand and moderate the intensity of their anger responses, enables clients to learn and implement these skills effectively. Skills training usually involves some didactic presentation by the therapist (e.g., description of stages of problem solving; distinction between assertiveness and aggressiveness; modeling of open-ended rather than closed-ended questions for active listening), followed by in-session and between-session practice implementing these skills. The general goal is to provide clients with alternative strategies, other than explosive expressions of anger, for managing and preventing anger-provoking situations.

Components of cognitive-behavioral anger-management interventions have been extensively evaluated in controlled studies, individually and in combination, and with a variety of populations (e.g., Achmon, Granek, Golomb, & Hart, 1989; Deffenbacher, McNamara, Stark, & Sabadell, 1990; Deffenbacher & Stark, 1992; Moon & Eisler, 1983; Novaco, 1980). Overall, studies show that these interventions yield robust and lasting changes.

Cognitive-behavioral interventions are straightforward, but we must caution that they should not be used without a thorough and compassionate understanding of the client. The impact of a therapeutic intervention depends on the meaning that that intervention carries for the client (Butler & Strupp, 1986; Safran, 1990b). Safran, Vallis, Segal, and Shaw (1986) describe a case in which a cognitive intervention yielded a negative and unexpected reaction because the therapist did not have a clear understanding of the client's view of himself and others or his pattern of relating. The client told his therapist that he consistently felt that others were uncaring toward him. The therapist noticed that the client had a rigid and demanding style of interacting. He used a cognitive approach to try to help the client lower what the therapist thought were excessive expectations of others and to help the client attend to instances in which others did behave in emotionally supportive ways. Following this intervention, the client canceled the next session and threatened suicide.

A subsequent and more helpful reformulation of this case suggested that because the client believed his own needs were unacceptable, he expected to be rejected or abandoned if he ever expressed them directly. He therefore tended to express his needs in an angry, blaming, or indirect manner, or not at all. This style of emotional communication made it difficult for others to respond warmly. The therapist's interventions aimed at lowering the client's expectations of others were experienced by the client as confirming his belief that expressions of vulnerability lead to rejection, and led the client to feel angry and hopeless.

Interpersonal Approaches to Anger Management

Cognitive-behavioral approaches to anger management usually focus on individual perceptions and behavior, but recent theorizing concerning the relationship between anger and cardiovascular disease has focused on interpersonal processes. Drawing from Bandura's (1977) notion that personal characteristics and social environment are reciprocally determined, Smith and Pope (1990) propose a transactional model of anger. They argue that chronically angry people create hostile interpersonal environments through their thoughts and actions, and these hostile environments, in turn, maintain their anger. Chronically angry clients tend to have a general view of the world as a hostile place. They mistrust others, expect mistreatment, and assume malicious intent. Given these expectations, their antagonistic or defensive behavior seems reasonable and even prudent, but it may inadvertently create the interpersonal conditions they fear. Their expressions of anger, hostility, and aggression increase interpersonal conflict and undermine social support. Their conflictual relations with others then confirm their initial expectations and maintain their anger. Thus these individuals experience more frequent, more intense, and more enduring anger reactions, with accompanying heightened levels of cardiovascular reactivity, which ultimately compromise their physical health.

Smith and Pope's formulation is very compatible with Safran's (1990a, 1990b; Safran & Segal, 1990) cognitive-interpersonal approach to psychotherapy. This approach involves using the therapeutic relationship as a means of understanding and modifying cognitive-interpersonal cycles. Safran describes *interpersonal schemas* as core beliefs representing self–other interactions. These interpersonal schemas activate and are maintained by *cognitive-interpersonal cycles,* in which individuals' initial schema-driven expectations lead them to behave in ways that elicit schema-consistent behavior from others (see Chapter 7). Clients with more rigid interpersonal schemas behave more similarly across different relationships, leading to less diversity in their interpersonal experiences. This means that individuals with rigid maladaptive schemas have little opportunity to encounter new interpersonal experiences that might modify their interpersonal schemas—all of their relationships turn out the same, unsatisfying way. For this reason, in cognitive-interpersonal therapy, the therapist tries to intervene in a way that elicits new adaptive behaviors from clients, which create positive interpersonal experiences and thereby help clients to disconfirm their dysfunctional interpersonal schemas.

In order to do this, the therapist uses his or her own feelings to identify *interpersonal markers,* which are specific client behaviors or communications that are problematic. Therapists' feelings are definitely not infallible indicators of problematic client behaviors, since some reactions may reflect idiosyncratic therapist sensitivities, but they can be an important source of clues concerning clients' styles of relating to others. As a participant–observer, the therapist notices the reactions that the client evoke in him or her, identifies the specific behaviors that evoke these reactions, then deliberately "unhooks" by refraining from following through on the action tendency automatically elicited by clients' interpersonal pull. For instance, a therapist may feel irritated by a client's quarrelsome expressions of hostility, but refrain from responding with hostility. By not responding in the expected way, the therapist provides this client with a new interpersonal experience, which can elicit new behaviors from the client. A therapist may also metacommunicate with clients about the reactions that they evoke in the therapist and provide specific feedback about the nonverbal or verbal expressive cues that lead to these reactions. Safran (1990b; Safran & Segal, 1990) notes that clients are often unaware of their impact on others or of what they do to elicit this reaction. Providing this type of feedback can help clients to decenter from their immediate experience so that they can begin to understand their own contribution to interpersonal interactions and to change aspects of their communication that maintain maladaptive cognitive-interpersonal cycles.

CONCLUSION

In this chapter we have described a number of expression-related interventions that can be helpful to medical patients. First we looked at the use of expression to enhance self-awareness and effective problem solving among psychosomatic patients. Then, we considered expression as a means of fostering social support among cancer patients. Finally we looked at ways of modifying maladaptive patterns of anger expression sometimes found among cardiac patients. These interventions address not just the overall quantity of expression but also the quality of expression. The goal of all of these interventions is to enable clients to engage in forms of expression that help them to effectively manage their distress in order to enhance their psychological well-being and perhaps even their physical health. In each case, we noted that understanding the meaning that emotional behavior carries for the client is critical for being able to design and implement appropriate interventions.

PART V

Conclusion

13

Balance in Emotional Behavior

INTRODUCTION

Emotional behavior is arguably the most fundamental and fascinating characteristic of human beings. As the link between internal experience and the outside world, it is intimately tied to who we are, how we feel, and how we relate to others. It has been studied in virtually every area of psychology, including developmental, personality, social, clinical, and health psychology.

In this book, we have explored our understanding of emotional behavior (i.e., expression or nonexpression) as a multifaceted process, influenced by intrapersonal and interpersonal feedback. The organizing framework for this book has been the process model of emotional expression that we presented in Chapter 1. This model illustrates how emotional experience, which occurs initially at a prereflective level, is processed through increasing levels of cognitive differentiation. This cognitive elaboration is guided by felt experience and also transforms that experience, in a dialectical process. People first become aware that they feel something, then they label what they feel, then they go on to determine the meaning of those feelings for themselves and others. Varieties of emotional expression and nonexpression arise because overt expression can occur *or* be blocked at any of these levels. We have described clinical interventions concerning emotional behavior that focus on the levels of attention, labeling, interpretation, social context, and overt behavior.

Throughout the book we have emphasized several key themes that are directly related to our model: (1) the distinction among the components of emotion (i.e., emotional expression, experience, arousal, and reflection), (2) the continuum of expressive awareness and control, (3) the interplay between cognition and emotion, and (4) the importance of the social context.

295

These themes are critical to understanding the relationship between emotional behavior and well-being and to designing effective interventions addressing maladaptive emotional behavior.

The central concern of this book has been the relationship between emotional behavior and well-being. We explained in Chapter 1 that emotional expression and nonexpression can take many forms, and that either can be adaptive or maladaptive. At this point, we would like to offer some guidelines concerning when and how emotional behavior is related to well-being. Consider the following hypothetical example:

Bella arrives home from work to be greeted by a huge pile of dirty dishes. She is tired. Tonight, like every Tuesday night, she worked late, and her husband was in charge of feeding the kids dinner, tucking them in bed, and tidying up. Bella hangs up her coat and walks over to assess the extent of the mess more closely. She notices a bowl from breakfast, with the remains of her husband's bran flakes, which have now turned to cement. She opens a cupboard and finds it empty. She will have to wash some dishes just to get a plate and a glass for her own dinner. She groans inwardly.

Bella is clearly feeling disgusted and annoyed. Should she express these feelings to her husband? Not necessarily. As most people in long-term, close relationships realize, sometimes the best response to minor or occasional irritations is to hold one's tongue. If tonight's dishes disaster is not typical, or if Bella suspects there might be mitigating circumstances (maybe the children were unusually ornery tonight), she might choose to ignore the dishes and find a paper plate for herself. She might even decide to surprise and delight her husband by tackling the dishes herself, even though it's his night, as an expression of love. On the other hand, if Bella finds a dirty kitchen particularly irksome, or if this scene is a regular occurrence, Bella may need to express her irritation to her husband. He is most likely to respond positively if Bella can express her feelings in a moderate, specific, nonaccusatory manner. But, what if Bella has already had four calm discussions with her husband about the dishes, to no avail? What if the problem is not just the dishes? Perhaps her husband agrees to share the household chores, but then laughs about his uncompleted chores and assumes Bella will pick up the slack. What if Bella has been feeling increasingly furious, resentful, and devalued? In this case, it may be important for Bella to express her feelings intensely so that her husband can understand the extent of her frustration and the importance of this issue to her. Then they can work out a compromise they can both live with. But first, maybe Bella should eat some dinner, so her level of irritation isn't exacerbated by hunger.

Even this simple example shows that there can be no blanket proscriptions regarding emotional behavior and well-being. Emotional behavior is not a yes/no question. The consequences of expression depend on what is expressed and how. Different responses may be most adaptive for different individuals or in different social contexts.

Although this example focuses on just a single incident, it is patterns of emotional behavior across time and across situations that are critical for understanding the effects of expression or nonexpression. Emotional behavior is most likely to influence well-being when it is associated with relatively intense, frequent, and/or enduring emotional states. Whether or not someone expresses an occasional feeling of mild annoyance is probably unimportant. On the other hand, repetitively harping about habitual irritation or chronically holding in feelings of intense rage can have serious consequences.

A FUNCTIONAL VIEW OF EMOTIONAL BEHAVIOR

So, what can we say, at this point, concerning the relationship between emotional behavior and well-being? In earlier chapters we suggested a number of possible mechanisms linking expression or nonexpression with physiological, psychological, and interpersonal adaptation. We now offer a summary of possible adaptive functions of emotional expression. We also describe ways that these functions can be derailed by either maladaptive nonexpression or maladaptive expression. We conclude this chapter and this book by describing what we believe are three characteristics of adaptive emotional behavior that can be used as broad guides to clinical interventions.

Table 13.1 presents a summary of possible adaptive functions of emotional expression. It also outlines ways that maladaptive emotional behavior, either excessive nonexpression or excessive expression, can interfere with these functions.

Arousal Regulation

One possible benefit of emotional expression is arousal regulation. Bodily arousal represents both a signal that something important is happening and a physiological preparedness to respond. Expression and nonexpression can influence arousal. Emotional behavior is adaptive when it facilitates the return of emotional arousal levels to baseline. It is maladaptive when it intensifies or prolongs arousal to an unhealthy extent.

Traditional psychosomatic models posit that nonexpression leads to emotions being "discharged" somatically, ultimately resulting in illness (e.g., Alexander, 1950). More modern theories emphasize the physiological "work" involved in suppressing or actively inhibiting expression (e.g., Pennebaker, 1992). Over time, the strain on the body of trying *not* to express may compromise health. Counteracting inhibition through emotional

TABLE 13.1. Possible Benefits and Costs of Emotional Behavior

Possible benefits of adaptive expression	Possible costs of maladaptive nonexpression	Possible costs of maladaptive expression
Arousal regulation	Suppression requires physiological work that may take a cumulative toll on the body.	Extreme or unrelenting expression may intensify or prolong arousal to an unhealthy extent.
Self-understanding	Lack of awareness of distress hinders initiation of appropriate coping efforts.	Being overwhelmed by emotion interferes with clear thinking and hinders the use of emotional responses as a source of information about the self and the environment.
Coping/emotional processing	Effortful preoccupation with holding in feelings impedes coping efforts and intensifies distress.	Passive preoccupation with emotion may interfere with ability to implement active coping efforts.
Adaptive social communication	Inability to communicate feelings may interfere with the development of intimate relationships and the marshaling of social support.	Inappropriate expression may drive away potential or existing social support. Violating social norms or personal values may evoke feelings of shame.

disclosure presumably alleviates this strain. Emotional disclosure of traumatic experiences has been linked to immunological changes consistent with better health (e.g., Esterling et al., 1994; K. J. Petrie et al., 1995), as well as less symptom reporting (e.g., Pennebaker & Beall, 1986).

On the other hand, emotional expression can also augment physiological arousal (Siegman, 1994). Expressing feelings often involves attending to feelings; focusing on feelings can intensify the experience of these feelings and their accompanying physiological arousal. When expression is excessive and unremitting, the associated bodily strain may compromise health. Research on affectively intense individuals, who characteristically experience intense emotions and tend to be highly expressive, suggests that these individuals are more likely than others to have physical health problems (R. J. Larsen & Diener, 1987). Just like an engine that revs too high wears out sooner than usual, unrelenting and intense emotional expression may take a toll on the body.

Self-Understanding

A second, very important function of emotional expression is enhancing self-understanding. Expression makes covert emotional experience overt. Therapists often encourage clients to express their feelings, in order to help clients recognize and understand these feelings. In daily life, as well, emotional expression can play an important role in interpreting inner experience. Putting emotional experience into words fleshes out the meaning of that experience. Observing one's own verbal and nonverbal emotional behavior can provide important clues about emotional experience, particularly when that experience is vague or confusing (Bem, 1972; Laird & Bresler, 1992).

The informative function of expression can be lost or thwarted by either excessive nonexpression or excessive expression. When nonexpression involves an inability to recognize or understand emotional experience, it's like going through life blindfolded. Individuals with these forms of nonexpression don't have available the potentially adaptive information contained in emotional experience. If they don't recognize when they are feeling distressed or why, they are less likely to initiate adaptive coping efforts.

Excessive expression can also impede understanding of emotional experience. Exploring feelings in a helpful way requires a "middle distance" from inner experience (e.g., Rice & Kerr, 1986; Scheff, 1979). If individuals are overdistanced from their emotional experience, they are unaware of it and are unable to access it as a source of information to guide their thoughts and behavior. If they are underdistanced, they are so flooded by feelings that they can't reflect upon their experience or modulate it. They express their emotions, but in an unfocused, spilling-over manner. To gain emotional understanding individuals need to be aware of their inner experience but not overwhelmed by it. They need to experience and express their feelings vividly, but with enough distance that they can thoughtfully examine and interpret these feelings.

Coping/Emotional Processing

A third possible function of expression is facilitating coping efforts and emotional processing. Expression can be a way of working through emotions, making sense of them, and drawing upon them to motivate adaptive behavior (Safran & Greenberg, 1991; Stanton et al., 1994). On the other hand, too little or too much expression can be paralyzing.

When nonexpression involves effortful suppression, individuals may become preoccupied with thoughts of trying to hold their feelings in. The more they try not to express, the more they think about whatever it is they are trying not to express (cf. Wegner & Gold, 1995; Wegner et al., 1987). This preoccupation with emotional expression and experience can intensify distress and interfere with other coping efforts. Just as someone with both hands tightly clasped over his mouth to keep from making any sound doesn't have free hands to do anything else, someone who is using all her energies to avoid expressing can't implement any other coping strategies.

Excessive expression can also derail coping efforts. This occurs when expression involves rumination or passive brooding about emotional experience (e.g., Nolen-Hoeksema, 1991). When expression is part of adaptive emotional processing, it carries a sense of movement and change, involving new, deeper understanding and readiness for action. In contrast, ruminative expression is stagnant. Repetitively expressing "I'm miserable; I'm always miserable; I'm just plain miserable" doesn't enhance coping. Instead it rehearses and intensifies distress, and it interferes with the implementation of active coping strategies.

Adaptive Social Communication

So far our discussion of the adaptive functions of expression has focused on responses within an individual. However, expression usually takes place in a social context and the social functions of expression are critically important for well-being. Ideally, expression leads to intimacy, a sense of connection with others, and the availability of practical and emotional support.

Nonexpression can interfere with the development of intimacy and the marshaling of social support. True interpersonal connection requires the ability to express both positive and negative feelings. A woman might express tender feelings toward her fiancé, but how can he really know her or build a life with her if she only lets him see her when her hair is curled and she is feeling perky? How can a man's family and friends know he needs their support and comfort unless he tells them? How likely are they to sustain support efforts unless he can acknowledge these efforts and express his appreciation for them? Thus, maladaptive nonexpression can involve a breakdown in the emotional communications that build and sustain close relationships.

On the other hand, maladaptive expression can actively destroy relationships. Frequent and uncontrolled outbursts of emotion can drive away potential or existing social support. Intense and enduring expressions of distress may be more than significant others can cope with (Coates & Winston, 1987; Coyne et al., 1988; Gottlieb & Wagner, 1991). Angry tirades are more likely to be met with counterattack than with understanding or acceptance (e.g., Tavris, 1989). Moreover, inappropriate expression that violates social norms and elicits negative responses from others can evoke shame in the expresser.

To summarize, the four main functions of emotional expression are arousal regulation, self-understanding, coping/emotional processing, adaptive and social communication. These functions can occur individually or in combination. They can be thwarted by either maladaptive nonexpression or maladaptive expression.

CHARACTERISTICS OF ADAPTIVE EXPRESSION

By now, it should be clear that when it comes to emotional behavior, the answer is *balance*: balance between indiscriminate venting of feelings and deadening emotional silence; balance between following one's own impulses and considering the impact on others (cf. Gross & Muñoz, 1995). More specifically, we believe that adaptive emotional expression has three characteristics, which can serve as guides for clinical interventions.

Integration

Ideally, emotional expression reflects and enhances an integration between experiential and cognitive response systems. The integration between these two response systems is evident in two ways: First, individuals are able to label and interpret their affective experience. Second, individuals accept and feel comfortable with their emotional experience and expression.

The first aspect of integration in emotional expression, involving labeling and interpretation, is illustrated by R. D. Lane and Schwartz's (1987) description of levels of emotional understanding. These levels progress from crude awareness of bodily sensations all the way to highly differentiated understandings of the nuances of one's own and others' emotional experience. The extent to which people are able to draw upon their emotional experience and understand it determines how effectively they can use this information and communicate it to others. Merely saying "I feel bad" communicates very little information about how either the self or others ought to respond. More differentiated expressions, such as "I feel resentful and discouraged," point more precisely to the issues needing to be addressed. Thus this aspect of integration in emotional expression involves the ability to recognize and communicate sometimes subtle distinctions among affective states, in order to draw out the meaning of experience.

The second aspect of integration in emotional expression involves incorporating emotional expression within one's self-view. Geller (1984) argues that emotional well-being necessitates the ability to tolerate and even enjoy intense affects such as love, anxiety, grief, or shame. Without this capacity, individuals may experience a lack of authenticity or a troubling sense of disengagement. Strictly forbidding oneself to express certain emotions or rigidly confining oneself to only mild expressions is in some sense walling oneself off to life. Different individuals and different cultures have different ways of expressing their feelings, often guided by their particular beliefs or values. The specific form of expression is less important than that individuals have an ego-syntonic way of acknowledging, articulating, and communicating their feelings. This aspect of integration in emotional expression involves finding and using one's true emotional voice.

For experiential therapists, integration is the heart of therapy. Through empathic reflection, therapists encourage clients' emotional expression. This technique addresses both aspects of integration in emotional expression: It helps clients to flesh out the meaning of their experience by putting their feelings into words, thereby integrating their rational and emotional response. It also communicates to clients that their expressions of emotion are acceptable and valuable, thereby helping to integrate clients' emotional behavior with their self-view.

Cognitive-behavioral therapists usually place less emphasis on labeling experience, but they do sometimes address integration of emotional expression with self-views, such as when they help clients to modify extreme beliefs concerning emotional behavior. For instance, a therapist might help a client to recognize and consider the basis for his belief that "I must *never* express anger to people I care about or they will abandon me." The client might discuss the origins of this belief and consider whether the circumstances giving rise to this belief are still relevant. With the therapist's help, he might consider the personal consequences of adhering to this belief. He might come up with ways of testing this belief, perhaps starting with expressing mild irritation with a particularly trustworthy relative.

The importance of integration in emotional expression suggests that it is critical for therapists to understand and respect clients' individual and/or cultural values concerning emotional expression. Forcing clients who value stoicism to burst into tears is unlikely to be helpful. They are likely to experience this expression as coerced, alien, and shameful. These clients may prefer more subtle or symbolic forms of expression. Therapists need to be flexible in working with the client's preferred style of expression rather than routinely imposing their own preferred style. Although some clients readily engage in highly perceptive expression from the first session, other clients prefer a more gradual approach. They might need time to build trust in the therapist or to gradually become comfortable with openly acknowledging their feelings. They might simply process their emotional experience more slowly than others, in which case the therapist needs to allow them time and space for this processing rather than jumping in prematurely and perhaps inaccurately with a label for the clients' feelings. One client may find it easier to write about her feelings and then talk about what she has written with her therapist. Another client might use painting as a way of giving voice to his feelings and use this as a starting point in communicating his feelings to his therapist or significant others. Still another client may want the therapist's help in devising a personally meaningful ritual for expressing his feelings.

When circumstances or symptoms suggest that clients would benefit from altering their usual expressive style, sensitively and respectfully helping clients to examine the beliefs underlying their old style versus a new style and providing clients with a rationale for changing may be important precursors to behavioral change. Consider the example of a client who believes that expressing anger in a moderate way and calmly discussing problems in a close relationship is "being fake," and who prides herself on "being real." However, her husband, who is not interested in coming to therapy, adamantly refuses to stay in the same room with her when she uses her usual style of angry screaming. This client is unlikely to want to try another style of expression unless she can reconcile it with her view of herself. Through gentle questioning and discussion, the therapist might help this client to observe that screaming works very well with her mother, who speaks the same emotional language, but it doesn't work with her husband. She may decide that approaching her husband in a more moderate way isn't "being fake," it's being emotionally multilingual. It's getting her "real" point across in a way that he can understand.

Flexibility

The second characteristic of adaptive emotional expression is flexibility. People need to have the capacity to express a variety of emotions in a variety of ways. For instance, a woman who only knows how to "be nice" and express her feelings mildly may have an especially difficult time if a coworker makes an unwanted sexual overture and she can't bring herself to snarl at him, "Hands off!" A parent who always screams at a toddler for all transgressions, major or minor, may find that the child tunes him out and doesn't learn important distinctions, such as that kicking the baby is much worse than spilling milk.

Many therapeutic interventions are aimed at enhancing the flexibility of emotional behavior. Interpersonal therapists (e.g., Kiesler, 1991; Safran & Segal, 1990) argue that people who have rigid, maladaptive ways of relating to others tend to elicit, over and over again, the same unsatisfying responses from others. These therapists focus on identifying patterns of relating and intervening within the therapeutic relationship to elicit new, adaptive behaviors from clients that can yield positive interpersonal experiences. Cognitive-behavioral therapists sometimes focus explicitly on expanding clients' behavioral repertoire through communication training, role playing, and *in vivo* practice. The idea here is that if clients are capable of expressing their feelings in a variety of ways, they are better able to choose how to respond and to adapt their behavior to their particular goals or circumstances.

Interpersonal Coordination

The final characteristic of adaptive emotional expression is interpersonal coordination. This involves the ability to get the point across in emotional communication. People need to be able to express their feelings in a way that produces the desired effect on others. To do this, they need to know not only what they want to communicate but also how they come across to others and how others are feeling. They must be able to clearly communicate their own feelings, while taking into account others' perspectives as well as relevant social norms. For instance, a man just beginning a relationship is more likely to evoke a positive response from his partner if he engages in gradually increasing and reciprocal self-disclosure, rather than plunging in and immediately revealing highly intimate feelings. (Lonely and depressed people often make this mistake. See review by Segrin, 1998.) A married couple is likely to get along better if they each communicate their expressions of affection in ways that the partner understands and appreciates.

Interpersonal coordination does *not* necessarily mean doing what other people want. The issue is not whether other people like the emotional message, but rather whether the individual is able to communicate the desired message in the desired way. Sometimes the desired impact of emotional communication is negative, as when someone wants to end an unsatisfying relationship and seeks to communicate this unambiguously. Other times, someone may want to communicate negative feelings gently but clearly, saying, for example, "I love you and I want to be with you, but I'm unhappy about X."

There are many ways of therapeutically addressing interpersonal coordination. Communication exercises, social skills training, or more general in-session practice describing one's feelings may be useful ways of helping clients learn to clearly articulate their feelings. Feedback from a therapist can be an important means of helping clients to become aware of unintended or ambiguous emotional communications. A therapist might comment, "I hear your words saying X, but your body seems to be saying something different. Try not to move for a moment, and tell me what you see your body saying."

The therapist can sometimes provide insight into others' likely responses. For example, one male client in his early 20s described having an angry scene at work, in front of his boss, when his lunch break was delayed because of the sudden arrival of many customers. The therapist asked how the client thought his boss understood his expression of anger. "That I care about my job?" the client suggested. He was astonished to hear the therapist's guess that the boss saw this as an expression of concern about lunch rather than the job. Insight into others' likely responses to emotional communication might also be fostered through having the client adopt the other's part during role play or through an experiential two-chair technique in which clients are urged to express both their own and the other's feelings.

Couples therapy provides an ideal format for exploring differences in intent and impact in emotional communication. Therapists can encourage clients to reflect back to each other their understanding of their partner's verbal expressions of emotion. "What I hear you saying is that you feel X." Partners can then either agree that that was the intended message or clarify their intent. "No, that's not what I meant at all. What I was trying to express was. . . . " Nonverbal expressions of emotion may also require clarification. For example, a therapist might observe, "Sally, I noticed that when Doug was talking just now, you rolled your eyes upward. Were you aware of doing that? . . . Why don't you do it again, now, and pay attention to how you feel as you do it. What is going on for you as you roll your eyes? . . . Doug, how do you experience Sally's rolling her eyes?" In this case, Sally's eye rolling may have been a sign of anxiety or even shame, but Doug might have understood it as disinterest or dismissal.

SUMMARY AND CONCLUSION

In this chapter, we outlined four key functions of emotional expression. We described how expression can promote arousal regulation, foster self-understanding, enhance coping, and improve interpersonal relationships. Our suggestion that these adaptive functions can be undermined by either maladaptive expression or maladaptive nonexpression underscores the complexity of emotional behavior. Neither expression nor nonexpression is universally beneficial or desirable. Neither is uniformly problematic. What type of emotional behavior is most adaptive in particular circumstances depends on characteristics of the individual and the situation.

We also argued that adaptive emotional behavior is characterized by integration, flexibility, and interpersonal coordination. We believe that the goal of clinical interventions should not be to uniformly increase or decrease clients' expression of emotion, but rather to help clients to achieve balance in their emotional behavior. Ideally, expression involves creating a delicate balance between our emotional, rational, and social selves, like a mobile that harmonizes its elements in a fluid whole.

References

Abbey, A., & Melby, C. (1986). The effects of nonverbal cues on gender differences in perceptions of sexual interest. *Sex Roles, 15,* 283–298.

Achmon, J., Granek, M., Golomb, M., & Hart, J. (1989). Behavioral treatment of essential hypertension: A comparison between cognitive therapy and biofeedback of heart rate. *Psychosomatic Medicine, 51,* 152–164.

Acklin, M. W., & Alexander, G. (1988). Alexithymia and somatization. *Journal of Nervous and Mental Diseases, 176,* 343–350.

Adams, G. R., & Shea, J. A. (1981). Talking and loving: A cross-lagged panel investigation. *Basic and Applied Social Psychology, 2,* 81–88.

Adelman, M. B. (1989, November). *Play and incongruity: Framing safe-sex talk.* Paper presented at the meeting of the Speech Communication Association, San Francisco, CA.

Adler, N., & Matthews, K. (1994). Health psychology: Why do some people get sick and some stay well? *Annual Review of Psychology, 45,* 229–259.

Ainsworth, M. D. S., Blehar, M. C., Waters, E., & Wall, S. (1978). *Patterns of attachment: A psychological study of the strange situation.* Hillsdale, NJ: Erlbaum.

Alberts, J. (1988). An analysis of couples' conversational complaints. *Communication Monographs, 55,* 184–197.

Albrecht, T. L., Burleson, B. R., & Goldsmith, D. (1994). Supportive communication. In M. L. Knapp & G. R. Miller (Eds.), *Handbook of interpersonal communication* (2nd ed., pp. 419–449). Thousand Oaks, CA: Sage.

Alexander, F. (1950). *Psychosomatic medicine: Its principles and applications.* New York: Norton.

Allen, J. G., & Hamsher, J. H. (1974). The development and validation of a test of emotional styles. *Journal of Consulting and Clinical Psychology, 42,* 663–668.

Alloy, L. B., Fedderly, S. S., Kennedy-Moore, E., & Cohan, C. L. (1998). Dysphoria and social interaction: An integration of behavioral confirmation and interpersonal perspectives. *Journal of Personality and Social Psychology, 74,* 1566–1579.

Altman, I., & Taylor, D. A. (1973). *Social penetration: The development of interpersonal relationships.* New York: Holt, Rinehart, & Winston.

Amato, P. R. (1993). Children's adjustment to divorce: Theories, hypotheses, and empirical support. *Journal of Marriage and the Family, 55,* 23–38.

Andersen, B. L. (1992). Psychological interventions for cancer patients to enhance the quality of life. *Journal of Consulting and Clinical Psychology, 60,* 552–568.

Andersen, P. A. (1985). nonverbal immediacy in interpersonal communication. In A. W.

Siegman & S. Feldstein (Eds.), *Multichannel integrations of nonverbal behavior* (pp. 1–36). Hillsdale, NJ: Erlbaum.

Andersen, P. A., & Guerrero, L. K. (1998). Principles of communication and emotion in social interaction. In P. A. Andersen & L. K. Guerrero (Eds.), *Handbook of communication and emotion: Research, theory, applications, and contexts* (pp. 49–96). San Diego, CA: Academic Press.

Anderson, C. D. (1981). Expression of affect and physiological response in psychosomatic patients. *Journal of Psychosomatic Research, 25,* 143–150.

Angus, L. E., & Rennie, D. L. (1988). Therapist participation in metaphor generation: Collaborative and non-collaborative styles. *Psychotherapy, 25,* 552–560.

Aries, E. (1996). *Men and women in interaction: Reconsidering the differences.* New York: Oxford University Press.

Arnkoff, D., & Glass, C. (1992). Cognitive therapy and psychotherapy integration. In D. Freedheim (Ed.), *History of psychotherapy: A century of change* (pp. 658–694). Washington, DC: American Psychological Association.

Aron, A., & Aron, E. N. (1991). Love and sexuality. In K. McKinney & S. Sprecher (Eds.), *Sexuality in close relationships* (pp. 25–48). Hillsdale, NJ: Erlbaum.

Asendorpf, J. B., & Scherer, K. R. (1983). The discrepant repressor: Differentiation between low anxiety, high anxiety, and repression of anxiety by autonomic–facial–verbal patterns of behavior. *Journal of Personality and Social Psychology, 45,* 1334–1346.

Averill, J. R. (1968). Grief: Its nature and significance. *Psychological Bulletin, 70,* 721–748.

Averill, J. R., & Nunley, E. P. (1992). *Voyages of the heart: Living an emotionally creative life.* New York: Free Press.

Bagby, R. M., Parker, J. D. A., & Taylor, G. J. (1994). The twenty-item Toronto Alexithymia Scale—I. Item selection and cross-validation of the factor structure. *Journal of Psychosomatic Research, 38,* 23–32.

Bagby, R. M., Taylor, G. J., & Parker, J. D. A. (1994). The twenty-item Toronto Alexithymia Scale—II. Convergent, discriminant, and concurrent validity. *Journal of Psychosomatic Research, 38,* 33–40.

Bandura, A. (1977). *Social learning theory.* Englewood Cliffs, NJ: Prentice-Hall.

Barbee, A. P., Rowatt, T. L., & Cunningham, M. R. (1998). When a friend is in need: Feelings about seeking, giving, and receiving social support. In P. A. Andersen & L. K. Guerrero (Eds.), *Handbook of communication and emotion: Research, theory, applications, and contexts* (pp. 281–301). San Diego, CA: Academic Press.

Barrett-Lennard, G. T. (1997). The recovery of empathy: Toward others and self. In A. Bohart & L. S. Greenberg (Eds.), *Empathy reconsidered* (103–121). Washington, DC: APA Books.

Bartholomew, K. (1990). Avoidance of intimacy: An attachment perspective. *Journal of Social and Personal Relationships, 7,* 147–178.

Bartholomew, K. (1993). From childhood to adult relationships: Attachment theory and research. In S. Duck (Ed.), *Learning about relationships* (pp. 30–62). Newbury Park, CA: Sage.

Bartholomew, K., & Horowitz, L. M. (1991). Attachment styles among young adults: A test of a four-category model. *Journal of Personality and Social Psychology, 61,* 226–244.

Baucom, D. H., Epstein, N., & Rankin, L. A. (1995). Cognitive aspects of cognitive-behavioral marital therapy. In N. S. Jacobson & A. S. Gurman (Eds.), *Clinical handbook of couple therapy* (pp. 65–90). New York: Guilford Press.

Baum, A., Newman, S., Weinman, J., West, R., & McManus, C. (Eds.). (1997) *Cambridge handbook of psychology, health and medicine.* New York: Cambridge University Press.

Baumeister, R. F. (1990a). Anxiety and deconstruction: On escaping the self. In J. M. Olson & M. P. Zanna (Eds.), *Self-inference processes: The Ontario Symposium* (Vol. 6, pp. 259–291). Hillsdale, NJ: Erlbaum.

Baumeister, R. F. (1990b). Suicide as escape from self. *Psychological Review, 97*, 90–113.

Baumeister, R. F., Stillwell, A., & Wotman, S. R. (1990). Victim and perpetrator accounts of interpersonal conflict: Autobiographical narratives about anger. *Journal of Personality and Social Psychology, 59*, 994–1005.

Baumeister, R. F., & Wotman, S. R. (1992). *Breaking hearts: The two sides of unrequited love.* New York: Guilford Press.

Bavelas, J. B., Black, A., Chovil, N., Lemery, C. R., & Mullet, J. (1988). Form and function in motor mimicry: Topographic evidence that the primary function is communicative. *Human Communication Research, 14*, 275–299.

Bavelas, J. B., Black, A., Lemery, C. R., & Mullet, J. (1986). "I show how you feel": Motor mimicry as a communicative act. *Journal of Personality and Social Psychology, 50*, 322–329.

Baxter, L. A. (1987). Self-disclosure and relationship disengagement. In V. J. Derlega & J. H. Berg (Eds.), *Self-disclosure: Theory, research, and therapy* (pp. 155–174). New York: Plenum Press.

Baxter, L. A. (1988). A dialectical perspective on communication strategies in relationship development. In S. W. Duck (Ed.), *Handbook of personal relationships: Theory, research, and interventions* (pp. 257–273). London: Wiley.

Baxter, L. A. (1990). Dialectical contradictions in relationship development. *Journal of Social and Personal Relationships, 7*, 69–88.

Baxter, L. A., & Wilmot, W. W. (1985). Taboo topics in close relationships. *Journal of Social and Personal Relationships, 2*, 253–269.

Baxter, L. A., & Wilmot, W. W. (1986). Interaction characteristics of disengaging, stable, and growing relationships. In R. Gilmour & S. W. Duck (Eds.), *The emerging field of personal relationships* (pp. 145–159). Hillsdale, NJ: Erlbaum.

Beach, S. R. H., & Fincham, F. D. (1994). Toward an integrated model of negative affectivity in marriage. In S. M. Johnson & L. S. Greenberg (Eds.), *The heart of the matter: Perspectives on emotion in marital therapy* (pp. 227–256). New York: Brunner/Mazel.

Beach, S. R. H., Sandeen, E. E., & O'Leary, K. D. (1990). *Depression in marriage: A model for etiology and treatment.* New York: Guilford Press.

Beck, A. T. (1983). Cognitive therapy of depression: New perspectives. In P. J. Clayton & J. E. Barrett (Eds.), *Treatment of depression: Old controversies and new approaches* (pp. 265–290). New York: Raven Press.

Beck, A. T. (1988). *Love is never enough.* New York: Harper & Row.

Beck, A. T., Rush, A. J., Shaw, B. F., & Emery, G. (1979). *Cognitive therapy of depression.* New York: Guilford Press.

Becker, R. E. & Heimberg, R. G. (1985). Social skills training approaches. In M. Hersen & A. S. Bellack (Eds.), *Handbook of clinical behavior therapy with adults* (pp. 201–228). New York: Plenum Press.

Bell, R. A., Buerkel-Rothfuss, N., & Gore, K. (1987). "Did you bring the yarmulke for the cabbage patch kid?": The idiomatic communication of young lovers. *Human Communication Research, 14*, 47–67.

Bem, D. J. (1972). Self-perception theory. In L. Berkowitz (Ed.), *Advances in experimental social psychology* (Vol. 6, pp. 1–62). New York: Academic Press.

Benjamin, L. S. (1996). Introduction to the special section on structural analysis of social behavior. *Journal of Consulting and Clinical Psychology, 64*, 1203–1212.

Bennet, P., Wallace, L., Carroll, D., & Smith, N. (1991). Treating Type A behaviors and mild hypertension in middle-aged men. *Journal of Psychosomatic Research, 35*, 209–223.

Berkowitz, L. (1970). Experimental investigations of hostility catharsis. *Journal of Consulting and Clinical Psychology, 35,* 1–7.

Berkowitz, L. (1983). Aversively stimulated aggression: Some parallels and differences in research with animals and humans. *American Psychologist, 38,* 1135–1144.

Berman, W. H., & Sperling, M. B. (1994). The structure and function of adult attachment. In M. B. Sperling & W. H. Berman (Eds.), *Attachment in adults: Clinical and development perspectives* (pp. 2–28). New York: Guilford Press.

Bernieri, F., Resnick, J. S., & Rosenthal, R. (1988). Synchrony, pseudosynchrony, and dissynchrony: Measuring the entrainment process in mother–infant dyads. *Journal of Personality and Social Psychology, 54,* 243–253.

Berscheid, E., & Walster, E. H. (1978). *Interpersonal attraction* (2nd ed.). Reading, MA: Addison-Wesley.

Bettes, B. A. (1988). Maternal depression and motherese: Temporal and intonational features. *Child Development, 59,* 1089–1096.

Biaggio, M. K. (1987). A survey of psychologists' perspective on catharsis. *Journal of Psychology, 121,* 243–248.

Biglan, A., & Thorensen, C. (1987). *Coercive interactions between women in chronic pain and their spouses.* Unpublished manuscript, Oregon Research Institute, Eugene, OR.

Birdwhistell, R. L. (1970). *Kinesics and context.* Philadelphia: University of Pennsylvania Press.

Blascovich, J. (1992). A biopsychosocial approach to arousal regulation. *Journal of Social and Clinical Psychology, 11,* 213–237.

Blechman, E. A. (1990). A new look at emotions and the family. In E. A. Blechman (Ed.), *Emotions and the family: For better or for worse* (pp. 201–224). Hillsdale, NJ: Erlbaum.

Blumstein, P., & Schwartz, P. (1983). *American couples: Money, work, sex.* New York: Morrow.

Bohart, A. C. (1977). Role playing and interpersonal-conflict reduction. *Journal of Counseling Psychology, 24,* 15–24.

Bohart, A. C. (1980). Toward a cognitive theory of catharsis. *Psychotherapy: Theory, Research, and Practice, 17,* 192–201.

Bohart, A. C. (1993). Experiencing: The basis of psychotherapy. *Journal of Psychotherapy Integration, 3,* 51–67.

Bohart, A. C., & Greenberg, L. S. (Eds.). (1997). *Empathy reconsidered.* Washington, DC: APA Books.

Bohart, A. C., & Tallman, K. (1997). Empathy and the active agent: An integrative cognitive–experiential approach. In A. C. Bohart & L. S. Greenberg (Eds.), *Empathy reconsidered* (pp. 393–415). Washington, DC: APA Books.

Bohart, A. C., & Tallman, K. (1998). The person as active agent in experiential therapy. In L. S. Greenberg, J. C. Watson, & G. Lietaer (Eds.), *Handbook of experiential psychotherapy* (pp. 178–200). New York: Guilford Press.

Bonanno, G. A., Keltner, D., Holen, A., & Horowitz, M. J. (1995). When avoiding unpleasant emotions might not be such a bad thing: Verbal–autonomic response dissociation and midlife conjugal bereavement. *Journal of Personality and Social Psychology, 69,* 975–989.

Bonanno, G. A., & Singer, J. L. (1990). Repressor personality style: Theoretical and methodological implications for health and pathology. In J. L. Singer (Ed.), *Repression and dissociation* (pp. 435–470). Chicago: University of Chicago Press.

Borkovec, T. D., & Costello, E. (1993). Efficacy of applied relaxation and cognitive-behavioral therapy in the treatment of generalized anxiety disorder. *Journal of Consulting and Clinical Psychology, 61,* 611–619.

Bowen, M. (1966). The use of family theory in clinical practice. *Comprehensive Psychiatry, 7,* 345–374.

Bowen, M. (1978). *Family therapy in clinical practice.* New York: Aronson.

Bowlby, J. (1969). *Attachment and loss: Vol. 1. Attachment.* New York: Basic Books.

Bowlby, J. (1973). *Attachment and loss: Vol. 1. Separation: Anxiety and anger.* New York: Basic Books.

Bradbury, T. M., & Fincham, F. K. (1990). Attributions in marriage: Review and critique. *Psychological Bulletin, 107,* 3–33.

Brehm, J. W. (1972). *Responses to loss of freedom: A theory of psychological reactance.* Morristown, NJ: General Learning Press.

Brehm, S. (1985). *Intimate relationships.* New York: Random House.

Bretherton, I. (1985). Attachment theory: Retrospect and prospect. In I. Bretherton & E. Waters (Eds.), Growing points of attachment theory and research. *Monographs of the Society for Research in Child Development, 50*(1–2, Serial No. 209), 3–35.

Briere, J. (1989). *Therapy for adults molested as children: beyond survival.* New York: Springer.

Brigman, B., & Knox, D. (1992). University students' motivations to have intercourse. *College Student Journal, 26,* 406–408.

Brody, L. R., & Landau, L. B. (1984, August). *Mothers' emotional styles and preschoolers' emotional attributions.* Paper presented at the meeting of the American Psychological Association, Toronto, Ontario, Canada.

Brokaw, D. W., & McLemore, C. W. (1991). Interpersonal models of personality and psychopathology. In D. G. Gilbert & J. J. Connolly (Eds.), *Personality, social skills, and psychopathology: An individual differences approach* (pp. 49–83). New York: Plenum Press.

Brown, G. W., & Harris, T. (1987). *Social origins of depression.* New York: Free Press.

Brown, M., & Auerback, A. (1981). Communication patterns in initiation of marital sex. *Medical Aspects of Human Sexuality, 15,* 101–117.

Brown, P., & Levinson, S. (1978). Universals in language use: Politeness phenomena. In E. Goody (Ed.), *Questions and politeness: Strategies in social interaction* (pp. 256–289). Cambridge, UK: Cambridge University Press.

Buck, R. (1980). Nonverbal behavior and the theory of emotion: The facial feedback hypothesis. *Journal of Personality and Social Psychology, 38,* 811–824.

Buck, R. (1988). *Human motivation and emotion* (2nd ed.). New York: Wiley.

Buck, R. (1989). Emotional communication in personal relationships: A developmental–interactionist view. In C. Hendrick (Ed.), *Review of personality and social psychology: Vol. 10. Close relationships* (pp. 144–163). Newbury Park, CA: Sage.

Buck, R. (1991). Temperament, social skills, and the communication of emotion: A developmental interactionist view. In D. G. Gilbert & J. J. Connolly (Eds.), *Personality, social skills, and psychopathology: An individual differences approach* (pp. 85–105). New York: Plenum Press.

Buck, R. (1993). Emotional communication, emotional competence, and physical illness: A developmental–interactionist view. In H. C. Traue & J. W. Pennebaker (Eds.), *Emotion, inhibition, and health* (pp. 32–56). Seattle, WA: Hogrefe & Huber.

Bugental, D. B. (1991). Affective and cognitive processes within threat-oriented family systems. In I. Siges, A. V. McGilicuddy-DeLisi, & J. J. Goodnow (Eds.), *Parental belief systems: The psychological consequences for children* (2nd ed., pp. 219–248). Hillsdale, NJ: Erlbaum.

Bugental, D. B., Blue, J., & Cruzcosa, M. (1989). Perceived control over caregiving outcomes: Implications for child abuse. *Developmental Psychology, 25,* 532–539.

Bugental, D. B., Blue, J., & Lewis, J. (1990). Caregiver beliefs and dysphoric affect directed to difficult children. *Developmental Psychology, 26,* 631–638.

Bugental, D. B., Mantyla, S. M., & Lewis, J. (1989). Parental attributions as moderators of affective communication to children at risk for physical abuse. In D. Cicchetti & V.

Carlson (Eds.), *Current research and theoretical advances in child maltreatment* (pp. 254–279). New York: Cambridge University Press.

Burgess, A. W., & Holmstrom, L. L. (1979). Adaptive strategies and recovery from rape. *American Journal of Psychiatry, 136,* 1278–1282.

Burgoon, J. K. (1985). Nonverbal signals. In M. Knapp & G. R. Miller (Eds.), *Handbook of interpersonal communications.* Beverly Hills, CA: Sage.

Burgoon, J. K., Buller, D. B., & Woodall, W. G. (1996). *Nonverbal communication: The unspoken dialogue.* New York: McGraw-Hill.

Burgoon, J. K., Stern, L. A., & Dillman, L. (1995). *Interpersonal adaptation: Dyadic interaction patterns.* New York: Cambridge University Press.

Burleson, B. R., Birch, J., & Kunkel, A. W. (1993). *Similarities in the cognitions of romantic partners.* Unpublished data, Department of Communication, Purdue University, West Lafayette, IN.

Burleson, B. R., & Denton, W. H. (1992). A new look at similarity and attraction in marriage: Similarities in social-cognitive and communication skills as predictors of attraction and satisfaction. *Communication Monographs, 59,* 268–287.

Burleson, B. R., & Goldsmith, D. J. (1998). How the comforting process works: Alleviating emotional distress through conversationally induced reappraisals. In P. A. Andersen & L. K. Guerrero (Eds.), *Handbook of communication and emotion: Research, theory, applications, and contexts* (pp. 245–280). San Diego, CA: Academic Press.

Burleson, B. R., & Samter, W. (1994). A social skills approach to relationship maintenance: How individual differences in communication skills affect the achievement of relationship functions. In D. J. Canary & L. Stafford (Eds.), *Communication and relational maintenance* (pp. 61–90). San Diego, CA: Academic Press.

Burns, D. D., & Nolen-Hoeksema, S. (1992). Therapeutic empathy and recovery from depression in cognitive-behavioral therapy: A structural equation model. *Journal of Consulting and Clinical Psychology, 60,* 441–449.

Buss, A. H., & Plomin, R. (1984). *Temperament: Early developing personality traits.* Hillsdale, NJ: Erlbaum.

Buss, D. M. (1988). Love acts: The evolutionary biology of love. In R. J. Sternberg & M. L. Barnes (Eds.), *The psychology of love* (pp. 100–117). New Haven, CT: Yale University Press.

Buss, D. M., & Schmitt, D. P. (1993). Sexual strategies theory: A contextual evolutionary analysis of human mating. *Psychological Review, 100,* 204–232.

Butler, S. F., & Strupp, H. H. (1986). Specific and nonspecific factors in psychotherapy: A problematic paradigm for psychotherapy research. *Psychotherapy, 23,* 30–40.

Byers, E. S. (1988). Effects of sexual arousal on men's and women's behavior in sexual disagreement situations. *Journal of Sex Research, 25,* 235–254.

Byers, E. S., & Heinlein, L. (1989). Predicting initiations and refusals of sexual activities in married and cohabiting heterosexual couples. *Journal of Sex Research, 26,* 210–231.

Cacioppo, J. T., & Tassinary, L. G. (1990). Inferring psychophysiological significance from physiological signals. *American Psychologist, 45,* 16–28.

Cacioppo, J. T., Uchino, B. N., Crites, S. L., Snydersmith, M. A., Smith, G., Berntson, G. G., & Lang, P. J. (1992). Relationship between facial expressiveness and sympathetic activation in emotion: A critical review, with emphasis on modeling underlying mechanisms and individual differences. *Journal of Personality and Social Psychology, 62,* 110–128.

Cahn, D. D. (1990). Confrontation behaviors, perceived understanding, and relationship growth. In D. D. Cahn (Ed.), *Intimates in conflict: A communications perspective* (pp. 153–165). Hillsdale, NJ: Erlbaum.

Caldwell, M. A., & Peplau, L. A. (1982). Sex differences in same-sex friendship. *Sex Roles, 8,* 721–732.

Campbell, J. D. (1990). Self-esteem and clarity of the self-concept. *Journal of Personality and Social Psychology, 59,* 538–549.

Camras, L. A., Ribordy, S., Hill, J., Martino, S., Sachs, V., & Spaccarelli, S., & Stefani, R. (1990). Maternal facial behavior and the recognition and production of emotional expression by maltreated and nonmaltreated children. *Developmental Psychology, 26,* 304–312.

Canary, D. J., Emmers-Sommer, T. M., & Faulkner, S. (1997). *Sex and gender differences in personal relationships.* New York: Guilford Press.

Canary, D. J., & Stafford, L. (1992). Relational maintenance strategies and equity in marriage. *Communication Monographs, 59,* 243–267.

Capella, J. N. (1981). Mutual influence in expressive behavior: Adult–adult and infant–adult dyadic interaction. *Psychological Bulletin, 89,* 101–132.

Capella, J. N. (1993). The facial feedback hypothesis in human interaction: Review and speculation. *Journal of Language and Social Psychology, 12,* 13–29.

Carlsen, M. B. (1996). Metaphor, meaning-making and metamorphosis. In K. T. Kuehlwein & H. Rosen (Eds.), *Cognitive therapies in action: Evolving innovative practice* (pp. 337–368). San Francisco: Jossey-Bass.

Cartensen, L. J. (1993). Motivation for social contact across the life span: A theory of socioemotional selectivity. In J. Jacobs (Ed.), *Nebraska Symposium on Motivation* (Vol. 40, pp. 209–254). Lincoln: University of Nebraska Press.

Cartensen, L. J., Gottman, J. M., & Levenson, R. W. (1995). Emotional behavior in longterm marriage. *Psychology and Aging, 10,* 140–149.

Carter, A. S., Little, C., & Garrity-Rokous, F. E. (1998, April). *Adapting the emotional availability scales for 4-month old infant–mother dyads: Associations with molecular coding and maternal psychopathology.* Paper presented at the 11th International Conference on Infancy Studies, Atlanta, GA.

Carver, C. S., Lawrence, J. W., & Scheier, M. F. (1996). A control-process perspective on the origins of affect. In L. L. Martin & A. Tesser (Eds.), *Striving and feeling: Interactions among goals, affect, and self-regulation* (pp. 11–52). Mahwah, NJ: Erlbaum.

Carver, C. S., Scheier, M. F., & Weintraub, J. K. (1989). Assessing coping strategies: A theoretically based approach. *Journal of Personality and Social Psychology, 56,* 267–283.

Caspi, A., Elder, G. H., & Bem, D. J. (1987). Moving against the world: Life-course patterns of explosive children. *Developmental Psychology, 23,* 308–313.

Cassidy, J., & Parke, R. D. (1989, April). Family expressiveness and children's social competence. In R. D. Parke (Chair), *Emotional expression in the family.* Symposium conducted at the meeting of the Society for Research in Child Development, Kansas City, MO.

Cate, R. M., & Lloyd, S. A. (1992). *Courtship.* Newbury Park, CA: Sage.

Cegala, D. J., Savage, G. T., Brunner, C. C., & Conrad, A. B. (1982). An elaboration of the meaning of interaction involvement: Toward the development of a theoretical concept. *Communication Monographs, 49,* 229–248.

Cherlin, A. J., Furstenberg, F. F., Chase-Lansdale, P. L., Kiernan, K. E., Robins, P. K., Morrison, D. R., & Teitler, J. O. (1991). Longitudinal studies of effects of divorce on children in Great Britain and the United States. *Science, 252,* 1386–1389.

Chodorow, N. (1978). *The reproduction of mothering.* Berkeley: University of California Press.

Choti, S. E., Marston, A. R., Holston, S. G., & Hart, J. T. (1987). Gender and personality variables in film-induced sadness and crying. *Journal of Social and Clinical Psychology, 5,* 535–544.

Christensen, A., & Heavey, C. L. (1990). Gender and social structure in the demand/withdraw pattern of marital conflict. *Journal of Personality and Social Psychology, 59,* 73–81.

Christensen, A., Jacobson, N. S., & Babcock, J. C. (1995). Integrative Behavioral Marital Therapy. In N. S. Jacobson & A. S. Gurman (Eds.), *Clinical handbook of couple therapy* (pp 31–64). New York: Guilford Press.

Christopher, F. S., & Cate, R. M. (1985). Premarital sexual pathways and relationship development. *Journal of Social and Personal Relationships, 2,* 271–288.

Christopher, F. S., & Frandsen, M. M. (1990). Strategies of influence in sex and dating. *Journal of Social and Personal Relationships, 7,* 89–105.

Clark, L. A., & Watson, D. (1991). General affective dispositions in physical and psychological health. In C. R. Snyder & D. R. Forsyth (Eds.), *Handbook of social and clinical psychology* (pp. 221–245). New York: Pergamon Press.

Clark, M. S., & Reis, H. T. (1988). Interpersonal processes in close relationships. *Annual Review of Psychology, 39,* 609–672.

Clark, R. D. (1990). The impact of AIDS on gender differences in willingness to engage in casual sex. *Journal of Applied Social Psychology, 20,* 771–782.

Clark, R. D., & Hatfield, E. (1989). Gender differences in receptivity to sexual offers. *Journal of Psychology and Human Sexuality, 2,* 39–55.

Coates, D., & Peterson, B. A. (1982). Depression and deviance. In G. Weary & H. L. Mirels (Eds.), *Integrations of clinical and social psychology* (pp 154–170.). New York: Oxford University Press.

Coates, D., & Winston, T. (1983). Counteracting the deviance of depression: Peer support groups for victims. *Journal of Social Issues, 39,* 169–194.

Coates, D., & Winston, T. (1987). The dilemma of distress disclosure. In V. J. Derlega & J. H. Berg (Eds.), *Self-disclosure: Theory, research, and therapy* (pp. 229–255). New York: Plenum Press.

Coates, D., & Wortman, C. B. (1980). Depression maintenance and interpersonal control. In A. Baum & J. Singer (Eds.), *Advances in environmental psychology* (Vol. 2, pp. 149–182). Hillsdale, NJ: Erlbaum.

Cohen, S., & Herbert, T. B. (1996). Health psychology: Psychological factors and physical disease from the perspective of human psychoneuroimmunology. *Annual Review of Psychology, 47,* 113–142.

Cohen, S., Lichtenstein, E., Mermelstein, R., Kingsolver, K., Baer, J. S., & Kamarck, T. W. (1988). Social support interventions for smoking cessation. In B. H. Gottlieb (Ed.), *Marshaling social support: Formats, processes, and effects* (pp. 211–240). Newbury Park, CA: Sage.

Cohen, S., & Rodriguez, M. S. (1995). Pathways linking affective disturbances and physical disorders. *Health Psychology, 14,* 364–380.

Cohen, S., & Wills, T. A. (1985). Stress, social support, and the buffering hypothesis. *Psychological Bulletin, 98,* 310–357.

Cohn, J. R., Campbell, S. B., Matias, R., & Hopkins, J. (1990). Face-to-face interactions of postpartum depressed and nondepressed mother–infant pairs at two months. *Developmental Psychology, 26,* 15–23.

Cole, P. M. (1986). Children's spontaneous control of facial expression. *Child Development, 57,* 1309–1321.

Collier, G. (1985). *Emotional expression.* Hillsdale, NJ: Erlbaum.

Collins, N. L., & Miller, L. C. (1994). Self-disclosure and liking: A meta-analytic review. *Psychological Bulletin, 116,* 457–475.

Collins, N. L., & Read, S. J. (1990). Adult attachment, working models, and relationship quality in dating couples. *Journal of Personality and Social Psychology, 58,* 644–663.

Collins, N. L., & Read, S. J. (1994). Cognitive representations of attachment: The structure and function of working models. In K. Bartholomew & D. Perlman (Eds.), *Advances in personal relationships: Vol. 5. Attachment processes in adulthood* (pp. 53–90). Bristol, PA: Kingsley.

Conte, H. R., Plutchik, R., Jung, B. B., Picard, S., Karasu, T. B., & Lotterman, A. (1990).

Psychological mindedness as a predictor of psychotherapy outcome: A preliminary report. *Comprehensive Psychiatry, 31,* 426–431.

Contrada, R. J., Leventhal, H., & O'Leary, A. (1990). Personality and health. In L. A. Pervin (Ed.), *Handbook of personality: Theory and research* (pp. 638–669). New York: Guilford Press.

Contreras, R., Hendrick, S. S., & Hendrick, C. (1996). Perspectives on marital love and satisfaction in Mexican American and Anglo-American couples. *Journal of Counseling and Development, 74,* 408–415.

Conway, M., & Giannopoulos, C. (1993). Self-esteem and specificity in self-focused attention. *Journal of Social Psychology, 133,* 121–123.

Conway, M., Giannopoulos, C., Csank, P., & Mendelson, D. (1993). Dysphoria and specificity in self-focused attention. *Personality and Social Psychology Bulletin, 19,* 265–268.

Cornelius, R. R. (1984). A rule model of emotional expression. In C. Z. Malatesta & C. E. Izard (Eds.), *Emotion in adult development* (pp. 213–233). Beverly Hills, CA: Sage.

Costa, P. T., Jr., & McCrae, R. R. (1988). Personality in adulthood: A six-year longitudinal study of self-ratings and spouse ratings on the NEO Personality Inventory. *Journal of Personality and Social Psychology, 54,* 853–863.

Courtois, C. A. (1988). *Healing the incest wound.* New York: Norton.

Cowan, P. A. (1996). Meta-thoughts on the role of meta-emotion in children's development: Comment on Gottman et al. (1996). *Journal of Family Psychology, 10,* 277–283.

Coyne, J. C. (1976a). Depression and the response of others. *Journal of Abnormal Psychology, 85,* 186–193.

Coyne, J. C. (1976b). Towards an interactional description of depression. *Psychiatry, 39,* 28–40.

Coyne, J. C. (1990). Interpersonal processes in depression. In G. I. Keitner (Ed.), *Depression and families: Impact and treatment* (pp. 33–53). Washington, DC: American Psychiatric Press.

Coyne, J. C., & Downey, G. (1991). Social factors and psychopathology: Stress, social support, and coping. *Annual Review of Psychology, 42,* 401–425.

Coyne, J. C., Wortman, C. B., & Lehman, D. R. (1988). The other side of support: Emotional overinvolvement and miscarried helping. In B. H. Gottlieb (Ed.), *Marshaling social support: Formats, processes, and effects* (pp. 305–330). Newbury Park, CA: Sage.

Creamer, M., Burgess, P., & Pattison, P. (1992). Reaction to trauma: A cognitive processing model. *Journal of Abnormal Psychology, 101,* 452–459.

Crester, G. A., Lombardo, W. K., Lombardo, B., & Mathis, S. (1982). Reactions to men and women who cry: A study of perceived societal attitudes versus personal attitudes. *Perceptual and Motor Skills, 55,* 479–486.

Crowne, D. P., & Marlowe, D. A. (1964). *The approval motive: Studies in evaluative dependence.* New York: Wiley.

Cummings, E. M., Iannotti, R. J., & Zahn-Waxler, C. (1985). Influence of conflict between adults on the emotions and aggression of young children. *Developmental Psychology, 21,* 495–507.

Cummings, E. M., Zahn-Waxler, C., & Radke-Yarrow, M. (1981). Young children's responses to expressions of anger and affection by others in the family. *Child Development, 52,* 1274–1282.

Cupach, W. R., & Comstock, J. (1990). Satisfaction with sexual communication in marriage: Links to sexual satisfaction and dyadic adjustment. *Journal of Social and Personal Relationships, 7,* 179–186.

Cupach, W. R., & Metts, S. (1991). Sexuality and communication in close relationships. In

K. McKinney & S. Sprecher (Eds.), *Sexuality in close relationships* (pp. 93–110). Hillsdale, NJ: Erlbaum.

Daldrup, R. J., Beutler, L. E., Engle, D., & Greenberg, L. S. (1988). *Focused expressive psychotherapy: Freeing the overcontrolled patient.* New York: Guilford Press.

Daly, E. M., Abramovitch, R., & Pliner, P. (1980). The relationship between mothers' encoding and their children's decoding of facial expressions of emotion. *Merrill–Palmer Quarterly, 26,* 25–33.

D'Augelli, A., & D'Augelli, J. F. (1985). The enhancement of sexual skills and competence: Promoting lifelong sexual unfolding. In L. L'Abate & M. A. Milan (Eds.), *Handbook of social skills training and research* (pp. 170–191). New York: Wiley.

Davidson, R. J., & Ekman, P. (1994). Afterword. In P. Ekman & R. J. Davidson (Eds.), *The nature of emotion: Fundamental questions* (pp. 232–234). New York: Oxford University Press.

Davis, J. D. (1978). When boy meets girl: Sex roles and the negotiation of intimacy in an acquaintance exercise. *Journal of Personality and Social Psychology, 36,* 684–692.

Davis, M. H., & Franzoi, S. L. (1986). Adolescent loneliness, self-disclosure, and private self-consciousness: A longitudinal investigation. *Journal of Personality and Social Psychology, 51,* 595–608.

Davis, M. H., & Franzoi, S. L. (1987). Private self-consciousness and self-disclosure. In V. J. Derlega & J. Berg (Eds.), *Self-disclosure: Theory, research, and therapy* (pp. 59–79). New York: Plenum Press.

Davison, K. P., & Petrie, K. J. (1997). Emotional expression and health. In A. Baum, S. Newman, J. Weinman, R. West, & C. McManus (Eds.), *Cambridge handbook of psychology, health and medicine* (pp. 103–106). New York: Cambridge University Press.

Dawes, R. M. (1996). *House of cards: Psychology and psychotherapy built on myth.* New York: Free Press.

Deaux, K., & Major, B. (1987). Putting gender into context: An interactive model of gender-related behavior. *Psychological Review, 94,* 369–389.

Deffenbacher, J. L. (1994). Anger reduction: Issues, assessment, and intervention strategies. In A. W. Siegman & T. W. Smith (Eds.), *Anger, hostility, and the heart* (pp. 239–269). Hillsdale, NJ: Erlbaum.

Deffenbacher, J. L., McNamara, K., Stark, R. S., & Sabadell, P. M. (1990). A combination of cognitive, relaxation, and behavioral coping skills in the reduction of general anger. *Journal of College Student Personnel, 31,* 351–358.

Deffenbacher, J. L., & Stark, R. S. (1992). Relaxation and cognitive-relaxation treatments of general anger. *Journal of Counseling Psychology, 39,* 158–167.

DeLamater, J. (1987). A sociological approach. In J. H. Geer & W. T. O'Donohue (Eds.), *Theories of human sexuality* (pp. 237–355). New York: Plenum Press.

DeLamater, J. D. (1991). Emotions and sexuality. In K. McKinney & S. Sprecher (Eds.), *Sexuality in close relationships* (pp. 49–70). Hillsdale, NJ: Erlbaum.

DeLamater, J. D., & MacCorquodale, P. (1979). *Premarital sexuality: Attitudes, relationships, behavior.* Madison: University of Wisconsin Press.

DeLongis, A., Wortman, C. B., Silver, R. C., & O'Brien, T. (1991). *The interpersonal dimensions of coping: The role of social relationships and support in emotional expression following a traumatic event.* Unpublished manuscript, University of British Columbia, Vancouver, British Columbia, Canada.

Derlega, V. J., & Berg, J. H. (Eds.). (1987). *Self-disclosure: Theory, research, and therapy.* New York: Plenum Press.

Derlega, V. J., Metts, S., Petronio, S., & Margulis, S. T. (1993). *Self-disclosure.* Newbury Park, CA: Sage.

Derlega, V. J., Winstead, B. A., Wong, P. T. P., & Hunter, S. (1985). Gender effects in an initial encounter: A case where men exceed women in disclosure. *Journal of Social and Personal Relationships, 2,* 25–44.

Descutner, C. J., & Thelen, M. H. (1991). Development and validation of a Fear of Intimacy Scale. *Psychological Assessment, 3,* 218–225.

Dickson, F. C. (1995). The best is yet to be: Research on long-lasting marriages. In J. T. Wood & S. Duck (Eds.), *Under-studied relationships: Off the beaten track* (pp. 22–50). Thousand Oaks, CA: Sage.

Dindia, K. (1994). A multiphasic view of relationship maintenance strategies. In D. J. Canary & L. Stafford (Eds.), *Communication and relational maintenance* (pp. 91–112). San Diego, CA: Academic Press.

Dindia, K., & Allen, M. (1992). Sex differences in self-disclosure: A meta-analysis. *Psychological Bulletin, 112,* 106–124.

Dindia, K., & Baxter, L. A. (1987). Strategies for maintaining and repairing marital relationships. *Journal of Social and Personal Relationships, 4,* 143–158.

Doi, S. C., & Thelen, M. H. (1993). The Fear of Intimacy Scale: Replication and extension. *Psychological Assessment, 5,* 377–383.

Donnelly, D. A., & Murray, E. J. (1991). Cognitive and emotional changes in written essays and therapy interviews. *Journal of Social and Clinical Psychology, 10,* 334–350.

Downey, G., & Coyne, J. C. (1990). Children of depressed parents: An integrative review. *Psychological Bulletin, 108,* 50–76.

Dozier, M., Cue, K. L., & Barnett, L. (1994). Clinicians as caregivers: Role of attachment organization in treatment. *Journal of Consulting and Clinical Psychology, 62,* 793–800.

Duck, S. (1991). Afterword: Couples and coupling. In K. McKinney & S. Sprecher (Eds.), *Sexuality in close relationships* (pp. 193–205). Hillsdale, NJ: Erlbaum.

Duck, S. (1994). Steady as (s)he goes: Relational maintenance as a shared meaning system. In D. J. Canary & L. Stafford (Eds.), *Communication and relational maintenance* (pp. 45–60). San Diego, CA: Academic Press.

Duck, S., Rutt, D. J., Hurst, M., & Strejc, H. (1991). Some evident truths about communication in everyday relationships: All communication is not created equal. *Human Communication Research, 18,* 228–267.

Duncan, S. D., Jr., & Fiske, D. W. (1977). *Face-to-face interaction: Research, methods, and theory.* Hillsdale, NJ: Erlbaum.

Dunn, J. (1994). Experience and understanding of emotions, relationships, and membership in a particular culture. In P. Ekman & R. J. Davidson (Eds.), *The nature of emotion: Fundamental questions* (pp. 352–355). New York: Oxford University Press.

Eagle, M. N. (1984). *Recent development in psychoanalysis: A critical evaluation.* Toronto, Ontario, Canada: McGraw-Hill.

Eagley, A. H., & Wood, W. (1991). Explaining sex differences in social behavior: A meta-analytic perspective. *Personality and Social Psychology Bulletin, 17,* 306–315.

Ebbesen, E. B., Duncan, B., & Konecni, V. J. (1975). Effects of content of verbal aggression on future verbal aggression: A field study. *Journal of Experimental Social Psychology, 11,* 192–204.

Efran, J. S., & Spangler, T. J. (1979). Why grown-ups cry: A two-factor theory and evidence from "The Miracle Worker." *Motivation and Emotion, 3,* 63–72.

Eisenberg, N., & Fabes, R. A. (1992). Emotion, regulation, and the development of social competence. In M. S. Clark (Ed.), *Review of personality and social psychology: Vol. 14. Emotion and social behavior* (pp. 119–150). Newbury Park, CA: Sage.

Eisenberg, N., & Fabes, R. A. (1994). Mothers' reactions to children's negative emotions: Relations to children's temperament and anger behavior. *Merrill–Palmer Quarterly, 40,* 138–156.

Eisenberg, N., Fabes, R. A., & Murphy, B. C. (1996). Parents' reactions to children's negative emotions: Relations to children's social competence and comforting behavior. *Child Development, 67,* 2227–2247.

Eisenberg, N., Fabes, R. A., Schaller, M., & Miller, P. A. (1989). Sympathy and personal distress: Development, gender differences, and interrelations of indices. In N.

Eisenberg (Ed.), *New directions in child development* (Vol. 44, pp. 107–126). San Francisco: Jossey-Bass.

Eisler, R. M., & Blalock, J. A. (1991). Masculine gender role stress: Implications for assessment of men. *Clinical Psychology Review, 11,* 45–60.

Ekman, P. (1972). Universals and cultural differences in facial expression of emotion. In J. Cole (Ed.), *Nebraska Symposium on Motivation* (Vol. 19, pp. 207–283). Lincoln: University of Nebraska Press.

Ekman, P. (1977). Biological and cultural contributions to body and facial movement. In J. Blacking (Ed.), *The anthropology of the body* (pp. 39–84). London: Academic Press.

Ekman, P. (1993). Facial expression and emotion. *American Psychologist, 48,* 384–392.

Ekman, P. (1994). Antecedent events and emotion metaphors. In P. Ekman & R. J. Davidson (Eds.), *The nature of emotion: Fundamental questions* (pp. 146–149). New York: Oxford University Press.

Ekman, P., & Friesen, W. V. (1969). Nonverbal leakage and clues to deception. *Psychiatry, 32,* 88–105.

Elliott, R., & Greenberg, L.S. (1993). Experiential therapy in practice: The process-experiential approach. In B. Bongar & L. Beutler (Eds.), *Comprehensive textbook of psychotherapy* (pp. 123–139). New York: Oxford University Press.

Elliott, R., Suter, P., Manford, J., Radpour-Markert, L., Siegel-Hinson, R., Layman, C., & Davis, K. (1996). A process–experiential approach to the treatment of post-traumatic stress disorder. In R. Hutterer, G. Pawlowsky, P. Schmid, & R. Stipsits (Eds.), *Client-centered and experiential psychotherapy: A paradigm in motion* (pp. 235–254). Vienna: Peter Lang.

Ellis, A. (1977). *Anger: How to live with and without it.* New York: Reader's Digest Press.

Ellis, A. (1991). The revised ABC's of rational-emotive therapy (RET). *Journal of Rational-Emotive and Cognitive-Behavioral Therapy, 9,* 139–172.

Ellsworth, P. C. (1994). Levels of thought and levels of emotion. In P. Ekman & R. J. Davidson (Eds.), *The nature of emotion: Fundamental questions* (pp. 192–196). New York: Oxford University Press.

Emmons, R. A. (1986). Personal strivings: An approach to personality and subjective well-being. *Journal of Personality and Social Psychology, 51*(5), 1058–1068.

Emmons, R. A. (1989). The personal striving approach to personality. In L. A. Pervin (Ed.), *Goal concepts in personality and social psychology* (pp. 87–126). Hillsdale, NJ: Erlbaum.

Emmons, R. A. (1992). Abstract versus concrete goals: Personal striving level, physical illness, and psychological well-being. *Journal of Personality and Social Psychology, 62,* 292–300.

Emmons, R. A., & King, L. A. (1988). Personal striving conflict: Immediate and long-term implications for psychological and physical well-being. *Journal of Personality and Social Psychology, 54,* 1040–1048.

Emmons, R. A., King, L. A., & Sheldon, K. (1993). Goal conflict and the self-regulation of action. In D. M. Wegner & J. W. Pennebaker (Eds.), *Handbook of mental control* (pp. 528–551). Englewood Cliffs, NJ: Prentice-Hall.

Engebretson, T. O., Matthews, K. A., & Scheier, M. F. (1989). Relations between anger expression and cardiovascular reactivity: Reconciling inconsistent findings through a matching hypothesis. *Journal of Personality and Social Psychology, 57,* 513–521.

Epstein, N., & Baucom, N. (1988). *Cognitive-behavioral marital therapy.* New York: Brunner/Mazel.

Epstein, S. (1990). Cognitive–experiential self theory. In L. A. Pervin (Ed.), *Handbook of personality: Theory and research* (pp. 165–192).

Epstein, S. (1994). Integration of the cognitive and the psychodynamic unconscious. *American Psychologist, 49,* 709–724.

Esterling, B. A., Antoni, M. H., Fletcher, M. A., Margulies, S., & Schneiderman, N. (1994).

Emotional disclosure through writing or speaking modulates latent Epstein–Barr virus antibody titers. *Journal of Consulting and Clinical Psychology, 62,* 130–140.

Eysenck, H. J. (1973). A short questionnaire for the measurement of two dimensions of personality. In H. J. Eysenck, *Eysenck on extraversion* (pp. 31–37). New York: Halsted.

Eysenck, H. J. (1985). Personality, cancer, and cardiovascular disease: A causal analysis. *Personality and Individual Differences, 6,* 535–556.

Eysenck, H. J. (1987). Arousal and personality: The origins of a theory. In J. Strelau & H. J. Eysenck (Eds.), *Personality dimensions and arousal* (pp. 1–13). New York: Plenum Press.

Eysenck, H. J. (1991a). Personality, stress, and disease: An interactionist perspective. *Psychological Inquiry, 2,* 221–232.

Eysenck, H. J. (1991b). Reply to criticisms of the Grossarth-Maticek studies. *Psychological Inquiry, 2,* 297–323.

Eysenck, H. J., & Eysenck, M. W. (1985). *Personality and individual differences: A natural science approach.* New York: Plenum Press.

Fairbank, J. A., Hansen, D. J., & Fitterling, J. M. (1991). Patterns of appraisal and coping across different stressor conditions among former prisoners of war with and without posttraumatic stress disorder. *Journal of Consulting and Clinical Psychology, 62,* 130–140.

Falbo, T., & Peplau, L. A. (1980). Power strategies in intimate relationships. *Journal of Personality and Social Psychology, 38,* 618–628.

Fawzy, F. I., Fawzy, N. W., Hyun, C. S., Elashoff, R., Guthrie, D., Fahey, J. L., & Morton, D. L. (1993). Malignant melanoma: Effects of an early structured psychiatric intervention, coping, and affective state on recurrence and survival six years later. *Archives of General Psychiatry, 50,* 681–689.

Feeney, J. A. (1995). Adult attachment and emotional control. *Personal Relationships, 2,* 143–159.

Feeney, J. A., Noller, P., & Callan, V. J. (1994). Attachment style, communication and satisfaction in the early years of marriage. *Advances in Personal Relationships, 5,* 269–308.

Feeney, J. A., Noller, P., & Roberts, N. (1998). Emotion, attachment, and satisfaction in close relationships. In P. A. Andersen & L. K. Guerrero (Eds.), *Handbook of communication and emotion: Research, theory, applications, and contexts* (pp. 473–505). San Diego, CA: Academic Press.

Fehr, B. (1988). Prototype analysis of the concepts of love and commitment. *Journal of Personality and Social Psychology, 55,* 557–579.

Feldstein, S., & Welkowitz, J. (1987). A chronography of conversation: in defense of an objective approach. In A. W. Siegman & S. Feldstein (Eds.), *Nonverbal behavior and communication* (pp. 435–500). Hillsdale, NJ: Erlbaum.

Fenigstein, A., Scheier, M. F., & Buss, A. H. (1975). Public and private self-consciousness: Assessment and theory. *Journal of Consulting and Clinical Psychology, 43,* 522–527.

Fernandez, A., Sriram, T. G., Rajkumar, A. N., & Chandrasekar, A. N. (1989). Alexithymic characteristics in rheumatoid arthritis: A controlled study. *Psychotherapy and Psychosomatics, 51,* 45–50.

Fichten, C. S., Taglakis, V., Judd, D., Wright, J., & Amsel, R. (1992). Verbal and nonverbal communication cues in daily conversations and dating. *Journal of Social Psychology, 132,* 751–769.

Field, T. M. (1982). Individual differences in the expressivity of neonates and young children. In R. S. Feldman (Ed.), *Development of nonverbal behavior in children* (pp. 279–298). New York: Springer-Verlag.

Field, T. M. (1984). Early interactions between infants and their postpartum depressed mothers. *Infant Behavior and Development, 7,* 517–522.

Field, T. M., Healy, B., Goldstein, S., & Guthertz, M. (1990). Behavior state matching in mother–infant interactions of nondepressed versus depressed mother–infant dyads. *Developmental Psychology, 26,* 7–14.

Field, T. M., Sandberg, D., Garcia, R., Vega-Lahr, N., Goldstein, S., & Guy, L. (1985). Pregnancy problems, postpartum depression, and early mother–infant interactions. *Developmental Psychology, 21,* 1152–1156.

Filsinger, E., & Thoma, S. (1988). Behavioral antecedents of relationship stability and adjustment: A five-year longitudinal study. *Journal of Marriage and the Family, 50,* 785–795.

Fincham, F. D., & Bradbury, T. N. (1993). Marital satisfaction, depression, and attributions: A longitudinal analysis. *Journal of Personality and Social Psychology, 64,* 442–452.

Fine, G. A., Stitt, J. L., & Finch, M. (1984). Couple tie-signs and interpersonal threat: A field experiment. *Social Psychology Quarterly, 47,* 282–286.

Fisher, J. D., Goff, B. A., Nadler, A., & Chinsky, J. M. (1988). Social psychological influences on help seeking and support from peers. In B. H. Gottlieb (Ed.), *Marshaling social support: Formats, processes and effects* (pp. 267–304). Newbury Park, CA: Sage.

Fitzpatrick, M. A. (1987). Marriage and verbal intimacy. In V. J. Derlega & J. H. Berg (Eds.), *Self-disclosure: Theory, research, and therapy* (pp. 131–154). New York: Plenum Press.

Fitzpatrick, M. A. (1988). *Between husbands and wives: Communication in marriage.* Newbury Park, CA: Sage.

Florin, I., Nostadt, A., Reck, C., Franzen, U., & Jenkins, M. (1992). Expressed emotion in depressed patients and their partners. *Journal of Family Process, 31,* 163–172.

Foa, E. B., & Kozak, M. J. (1986). Emotional processing of fear: Exposure to corrective information. *Psychological Bulletin, 99,* 20–35.

Foa, E. B., Rothbaum, B. O., Riggs, D. S., & Murdock, T. B. (1991). Treatment of post traumatic stress disorder in rape victims: A comparison between cognitive-behavioral procedures and counseling. *Journal of Consulting and Clinical Psychology, 59,* 715–723.

Foa, E. B., Steketee, G., & Rothbaum, B. O. (1989). Behavioral/cognitive conceptualizations of post-traumatic stress disorder. *Behavior Therapy, 20,* 155–176.

Folkman, S., Chesney, M. A., Cooke, M., Boccellari, A., & Collette, L. (1994). Caregiver burden in HIV-positive and HIV-negative partners of men with AIDS. *Journal of Consulting and Clinical Psychology, 62,* 746–756.

Forehand, R., & Smith, K. A. (1986). Who depressed whom? A look at the relationship of adolescent mood to maternal and paternal depression. *Child Study Journal, 16,* 19–23.

Fowles, D. C. (1980). The three arousal model: Implications of Gray's two-factor theory for heart rate, electrodermal activity, and psychopathy. *Psychophysiology, 17,* 87–104.

Fox, N. A. (1995). Of the way we were: Adult memories about attachment experiences and their role in determining infant–parent relationships: A commentary on van IJzendoorn (1995). *Psychological Bulletin, 117,* 404–410.

Foy, D. W. (1992). Introduction and Description of the Disorder. In D. W. Foy (Ed.), *Treating PTSD: Cognitive-behavioral strategies* (pp. 1–12). New York: Guilford Press.

Francis, M. E., & Pennebaker, J. W. (1992). Putting stress into words: The impact of writing on physiological, absentee, and self-reported emotional well-being measures. *American Journal of Health Promotion, 6,* 280–287.

Frandsen, M. M. (1989). *Attributional processes in premarital sexual interaction.* Unpublished master's thesis, Arizona State University, Tempe, AZ.

Franzoi, S. L. (1983). Self-concept differences as a function of private self-consciousness and social anxiety. *Journal of Research in Personality, 17,* 275–287.

Franzoi, S. L., Davis, M. H., & Markwiese, B. (1990). A motivational explanation for the existence of private self-consciousness differences. *Journal of Personality, 58,* 641–659.

Franzoi, S. L., Davis, M. H., & Young, R. D. (1985). The effects of private self-consciousness and perspective taking on satisfaction in close relationships. *Journal of Personality and Social Psychology, 48,* 1584–1594.

Freud, S. (1921). *Introductory lectures on psychoanalysis.* London: Allen & Irwin.

Freud, S. (1963). *Therapy and technique.* New York: MacMillan Company. (Original work published 1914)

Frey, W. H., II. (1985). *Crying: The mystery of tears.* Minneapolis, MN: Winston Press.

Frey, W. H., II, DeSota-Johnson, D., Hoffman, C., & McCall, J. T. (1981). Effect of stimulus on the chemical composition of human tears. *American Journal of Ophthalmology, 92,* 559–567.

Frey, W. H., II, Hoffman-Ahern, C., Johnson, R. A., Lykken, D. T., & Tuason, V. B., (1983). Crying behavior in the human adult. *Integrative Psychiatry, 1,* 94–100.

Fridlund, A. J. (1992). The behavioral ecology and sociality of human faces. In M. S. Clark (Ed.), *Review of personality and social psychology: Vol. 13. Emotion* (pp. 90–121). Newbury Park, CA: Sage.

Friedman, H. S. (1990). Where is the disease-prone personality? In H. S. Friedman (Ed.), *Personality and disease* (pp. 283–292). New York: Wiley.

Friedman, H. S. (1991). *The self-healing personality.* New York: Holt.

Friedman, H. S. (1992). Understanding hostility, coping, and health. In H. S. Friedman (Ed.), *Hostility, coping, and health* (pp. 3–9). Washington, DC: American Psychological Association.

Friedman, H. S., & Booth-Kewley, S. (1987a). The "disease-prone personality": A meta-analytic view of the construct. *American Psychologist, 42,* 539–555.

Friedman, H. S., & Booth-Kewley, S. (1987b). Personality, Type A behavior, and coronary heart disease: The role of emotional expression. *Journal of Personality and Social Psychology, 53,* 783–792.

Friedman, H. S., Hall, J. A., & Harris, M. J. (1985). Type A behavior, nonverbal expressive style, and health. *Journal of Personality and Social Psychology, 48,* 1299–1315.

Friedman, H. S., & Miller-Herringer, T. (1991). Nonverbal display of emotion in public and private: Self-monitoring, personality, and expressive cues. *Journal of Personality and Social Psychology, 61,* 766–775.

Friedman, H. S., Prince, L. M., Riggio, R. E., & DiMatteo, M. R. (1980). Understanding and assessing nonverbal expressiveness: The Affective Communication Test. *Journal of Personality and Social Psychology, 39,* 333–351.

Friedman, H. S., Tucker, J. S., Tomlinson-Keasey, C., Schwartz, J., Wingard, D., & Criqui, M. (1993). Does childhood personality predict longevity? *Journal of Personality and Social Psychology, 65,* 176–185.

Friedman, M., & Rosenman, R. H. (1974). *Type A behavior and your heart.* New York: Knopf.

Friedman, M., Thoresen, C. E., Gill, J., Ulmer, D., Powell, L. H., Price, V. A., Brown, B., Thompson, L., Rabin, D. D., Breall, W. S., Bourg, W., Levy, R., & Dixon, T. (1986). Alteration of Type A Behavior and its effect on cardiac recurrences in post myocardial infarction patients: Summary results of the Recurrent Coronary Prevention Project. *American Heart Journal, 112,* 653–665.

Frijda, N. H. (1986). *The emotions.* New York: Cambridge University Press.

Frijda, N. H. (1993). Moods, emotion episodes, and emotions. In M. Lewis & J. M. Haviland (Eds.), *Handbook of emotions* (pp. 381–404). New York: Guilford Press.

Frijda, N. H., Ortony, A., Sonnemans, J., & Clore, G. L. (1992). The complexity of intensity: Issues concerning the structure of emotion intensity. In M. S. Clark (Ed.), *Review of personality and social psychology: Vol. 13. Emotion* (pp. 60–89). Newbury Park, CA: Sage.

Fruzzetti, A. E., & Jacobson, N. S. (1990). Toward a behavioral conceptualization of adult intimacy: Implications for marital therapy. In E. A. Blechman (Ed.), *Emotions and the family: For better or for worse* (pp. 117–135). Hillsdale, NJ: Erlbaum.

Fuchs, D., & Thelen, M. (1988). Children's expected interpersonal consequences of communicating their affective state and reported likelihood of expression. *Child Development, 59,* 1314–1322.

Fuller, T. L., & Fincham, F. D. (1995). Attachment style in married couples: Relation to current marital functioning, stability over time, and method of assessment. *Personal Relationships, 2,* 17–34.

Gaelick, L., Bodenhausen, G. V., & Wyer, R. S. (1985). Emotional communication in close relationships. *Journal of Personality and Social Psychology, 49,* 1246–1265.

Gaensbauer, T. J. (1982). Regulation of emotional expression in infants from two contrasting caretaking environments. *Journal of the American Academy of Child Psychiatry, 21,* 163–171.

Gagnon, J. H., & Simon, W. (1973). *Sexual conduct: The social origins of human sexuality.* Chicago: Aldine.

Gano-Phillips, S., & Fincham, F. D. (1995). Family conflict, divorce, and children's adjustment. In M. A. Fitzpatrick & A. L. Vangelisti (Eds.), *Explaining family interaction* (pp. 206–231). Thousand Oaks, CA: Sage.

Geer, J. H., & Broussard, D. B. (1990). Scaling heterosexual behavior and arousal: Consistency and sex differences. *Journal of Personality and Social Psychology, 58,* 664–671.

Gelfand, D. M., & Teti, D. M. (1990). Children of depressed parents: An integrative review. *Psychological Bulletin, 108,* 50–76.

Geller, J. D. (1984). Moods, feelings, and the processing of affect information. In C. VanDyke, L. Temoshok, & L. S. Zegans (Eds.), *Emotions in health and illness: Applications to clinical practice* (pp. 171–186). New York: Grune & Stratton.

Gellert, G. A., Maxwell, R. M., & Siegel, B. S. (1993). Survival of breast cancer patients receiving adjunctive psychosocial support therapy: A 10-year follow-up study. *Journal of Clinical Oncology, 11,* 66–69.

Gendlin, E. T. (1974). Client-centered and experiential psychotherapy. In D. Wexler & L. N. Rice (Eds.), *Innovations in client-centered therapy* (pp. 211–246). New York: Wiley.

Gendlin, E. T. (1981). *Focusing* (2nd ed.). New York: Bantam Books.

George, C., Kaplan, N., & Main, M. (1985). *Adult Attachment Interview.* Unpublished manuscript, University of California, Berkeley.

Gilbert, D. G. (1991). A personality × personality × setting biosocial model of interpersonal affect and communication. In D. G. Gilbert & J. J. Connolly (Eds.), *Personality, social skills, and psychopathology: An individual differences approach* (pp. 107–135). New York: Plenum Press.

Gilbert, K. R. (1989). Interactive grief and coping in the marital dyad. *Death Studies, 13,* 605–626.

Gilbert, P. (1991). *Depression: The evolution of powerlessness.* New York: Guilford Press.

Giles, H. (1980). Accommodation theory: Some new directions. In S. De Silva (Ed.), *Aspects of linguistic behavior* (pp. 105–136). York, UK: University of York Press.

Gilligan, C. (1982). *In a different voice: Psychological theory and women's development.* Cambridge, MA: Harvard University Press.

Glaser, J., & Salovey, P. (1998). Affect in electoral politics. *Personality and Social Psychology Review, 2,* 156–172.

Goffman, E. (1972). *Relations in public.* New York: Harper & Row.

Goldfried, M. R. (1982). *Converging themes in psychotherapy: Trends in psychodynamic, humanistic, and behavioral practice.* New York: Springer.

Goldfried, M. R. (1995). *From cognitive-behavior therapy to psychotherapy integration: An evolving view.* New York: Springer.

Goldfried, M., De Canteceo, E. T., & Weinberg, L. (1974). Systematic rational restructuring as a self control technique. *Behavior Therapy, 5,* 247–254.

Goldman, S. L., Kraemer, D. T., & Salovey, P. (1996). Beliefs about mood moderate the relationship of stress to illness and symptom reporting. *Journal of Psychosomatic Research, 2,* 115–128.

Goleman, D. (1995). *Emotional intelligence.* New York: Bantam Books.

Gottlieb, B. H., & Wagner, F. (1991). Stress and support processes in close relationships. In J. Eckenrode (Ed.), *The social context of coping* (pp. 165–188). New York: Plenum Press.

Gottman, J. M. (1979). *Marital interaction: Experimental investigations.* New York: Academic Press.

Gottman, J. M. (1993a). *What predicts divorce: The relationship between marital processes and marital outcomes.* Hillsdale, NJ: Erlbaum.

Gottman, J. M. (1993b). The roles of conflict engagement, escalation, and avoidance in marital interaction: A longitudinal view of five types of couples. *Journal of Consulting and Clinical Psychology, 61,* 6–15.

Gottman, J. M. (1994). An agenda for marital therapy. In S.M. Johnson & L.S. Greenberg (Eds.), *The heart of the matter: Perspectives on emotion in marital therapy* (pp 256–296). New York: Brunner/Mazel.

Gottman, J. M., & Carrere, S. (1994). Why can't men and women get along? Developmental roots and marital inequities. In D. J. Canary & L. Stafford (Eds.), *Communication and relational maintenance* (pp. 203–229). San Diego, CA: Academic Press.

Gottman, J. M., Katz, L. F., & Hooven, C. (1996a). *Meta-emotion: How families communicate emotionally.* Mahwah, NJ: Erlbaum.

Gottman, J. M., Katz, L. F., & Hooven, C. (1996b). Parental meta-emotion philosophy and the emotional life of families: Theoretical models and preliminary data. *Journal of Family Psychology, 10,* 243–268.

Gottman, J. M., & Krokoff, L. J. (1989). Marital interaction and satisfaction: A longitudinal view. *Journal of Consulting and Clinical Psychology, 57,* 47–52.

Gottman, J. M., & Levenson, R. W. (1986). Assessing the role of emotion in marriage. *Behavioral Assessment, 8,* 31–48.

Gottman, J. M., & Levenson, R. W. (1988). The social psychophysiology of marriage. In P. Noller & M. A. Fitzpatrick (Eds.), *Perspectives on marital interactions* (pp. 183–200). Avon, UK: Multilingual Matters.

Gottman, J. M., Markman, H., & Notarius, C. (1977). The topography of marital conflict: A sequential analysis of verbal and nonverbal behavior. *Journal of Marriage and the Family, 39,* 461–477.

Gottman, J. M., & Parker, J. (Eds.). (1986). *Conversations of friends.* New York: Cambridge University Press.

Graham, T., & Ickes, W. (1997). When women's intuition isn't greater than men's. In W. Ickes (Ed.), *Empathic accuracy* (pp. 117–143). New York: Guilford Press.

Gray, J. (1995). *Mars and Venus in the bedroom.* New York: Harper Collins.

Green, R. A., & Murray, E. J. (1975). Expression of feeling and cognitive reinterpretation in the reduction of hostile aggression. *Journal of Consulting and Clinical Psychology, 43,* 375–383.

Greenberg, L. S., & Elliott, R. (1997). Varieties of empathic responding. In A. C. Bohart & L. S. Greenberg (Eds.), *Empathy reconsidered* (pp. 167–186). Washington, DC: APA Books.

Greenberg, L. S., & Johnson, S. M. (1988). *Emotionally focused therapy for couples.* New York: Guilford Press.

Greenberg, L. S., & Johnson, S. M. (1990). Emotional change processes in couples' therapy. In E. A. Blechman (Ed.), *Emotions and the family: For better or for worse* (pp. 137–153). Hillsdale, NJ: Erlbaum.

Greenberg, L. S., & Paivio, S. (1997). *Working with emotions in psychotherapy.* New York: Guilford Press.

Greenberg, L. S., Rice, L. N., & Elliott, R. (1993). *Facilitating emotional change: The moment-by-moment process.* New York: Guilford Press.

Greenberg, L. S., & Safran, J. D. (1987). *Emotion in psychotherapy: Affect, cognition, and the process of change.* New York: Guilford Press.

Greenberg, L. S., & Safran, J. D. (1989). Emotion in psychotherapy. *American Psychologist, 44,* 19–29.

Greenberg, L. S., Watson, J. C., & Goldman, R. (1998). Process–experiential therapy of depression. In L. S. Greenberg, J. C. Watson, & G. Lietaer (Eds.), *Handbook of experiential psychotherapy* (pp. 227–249). New York: Guilford Press.

Greenberg, L. S., Watson, J. C., & Lietaer, G. (Eds.). (1998). *Handbook of experiential psychotherapy.* New York: Guilford Press.

Greenberg, M. A. (1995). Cognitive processing of traumas: The role of intrusive thoughts and reappraisals. *Journal of Applied Social Psychology, 25,* 1262–1296.

Greenberg, M. A., & Stone, A. A. (1992). Emotional disclosure about traumas and its relation to health: Effects of previous disclosure and trauma severity. *Journal of Personality and Social Psychology, 63,* 75–84.

Greenberg, M. A., Wortman, C. B., & Stone, A. A. (1996). Emotional expression and physical health: Revising traumatic memories or fostering self-regulation? *Journal of Personality and Social Psychology, 71,* 588–602.

Greenberg, R. L. (1993). When the going gets tough the tough get going. In K. T. Kuehlwein & H. Rosen (Eds.), *Cognitive therapies in action: Evolving innovative practice* (pp. 126–142). San Francisco: Jossey-Bass.

Greer, S., & Watson, M. (1985). Towards a psychobiological model of cancer: Psychological considerations. *Social Science and Medicine, 20,* 773–777.

Griffin, D., & Bartholomew, K. (1994). The metaphysics of measurement: The case of adult attachment. In K. Batholomew & D. Perlman (Eds.), *Advances in personal relationships: Vol. 5. Attachment processes in adulthood* (pp. 17–52). London: Kingsley.

Gross, J. J. (1989). Emotional expression in cancer onset and progression. *Social Science and Medicine, 28,* 1239–1248.

Gross, J. J. (1998). Antecedent- and response-focused emotion regulation: Divergent consequences for experience, expression, and physiology. *Journal of Personality and Social Psychology, 74,* 224–237.

Gross, J. J., Fredrickson, B. L., & Levenson, R. W. (1994). The psychophysiology of crying. *Psychophysiology, 31,* 460–468.

Gross, J. J., & John, O. P. (1997). Revealing feelings: Facets of emotional expressivity in self-reports, peer ratings, and behavior. *Journal of Personality and Social Psychology, 72,* 435–448.

Gross, J. J., & Levenson, R. W. (1993). Emotional suppression: Physiology, self-report, and expressive behavior. *Journal of Personality and Social Psychology, 64,* 970–986.

Gross, J. J., & Levenson, R. W. (1997). Hiding feelings: The acute effects of inhibiting negative and positive emotion. *Journal of Abnormal Psychology, 106,* 95–103.

Gross, J. J., & Muñoz, R. F. (1995). Emotion regulation and mental health. *Clinical Psychology: Science and Practice, 2,* 151–164.

Grossarth-Maticek, R., Bastiaans, J., & Kanazir, D. T. (1985). Psychosocial factors as strong predictors of mortality from cancer, ischaemic heart disease and stroke: The Yugoslav prospective study. *Journal of Psychosomatic Research, 29,* 167–176.

Grossarth-Maticek, R., Kanazir, D. T., Schmidt, P., & Vetter, H. (1985). Psychosocial and organic variables as predictors of lung cancer, cardiac infarct and apoplexy: Some differential predictors. *Personality and Individual Differences, 6,* 313–321.

Grossarth-Maticek, R., Kanazir, D. T., Vetter, H., & Schmidt, P. (1983). Psychosomatic factors involved in the process of cancerogenesis: Preliminary results of the Yugoslav prospective study. *Psychotherapy and Psychosomatics, 40,* 191–210.

Grych, J. H., & Fincham, F. D. (1990). Marital conflict and children's adjustment: A cognitive-contextual framework. *Psychological Bulletin, 108,* 267–290.

Grych, J. H., & Fincham, F. D. (1993). Children's appraisals of marital conflict: Initial investigations of the cognitive-contextual framework. *Child Development, 64,* 1–17.

Guerney, B. G. (1994). The role of emotion in relationship enhancement marital/family therapy. In S. M. Johnson & L. S. Greenberg (Eds.), *The heart of the matter: Perspectives on emotion in marital therapy* (pp 124–150). New York: Brunner/Mazel.

Guerrero, L. K. (1996). Attachment-style differences in intimacy and involvement: A test of the four-category model. *Communication Monographs, 63,* 269–293.

Guerrero, L. K., & Andersen, P. A. (1991). The waxing and waning of relational intimacy: Touch as a function of relational stage, gender, and touch avoidance. *Journal of Social and Personal Relationships, 8,* 147–165.

Guerrero, L. K., & Andersen, P. A. (1994). Patterns of matching and initiation: Touch behavior and touch avoidance across romantic relationship stages. *Journal of Nonverbal Behavior, 18,* 137–153.

Guerrero, L. K., Eloy, S. V., & Wabnik, A. I. (1993). Linking maintenance strategies to relationship development and disengagement: A reconceptualization. *Journal of Social and Personal Relationships, 10,* 273–283.

Gur, R. C., & Sackeim, H. A. (1979). Self-deception: A concept in search of a phenomenon. *Journal of Personality and Social Psychology, 37,* 147–169.

Gurman, A. S., & Jacobson, N. S. (1995). Therapy with couples: A coming of age. In N. S. Jacobson & A. S. Gurman (Eds.), *Clinical handbook of couple therapy* (pp 1–10). New York: Guilford Press.

Haggard, E. A., & Isaacs, K. S. (1966). Micromomentary facial expressions as indicators of ego mechanisms in psychotherapy. In L. A. Gottschalk & A. H. Auerbach (Eds.), *Methods of research in psychotherapy* (pp.154–165). New York: Appleton-Century-Crofts.

Halberstadt, A. G. (1983). Family expressiveness styles and nonverbal communication skills. *Journal of Nonverbal Behavior, 8,* 14–26.

Halberstadt, A. G. (1985). Race, socioeconomic status, and nonverbal behavior. In A. Siegman & S. Feldstein (Eds.), *Nonverbal communication and interpersonal relations* (pp. 227–266). Hillsdale, NJ: Erlbaum.

Halberstadt, A. G. (1986). Family socialization of emotional expression and nonverbal communication styles and skills. *Journal of Personality and Social Psychology, 51,* 827–836.

Halberstadt, A. G. (1991). Toward an ecology of expressiveness: Family socialization in particular and a model in general. In R. S. Feldman & B. Rimé (Eds.), *Fundamentals of nonverbal behavior* (pp. 106–160). New York: Cambridge University Press.

Halberstadt, A. G., Fox, N. A., & Jones, N. A. (1993). Do expressive mothers have expressive children? The role of socialization in children's affect expression. *Social Development, 2,* 48–65.

Hall, J. A. (1984). *Nonverbal sex differences: Communication accuracy and expressive style.* Baltimore: Johns Hopkins University Press.

Hall, J. A. (1987). On explaining gender differences: The case of nonverbal communication. In P. Shaver & C. Hendrick (Eds.), *Review of personality and social psychology: Vol. 6. Sex and gender* (pp. 177–200). Newbury Park, CA: Sage.

Hall, J. A., & Veccia, E. M. (1990). More "touching" observations: New insights on men, women, and interpersonal touch. *Journal of Personality and Social Psychology, 59,* 1155–1162.

Hamilton, C. E. (1995, March). *Continuity and discontinuity of attachment from infancy through adolescence.* Paper presented at the meeting of the Society for Research in Child Development, Indianapolis, IN.

Hammen, C. L., Gordon, D., Burge, D., Adrian, C., Janicke, C., & Hiroto, D. (1987). Communication patterns of mothers with affective disorders and their relationship to children's status and social functioning. In K. Hahlweg & M. J. Goldstein (Eds.), *Understanding major mental disorder* (pp. 103–119). New York: Family Process Press.

Hanna, J. L. (1984). Black/white nonverbal differences, dance, and dissonance: Implications for desegregation. In A. Wolfgang (Ed.), *Nonverbal behavior: Perspectives, applications, intercultural insights* (pp. 373–409). Lewiston, NY: Hofgrefe.

Harburg, E., Blakelock, E. H., & Roeper, P. J. (1979). Resentful and reflective coping with arbitrary authority and blood pressure. *Psychosomatic Medicine, 41,* 189–202.

Harvey, J. H., Weber, A. L., Galvin, K. S., Huszti, H. C., & Garnick, N. N. (1986). Attribution and the termination of close relationships: A special focus on the account. In R. Gilmour & S. Duck (Eds.), *The emerging field of personal relationships* (pp. 189–201). Hillsdale, NJ: Erlbaum.

Hatfield, E. (1984). The dangers of intimacy. In V. J. Derlega (Ed.), *Communication, intimacy, and close relationships* (pp. 207–220). Orlando, FL: Academic Press.

Hatfield, E., Cacioppo, J. T., & Rapson, R. L. (1992). Primitive emotional contagion. In M. S. Clark (Ed.), *Review of personality and social psychology: Vol. 14. Emotion and social behavior* (pp. 119–150). Newbury Park, CA: Sage.

Hatfield, E., Cacioppo, J. T., & Rapson, R. L. (1994). *Emotional contagion.* New York: Cambridge University Press.

Hatfield, E., & Rapson, R. L. (1987). Gender differences in love and intimacy: The fantasy vs. the reality. *Journal of Social Work and Human Sexuality, 5,* 15–26.

Hatfield, E., & Sprecher, S. (1986). Measuring passionate love in intimate relations. *Journal of Adolescence, 9,* 383–410.

Haviland, J. M., & Lelwica, M. (1987). The induced affect response: 10-week old infants' responses to three emotion expressions. *Developmental Psychology, 23,* 97–104.

Hays, R. B. (1984). The development and maintenance of friendship. *Journal of Social and Personal Relationships, 1,* 75–98.

Hays, R. B. (1985). A longitudinal study of friendship development. *Journal of Personality and Social Psychology, 48,* 909–924.

Hazan, C., & Shaver, P. (1987). Romantic love conceptualized as an attachment process. *Journal of Personality and Social Psychology, 52,* 511–524.

Heatherton, T. F., & Baumeister, R. F. (1991). Binge eating as escape from self-awareness. *Psychological Bulletin, 110,* 86–108.

Hecht, M. L., Marston, P. J., & Larkey, L. K. (1994). Love ways conceptualized as an attachment process. *Journal of Social and Personal Relationships, 4,* 281–298.

Heise, D. R. (1989). Effects of emotion displays on social identification. *Social Psychology Quarterly, 52,* 10–21.

Helgeson, V. S., & Cohen, S. (1996). Social support and adjustment to cancer: Reconciling descriptive, correlational, and intervention research. *Health Psychology, 15,* 135–148.

Hendrick, C., & Hendrick, S. S. (1986). A theory and method of love. *Journal of Personality and Social Psychology, 50,* 392–402.

Hendrick, S. S. (1981). Self-disclosure and marital satisfaction. *Journal of Personality and Social Psychology, 40,* 1150–1159.

Hendrick, S. S., & Hendrick, C. (1987). Love and sexual attitudes, self-disclosure, and sensation-seeking. *Journal of Social and Personal Relationships, 4,* 281–297.

Hendrick, S. S., & Hendrick, C. (1992). *Romantic love.* Newbury Park, CA: Sage.

Hendrick, S. S., & Hendrick, C. (1995). Gender differences and similarities in sex and love. *Personal Relationships, 2,* 55–65.

Hendrick, S. S., Hendrick, C., Slapion-Foote, M. J., & Foote, F. H. (1985). Gender differences in sexual attitudes. *Journal of Personality and Social Psychology, 48,* 1630–1642.

Henley, N. M. (1977). *Body politics: Power, sex, and nonverbal communication.* Englewood Cliffs, NJ: Prentice-Hall.

Herman, J. (1988). Father–daughter incest. In F. Ochberg (Ed.), *Post-traumatic therapy and victims of violence* (pp. 175–195). New York: Brunner/Mazel.

Herman, J. (1992). *Trauma and recovery*. New York: Basic Books.

Hetherington, E. M., Cox, M., & Cox, R. (1982). Effects of divorce on parents and children. In M. Lamb (Ed.), *Nontraditional families* (pp. 233–288). Hillsdale, NJ: Erlbaum.

Higgins, E. T. (1997). Beyond pleasure and pain. *American Psychologist, 52,* 1280–1300.

Hill, C. E., Helms, J. E., Spiegel, S. B., & Tichenor, V. (1988). Development of a system for categorizing client reactions to therapist interventions. *Journal of Counseling Psychology, 35,* 27–36.

Hill, C. T., & Stull, D. E. (1987). Gender and self-disclosure: Strategies for exploring the issues. In V. J. Derlega & J. H. Berg (Eds.), *Self-disclosure: Theory, research, and therapy* (pp. 81–100). New York: Plenum Press.

Hinchliffe, M. K., Hooper, D., & Roberts, J. F. (1978). *The melancholy marriage; Depression in marriage and psychosocial approaches to therapy*. New York: Wiley.

Hinde, R. A. (1984). Why do the sexes behave differently in close relationships? *Journal of Social and Personal Relationships, 1,* 471–501.

Hochschild, A. (1983). *The managed heart: Commercialization of human feeling*. Berkeley: University of California Press.

Hokanson, J. E., & Rupert, M. P. (1991). Interpersonal factors in depression. In D. G. Gilbert & J. J. Connolly (Eds.), *Personality, social skills and psychopathology: An individual differences approach* (pp. 157–184). New York: Plenum Press.

Hollon, S. D., & Beck, A. T. (1979). Cognitive therapy of depression. In P. C. Kendall & S. D. Hollon (Eds.), *Cognitive-behavioral interventions: Theory, research and procedures* (pp. 153–204). New York: Academic Press.

Hollon, S. D., & Jacobsen, V. (1985). Cognitive approaches. In M. Hersen & A. S. Bellack (Eds.), *Handbook of clinical behavior therapy with adults* (pp. 169–200). New York: Plenum Press.

Hollon, S. D., Shelton, R. C., & Loosen, P. T. (1991). Cognitive therapy and pharmacotherapy for depression. *Journal of Consulting and Clinical Psychology, 59,* 88–99.

Hooley, J. M., Orley, J., & Teasdale, J. D. (1986). Levels of expressed emotion and relapse in depressed patients. *British Journal of Psychiatry, 148,* 642–647.

Hooley, J. M., & Teasdale, J. D. (1989). Predictors of relapse in unipolar depressives: Expressed emotion, marital distress, and perceived criticism. *Journal of Abnormal Psychology, 98,* 229–235.

Hoover-Dempsey, K. V., Plas, J. M., & Strudler Wallston, B. (1986). Tears and weeping among professional women: In search of new understanding. *Psychology of Women Quarterly, 10,* 19–34.

Hops, H., Biglan, A., Sherman, L., Arthur, J., Friedman, L., & Osteen, V. (1987). Home observation of family interactions of depressed women. *Journal of Consulting and Clinical Psychology, 55,* 341–346.

Horney, K. (1950). *Neurosis and human growth*. New York: Norton.

Horowitz, M. J. (1985). Disasters and psychological response to stress. *Psychiatric Annals, 15,* 161–167.

Horowitz, M. J. (1986). *Stress response syndromes* (2nd ed.). Northvale, NJ: Aronson.

Horowitz, M. J. (1991). *Person schemas and maladaptive interpersonal patterns*. Chicago: University of Chicago Press.

Horowitz, M. J., Stinson, C., Curtis, D., Ewert, M., Redington, D., Singer, J., Bucci, W., Mergenthaler, E., Milbrath, C., & Hartley, D. (1993). Topics and signs: Defensive control of emotional expression. *Journal of Consulting and Clinical Psychology, 61,* 421–430.

Horvath, A., & Greenberg, L. (Eds.). (1994). *The working alliance: Theory, research and practice*. New York: Wiley.

Hudgins, M. K. (1998). Experiential psychotherapy with sexual trauma. In L. S. Greenberg, J. C. Watson, & G. Lietaer (Eds.), *Handbook of experiential psychotherapy* (pp. 328–348). New York: Guilford Press.

Huston, T. L., McHale, S. M., & Crouter, A. C. (1986). When the honeymoon's over: Changes in the marriage relationship over the first year. In R. Gilmour & S. Duck (Eds.), *The emerging field of personal relationships* (pp. 109–132). Hillsdale, NJ: Erlbaum.

Huston, T. L., & Vangelisti, A. L. (1991). Socioemotional behavior and satisfaction in marital relationships: A longitudinal study. *Journal of Personality and Social Psychology, 6,* 721–733.

Ingram, R. E. (1990). Self-focused attention in clinical disorders: Review and a conceptual model. *Psychological Bulletin, 107,* 156–176.

Izard, C. E. (1992). Basic emotions, relations among emotions, and emotion–cognition relations. *Psychological Review, 99,* 561–564.

Jacobson, N. S. (1983). Beyond empiricism: The politics of marital therapy. *American Journal of Family Therapy, 11,* 11–24.

Jacobson, N. S. (1989). The politics of intimacy. *The Behavior Therapist, 12,* 29–32.

Jacobson, N. S., & Holtzworth-Munroe, A. (1986). Marital therapy: A social learning–cognitive perspective. In N. S. Jacobson & A. S. Gurman (Eds.), *Clinical handbook of marital therapy* (pp. 29–70). New York: Guilford Press.

Jacobson, N. S., & Margolin, G. (1979). *Marital therapy: Strategies based on social learning and behavior exchange principles.* New York: Brunner/Mazel.

Jacobson, N. S., Waldron, H., & Moore, D. (1980). Toward a behavioral profile of marital distress. *Journal of Consulting and Clinical Psychology, 48,* 696–703.

Jamison, K. R., Wellisch, D. K., & Pasnau, R. O. (1978). Psychosocial aspects of mastectomy: I. The woman's perspective. *American Journal of Psychiatry, 135,* 432–436.

Janoff-Bullman, K. (1992). *Shattered assumptions.* New York: Free Press.

Jenkins, C. D., Zyzanski, S. J., & Rosenman, R. H. (1979). *Jenkins Activity Survey.* New York: Psychological Corporation.

Jesser, C. J. (1978). Male responsiveness to direct verbal sexual initiatives of females. *Journal of Sex Research, 14,* 118–128.

Jesser, C. J. (1982, April). *Gender and crying among college students.* Paper presented at the meeting of the Midwest Sociological Society, Des Moines, IA.

Johnson, F., & Aries, E. (1983). Conversational patterns among same-sex pairs of late adolescent close friends. *Journal of Genetic Psychology, 142,* 225–238.

Johnson, K., & Edwards, R. (1991). The effects of gender and type of romantic touch on perceptions of relational commitment. *Journal of Nonverbal Behavior, 15,* 43–55.

Johnson, S. M., & Greenberg, L. S. (1994a). Emotion in intimate interactions: A synthesis. In S.M. Johnson & L. S. Greenberg (Eds.), *The heart of the matter: Perspectives on emotion in marital therapy* (pp. 297–324). New York: Brunner/Mazel.

Johnson, S. M., & Greenberg, L. S. (1994b). Emotion in intimate relationships: Theory and implications for therapy. In S. M. Johnson & L. S. Greenberg (Eds.), *The heart of the matter: Perspectives on emotion in marital therapy* (pp. 3–26). New York: Brunner/ Mazel.

Johnson, S., & Greenberg, L. S. (1995). The emotionally focused approach to problems in adult attachment. In N. S. Jacobson & A.S. Gurman (Eds.), *Clinical handbook of couple therapy* (pp. 121–141). New York: Guilford Press.

Johnston, D. W. (1992). The management of stress in the prevention of coronary heart disease. In S. Maes, H. Leventhal, & M. Johnston (Eds.), *International review of health psychology* (Vol. 1, pp. 57–83). Chichester, UK: Wiley.

Jones, H. E. (1950). The study of patterns of emotional expression. In M. L. Reymert (Ed.), *Feelings and emotions* (pp. 161–168). New York: McGraw-Hill.

Jones, H. E. (1960). The longitudinal method in the study of personality. In I. Iscoe & H. W. Stevenson, (Eds.), *Personality development in children* (pp. 3–27). Austin: University of Texas Press.

Joseph, S., Williams, R., Irwing, P., & Cammock, T. (1994). The preliminary development of a measure to assess attitudes towards emotional expression. *Personality and individual differences, 16,* 869–875.

Julien, D., Markman, H. J., & Lindahl, K. M. (1989). A comparison of a global and a microanalytic coding system: Implications for future trends in studying interaction. *Behavioral Assessment, 11,* 81–100.

Kagan, J. (1992). Temperamental contributions to emotion and social behavior. In M. S. Clark (Ed.), *Review of personality and social psychology: Vol. 14. Emotion and social behavior* (pp. 99–118). Newbury Park, CA: Sage.

Kagan, J., Reznick, J. S., & Snidman, N. (1987). The physiology and psychology of behavioral inhibition in children. *Child Development, 58,* 1459–1473.

Kahn, J., Coyne, J. C., & Margolin, G. (1985). Depression and marital conflict: The social construction of despair. *Journal of Social and Personal Relationships, 2,* 447–462.

Katkin, E. S. (1984). Blood, sweat, and tears: Individual differences in autonomic self-perception. *Psychophysiology, 22,* 125–137.

Katz, L. F., & Gottman, J. M. (1993). Patterns of marital conflict predict children's internalizing and externalizing behaviors. *Developmental Psychology, 29,* 940–950.

Katz, L. F., Gottman, J. M., & Hooven, C. (1996). Meta-emotion philosophy and family functioning: Reply to Cowan (1996) and Eisenberg (1996). *Journal of Family Psychology, 10,* 284–291.

Keinan, G., Ben-zur, H., Zilka, M., & Carel, R. S. (1992). Anger in or out, which is healthier? An attempt to reconcile inconsistent findings. *Psychology and Health, 7,* 83–98.

Kellner, R. (1990). Somatization: The concept and its clinical application. *Journal of Nervous and Mental Disease, 178,* 150–160.

Kelly, A. E., & McKillop, K. J. (1996). Consequences of revealing personal secrets. *Psychological Bulletin, 120,* 450–465.

Keltner, D., & Kring, A. M. (1998). Emotion, social function, and psychopathology. *Review of General Psychology, 2,* 320–324.

Kennedy-Moore, E. (1999). *Mood attributions and mood regulation: Beliefs about why we feel the way we feel.* Manuscript submitted for publication.

Kennedy-Moore, E., Greenberg, M. A., & Wortman, C. B. (1991, August). *Varieties of nonexpression: A review of self-report measures of emotional control.* Paper presented at the meeting of the American Psychological Association, San Francisco, CA.

Kennedy-Moore, E., & Stone, A. A. (1999). *Expression, experience, and attitude toward emotion: Mental and physical correlates.* Manuscript submitted for publication.

Kernberg, O. F. (1993). Convergences and divergences in contemporary psychoanalytic technique. *International Journal of Psycho-Analysis, 74,* 659–673.

Kiecolt, J., & McGrath, E. (1979). Social desirability responding in the measurement of assertive behavior. *Journal of Consulting and Clinical Psychology, 47,* 640–642.

Kiecolt-Glaser, J. K., & Murray, J. A. (1980). Social desirability bias in self-monitoring data. *Journal of Behavioral Assessment, 2,* 239–247.

Kiesler, D. J. (1991). Interpersonal methods of assessment and diagnosis. In C. R. Snyder & D. R. Forsyth (Eds.), *Handbook of social and clinical psychology: The health perspective* (pp. 438–468). New York: Pergamon Press.

King, C. E., & Christensen, A. (1983). The Relationship Events Scale: A Guttman scaling of progress in courtship. *Journal of Marriage and the Family, 45,* 671–678.

King, L. A., & Emmons, R. A. (1990). Conflict over emotional expression: Psychological and physical correlates. *Journal of Personality and Social Psychology, 58,* 864–877.

King, L. A., Emmons, R. A., & Woodley, S. (1992). The structure of inhibition. *Journal of Research in Personality, 26,* 85–102.

Kirsch, I., Mearns, J., & Catanzaro, S. J. (1990). Mood regulation expectancies as determinants of dysphoria in college students. *Journal of Counseling Psychology, 37,* 306–312.

Kitayama, S., & Markus, H. R. (Eds.). *(1996). Emotion and culture*. Washington, DC: American Psychological Association.

Klein, M. H., Mathieu-Coughlan, P., & Kiesler, D. J. (1986). The experiencing scales. In L. S. Greenberg & W. M. Pinsof (Eds.), *The psychotherapeutic process: A research handbook* (pp. 21–71). New York: Guilford Press.

Klerman, G. L., Weissman, M. M., Rounsaville, B. J., & Chevron, E. S. (1984). *Interpersonal psychotherapy of depression*. New York: Basic Books.

Klinnert, M. D., Campos, J. J., Sorce, J. F., Emde, R. N., & Svejda, M. (1983). Emotions as behavior regulators: Social referencing in infancy. In R. Plutchik & H. Kellerman (Eds.), *Emotion, theory, research, and experience: Vol. 2. Emotions in early development* (pp. 57–86). New York: Academic Press.

Knapp, M. L. (1984). *Interpersonal communication and human relationships*. Boston: Allyn & Bacon.

Kobak, R., & Hazan, C. (1991). Attachment in marriage: Effects of security and accuracy of working models. *Journal of Personality and Social Psychology, 60,* 861–869.

Koeppel, L. B., Montagne-Miller, Y., O'Hair, E., & Cody, M. J. (1993). Friendly? Flirting? Wrong? In P. J. Kalbfleisch (Ed.), *Interpersonal communication: Evolving interpersonal relationships* (pp. 13–32). Hillsdale, NJ: Erlbaum.

Koerner, K., & Jacobson, N. (1994). Emotion and behavioral couple therapy. In S. M. Johnson & L. S. Greenberg (Eds.), *The heart of the matter: Perspectives on emotion in marital therapy* (pp 207–226). New York: Brunner/Mazel.

Kosmicki, F. X., & Glickauf-Hughes, C. (1997). Catharsis in psychotherapy. *Psychotherapy, 34,* 154–159.

Kottler, J. (1996). *The language of tears*. San Francisco: Jossey-Bass.

Kraemer, D. L., & Hastrup, J. L. (1986). Crying in natural settings: Global estimates, self-monitored frequencies, depression, and sex differences in an undergraduate population. *Behaviour Research and Therapy, 24,* 371–373.

Kraemer, D. L., & Hastrup, J. L. (1988). Crying in adults: Self-control and autonomic correlates. *Journal of Social and Clinical Psychology, 6,* 53–68.

Krantz, A. M., & Pennebaker, J. W. (1996). *Bodily versus written expression of traumatic experience*. Unpublished manuscript, Southern Methodist University, Dallas, TX.

Kring, A. M., Smith, D. A., & Neale, J. M. (1994). Individual differences in dispositional expressiveness: Development and validation of the Emotional Expressivity Scale. *Journal of Personality and Social Psychology, 66,* 934–949.

Krystal, H. (1978). Trauma and affects. *Psychoanalytic Study of the Child, 33,* 81–117.

Krystal, H. (1988). *Integration and self-healing: Affect, trauma, alexithymia*. Hillsdale, NJ: Analytic Press.

Kübler-Ross, E. (1969). *On death and dying*. New York: Springer.

Kuiken, D., Carey, R., Nielsen, T. (1987). Moments of affective insight: Their phenomenon and relations to selected individual differences. *Imagination, Cognition, and Personality, 6,* 341–364.

Kuipers, L. (1979). Expressed emotion: A review. *British Journal of Social and Clinical Psychology, 18,* 237–243.

Labott, S. M., Ahleman, S., Wolever, M. E., & Martin, R. B. (1990). The physiological and psychological effects of the expression and inhibition of emotion. *Behavioral Medicine, 16,* 182–189.

Labott, S. M., Elliot, R., & Eason, P. S. (1992). "If you love someone, you don't hurt them": A comprehensive process analysis of a weeping event in therapy. *Psychiatry, 55,* 49–62.

Labott, S. M., & Martin, R. B. (1988). Weeping: Evidence for a cognitive theory. *Motivation and Emotion, 12,* 205–216.

Labott, S. M., & Martin, R. B. (1990). Emotional coping, age, and physical disorder. *Behavioral Medicine, 16,* 53–61.

Labott, S. M., Martin, R. B., Eason, P. S., & Berkey, E. Y. (1991). Social reactions to the expression of emotion. *Cognition and Emotion, 5*, 397–417.

Labott, S. M., & Teleha, M. K. (1996). Weeping propensity and the effects of laboratory expression or inhibition. *Motivation and Emotion, 20*, 273–284.

Labouvie-Vief, G., & DeVoe, M. (1991). Emotional regulation in adulthood and later life: A developmental view. *Annual Review of Gerontology and Geriatrics, 11*, 172–194.

Lacey, J. I. (1956). The evaluation of autonomic responses: Toward a general solution. *Annals of the New York Academy of Sciences, 67*, 123–163.

Lacey, J. I. (1967). Somatic response patterning and stress: Some revisions of activation theory. In M. H. Appley & R. Tumbull (Eds.), *Psychological stress: Issues in research* (pp. 14–44). New York: Appleton-Century-Crofts.

LaFrance, M. (1979). Nonverbal synchrony and rapport: Analysis by the cross-lag panel technique. *Social Psychology Quarterly, 42*, 66–70.

LaFrance, M. (1985). Postural mirroring and intergroup relations. *Personality and Social Psychology Bulletin, 11*, 207.

Laird, J. D. (1974). Self-attribution of emotion: The effects of expressive behavior on the quality of emotional experience. *Journal of Personality and Social Psychology, 29*, 475–486.

Laird, J. D., & Bresler, C. (1992). The process of emotional experience: A self-perception theory. In M. S. Clark (Ed.), *Review of personality and social psychology: Vol. 13. Emotion* (pp. 213–234). Newbury Park, CA: Sage.

Lane, C., & Hobfoll, S. E. (1992). How loss affects anger and alienates potential supporters. *Journal of Consulting and Clinical Psychology, 60*, 935–942.

Lane, R. D., Merikangas, K. R., Schwartz, G. E., Huang, S. S., & Prusoff, B. A. (1990). Inverse relationship between defensiveness and lifetime prevalence of psychiatric disorder. *American Journal of Psychiatry, 147*, 573–578.

Lane, R. D., Quinlan, D. M., Schwartz, G. E., Walker, P. A., & Zeitlin, S. B. (1990). The levels of emotional awareness scale: A cognitive-developmental measure of emotion. *Journal of Personality Assessment, 55*, 124–134.

Lane, R. D., & Schwartz, G. E. (1987). Levels of emotional awareness: A cognitive-developmental theory and its application to psychopathology. *American Journal of Psychiatry, 144*, 133–143.

Lane, R. D., & Schwartz, G. E. (1992). Levels of emotional awareness: Implications for psychotherapeutic integration. *Journal of Psychotherapy Integrations, 2*, 1–18.

Lang, P. J. (1994). The varieties of emotional experience: A meditation on James–Lange theory. *Psychological Review, 101*, 211–221.

Lang, P. J., Levin, D. N., Miller, G. A., & Kozak, M. J. (1983). Fear behavior, fear imagery, and the psychophysiology of emotion: The problem of affective response integration. *Journal of Abnormal Psychology, 92*, 276–306.

Langston, C. A. (1994). Capitalizing on and coping with daily-life events: Expressive responses to positive events. *Journal of Personality and Social Psychology, 67*, 1112–1125.

Lanzetta, J. T., Cartwright-Smith, J., & Kleck, R. E. (1976). Effects of nonverbal dissimulation on emotional experience and autonomic arousal. *Journal of Personality and Social Psychology, 33*, 354–370.

Lanzetta, J. T., & Kleck, R. E. (1970). Encoding and decoding of nonverbal affect in humans. *Journal of Personality and Social Psychology, 16*, 12–19.

Larsen, D., & Chastain, R. L. (1990). Self-concealment: Conceptualization, measurement, and health implications. *Journal of Social and Clinical Psychology, 9*, 439–455.

Larsen, R. J., & Diener, E. (1987). Affect intensity as an individual difference characteristic: A review. *Journal of Research in Personality, 21*, 1–39.

Larsen, R. J., Diener, E., & Cropanzano, R. S. (1987). Cognitive operations associated with individual differences in affect intensity. *Journal of Personality and Social Psychology, 53*, 767–774.

Larsen, R. J., Diener, E., & Emmons, R. A. (1986). Affect intensity and reactions to daily life events. *Journal of Personality and Social Psychology, 51,* 803–814.

Larsen, R. J., & Zarate, M. A. (1991). Extending the reducer/augmenter theory into the emotion domain: The role of affect in regulating stimulation level. *Personality and Individual Differences, 12,* 713–723.

Lawton, M. P., Kleban, M. H., Rajagopal, D., & Dean, J. (1992). Dimensions of affective experience in three age groups. *Psychology and Aging, 7,* 171–184.

Lazarus, R. S. (1984). On the primacy of cognition. *American Psychologist, 39,* 124–129.

Lazarus, R. S. (1991). *Emotion and adaptation.* New York: Oxford University Press.

Lazarus, R. S. (1995). Vexing research problems inherent in cognitive-mediational theories of emotion—and some solutions. *Psychological Inquiry, 6,* 183–196.

Lazarus, R. S., & Folkman, S. (1984). *Stress, appraisal, and coping.* New York: Springer.

LeDoux, J. E. (1989). Cognitive–emotional interactions in the brain. *Cognition and Emotion, 3,* 267–289.

LeDoux, J. E. (1994). Cognitive–emotional interactions in the brain. In P. Ekman & R. J. Davidson (Eds.), *The nature of emotion: Fundamental questions* (pp. 216–223). New York: Oxford University Press.

LeDoux, J. E. (1996). *The emotional brain: The mysterious underpinnings of emotional life.* New York: Simon & Schuster.

Leijssen, M. (1990). On focusing and the necessary conditions of therapeutic personality change. In G. Lietaer, J. Rombauts, & R. Van Balen (Eds.), *Client-centered and experiential psychotherapy in the nineties* (pp. 225–250). Leuven, Belgium: Leuven University Press.

Lemerise, E. A., & Dodge, K. A. (1993). The development of anger and hostile interaction. In M. Lewis & J. M. Haviland (Eds.), *Handbook of emotions* (pp. 537–546). New York: Guilford Press.

Lepore, S. J., Silver, R. C., Wortman, C. B., & Wayment, H. A. (1996). Social constraints, intrusive thoughts, and depressive symptoms among bereaved mothers. *Journal of Personality and Social Psychology, 70,* 271–282.

Levenson, R. W. (1994). Emotional control: Variation and consequences. In P. Ekman & R. J. Davidson (Eds.), *The nature of emotion: Fundamental questions* (pp. 273–279). New York: Oxford University Press.

Levenson, R. W., Cartensen, L. L., & Gottman, J. M. (1993). Long-term marriage: Age, gender and satisfaction. *Psychology and Aging, 8,* 301–313.

Levenson, R. W., & Gottman, J. M. (1983). Marital interaction: Physiological and affective exchange. *Journal of Personality and Social Psychology, 45,* 587–597.

Levenson, R. W., & Mades, L. L. (1980, October). *Physiological response, facial expression, and trait anxiety: Two methods for improving consistency.* Paper presented at the meeting of the Society for Psychophysiological Research, Vancouver, British Columbia, Canada.

Leventhal, H. (1984). A perceptual–motor theory of emotion. In L. Berkowitz (Ed.), *Advances in experimental social psychology* (Vol. 17, pp. 117–182). New York: Academic Press.

Leventhal, H. (1991). Emotion: Prospects for conceptual and empirical development. In R. G. Lister & H. J. Weingartner (Eds.), *Perspective on cognitive neuroscience* (pp. 325–348). Oxford, UK: Oxford University Press.

Leventhal, H., & Patrick-Miller, L. (1993). Emotion and illness: The mind is in the body. In M. Lewis & J. M. Haviland (Eds.), *Handbook of emotions* (pp. 365–379). New York: Guilford Press.

Lewin, M. (1985). Unwanted intercourse: The difficulty of saying no. *Psychology of Women Quarterly, 9,* 184–192.

Lewinsohn, P. H. (1974). A behavioral approach to depression. In R. J. Friedman & M. M. Katz (Eds.), *The psychology of depression: Contemporary theory and research* (pp. 157–185). Washington, DC: Winston.

Lewis, M. (1992). *Shame: The exposed self.* New York: Free Press.

Lieberman, M. A., Yalom, I. D., & Miles, M. B. (1973). *Encounter groups: First facts.* New York: Basic Books.

Lindahl, K. M., & Markman, H. J. (1990). Communication and negative affect regulation in the family. In E. A. Blechman (Ed.), *Emotions and the family: For better or for worse* (pp. 99–115). Hillsdale, NJ: Erlbaum.

Linehan, M. (1997). Empathy in cognitive-behavioral therapy. In A. C. Bohart & L. S. Greenberg (Eds.), *Empathy reconsidered* (pp. 353–392). Washington: APA Books.

Litz, B. T. (1992). Emotional numbing in combat-related post-traumatic stress disorder: A critical review and reformulation. *Clinical Psychology Review, 12,* 417–432.

Lloyd, C. (1980). Life events and depressive disorder reviewed. *Archives of General Psychiatry, 37,* 529–548.

Loiselle, C. G., & Dawson, C. (1988). Toronto Alexithymia Scale: Relationships with measures of patient self-disclosure and private self-consciousness. *Psychotherapy and Psychosomatics, 50,* 109–116.

Lutgendorf, S. K., Antoni, M. H., Kumar, M., & Schneiderman, N. (1994). Changes in cognitive coping strategies predict EBV-antibody titre change following a stressor disclosure induction. *Journal of Psychosomatic Research, 38,* 63–78.

Maccoby, E. E. (1990). Gender and relationships: A developmental account. *American Psychologist, 45,* 513–520.

Magai, C., & McFadden, S. H. (1995). *The role of emotions in social and personality development: History, theory, and research.* New York: Wiley.

Mahoney, M. J. (1993). Theoretical development in the cognitive psychotherapies. *Journal of Consulting and Clinical Psychology, 61,* 187–193.

Mahoney, M. J. (1995). *Human change processes.* New York: Basic Books.

Main, M. (1995). Discourse, prediction and recent studies in attachment: Implications for psychoanalysis. In T. Shapiro & R. N. Emde (Eds.), *Research in psychoanalysis: Process, development, outcome* (pp. 209–244). Madison, CT: International Universities Press.

Main, M. (1996). Introduction to the special section on attachment and psychopathology: 2. Overview of the field of attachment. *Journal of Consulting and Clinical Psychology, 64,* 237–243.

Main, M., & Goldwyn, R. (1991). *Adult Attachment Classification System, Version 5.* Unpublished manuscript, University of California, Berkeley.

Main, M., & Goldwyn, R. (in press). Adult attachment rating and classification system. In M. Main (Ed.), *A typology of human attachment organization assessed in discourse, drawings and interviews.* New York: Cambridge University Press.

Malatesta, C. Z., Grigoryev, P., Lamb, C., Albin, M., & Culver, C. (1986). Emotion socialization and expressive development in preterm and full-term infants. *Child Development, 57,* 316–330.

Malatesta, C. Z., & Haviland, J. M. (1982). Learning display rules: The socialization of emotion expression in infancy. *Child Development, 53,* 991–1003.

Mandler, G. M., Mandler, J. M., Kremen, J., & Sholiton, R. D. (1961). The response to threat: Relations among verbal and physiological indices. *Psychological Monographs, 75*(9, Whole No. 513).

Manstead, A. S. R. (1991). Expressiveness as an individual difference. In R. S. Feldman & B. Rimé, (Eds.), *Fundamentals of nonverbal behavior* (pp. 285–328). New York: Cambridge University Press.

Marcus, D. K., & Nardone, M. E. (1992). Depression and interpersonal rejection. *Clinical Psychology Review, 12,* 433–449.

Margolin, G., & Fernandez, V. (1985). Marital dysfunction. In M. Hersen & A. S. Bellack (Eds.), *Handbook of clinical behavior therapy with adults* (pp. 693–728). New York: Plenum Press.

Marston, P. J., & Hecht, M. L. (1994). Love ways: An elaboration and application to relational maintenance. In D. J. Canary & L. Stafford (Eds.), *Communication and relational maintenance* (pp. 187–202). San Diego, CA: Academic Press.

Marston, P. J., Hecht, M. L., & Robers, T. (1987). "True love ways": The subjective experience and communication of romantic love. *Journal of Social and Personal Relationships, 4,* 387–407.

Martin, J., Martin, W., Mayer, M., & Sleman, A. (1986). Empirical investigations of the cognitive mediational paradigm for research on counseling. *Journal of Counseling Psychology, 33,* 115–123.

Martin, J. B., & Pihl, R. (1986). Influence of alexithymic characteristics on physiological and subjective stress responses in normal individuals. *Psychotherapy and Psychosomatics, 45,* 66–77.

Martin, L. L., & Tesser, A. (Eds.). (1996). *Striving and feeling: Interactions among goals, affect, and self-regulation.* Mahwah, NJ: Erlbaum.

Martin, R. B., & Labott, S. M. (1991). Mood following emotional crying: Effects of the situation. *Journal of Research in Personality, 25,* 218–244.

Matsumoto, D. (1993). Ethnic differences in affect intensity, emotion judgments, display rule attitudes, and self-reported emotional expression in an American sample. *Motivation and Emotion, 17,* 107–123.

Mayer, J. D., & Gaschke, Y. N. (1988). the experience and meta-experience of mood. *Journal of Personality and Social Psychology, 52,* 102–111.

Mayer, J. D., & Salovey, P. (1997). What is emotional intelligence? In P. Salovey & D. Sluyter (Eds.), *Emotional development and emotional intelligence* (pp. 3–34). New York: Basic Books.

Mayer, J. D., Salovey, P., Gomberg-Kaufman, S., & Blainey, K. (1991). A broader conception of mood experience. *Journal of Personality and Social Psychology, 60,* 100–111.

McCann, I. L., & Pearlman, L. A. (1990). *Psychological trauma and the adult survivor: theory, therapy and transformation.* New York: Brunner/Mazel.

McCormick, N. B. (1979). Come-ons and put-offs: Unmarried students' strategies for having and avoiding sexual intercourse. *Psychology of Women Quarterly, 4,* 194–211.

McCoy, C. L., & Masters, J. C. (1985). The development of children's strategies for the social control of emotion. *Child Development, 56,* 1214–1222.

Mehrabian, A., & Wiener, M. (1967). Decoding of inconsistent communications. *Journal of Personality and Social Psychology, 6,* 109–114.

Meichenbaum, D. (1990). *Cognitive-behavior modification: An integrative approach.* New York: Plenum Press.

Meichenbaum, D., & Fong, G. T. (1993). How individuals control their own minds: A constructive narrative perspective. In D. M. Wegner & J. W. Pennebaker (Eds.), *Handbook of mental control* (pp. 473–490). Englewood Cliffs, NJ: Prentice Hall.

Meleshko, K. G. A., & Alden, L. E. (1993). Anxiety and self-disclosure: Toward a motivational model. *Journal of Personality and Social Psychology, 64,* 1000–1009.

Menaghan, E. (1982). Measuring coping effectiveness: A panel analysis of marital problems and coping efforts. *Journal of Health and Social Behavior, 23,* 220–234.

Mendolia, M., & Kleck, R. E. (1993). Effects of talking about a stressful event on arousal: Does what we talk about make a difference? *Journal of Personality and Social Psychology, 64,* 817–826.

Mergenthaler, E. (1996). Emotion-abstraction patterns in verbatim protocols: A new way of describing psychotherapeutic processes. *Journal of Consulting and Clinical Psychology, 64,* 1306–1315.

Mesquita, B., & Frijda, N. H. (1992). Cultural variations in emotions: A review. *Psychological Bulletin, 112,* 179–204.

Metts, S., & Cupach, W. R. (1987, July). *Sexual themes and marital adjustment.* Paper presented at the Third International Conference on Social Psychology and Language, Bristol, UK.

Metts, S., & Cupach, W. R. (1989). The role of communication in human sexuality. In K. McKinney & S. Sprecher (Eds.), *Human sexuality: The societal and interpersonal context* (pp. 139–161). Norwood, NJ: Ablex.

Metts, S., Sprecher, S., & Regan, P. C. (1998). Communication and sexual desire. In P. A. Andersen & L. K. Guerrero (Eds.), *Handbook of communication and emotion: Research, theory, applications, and contexts* (pp. 353–377). San Diego, CA: Academic Press.

Meyer, T. J., & Mark, M. M. (1995). Effects of psychosocial interventions with adult cancer patients: A meta-analysis of randomized experiments. *Health Psychology, 14,* 101–108.

Miller, L. C., & Berg, J. H. (1984). Selectivity and urgency in interpersonal exchange. In V. J. Derlega (Ed.), *Communication, intimacy, and close relationships* (pp. 161–206). New York: Academic Press.

Miller, L. C., Berg, J. H., & Archer, R. L. (1983). Openers: Individuals who elicit intimate self-disclosure. *Journal of Personality and Social Psychology, 44,* 1234–1244.

Miller, L. C., & Read, S. J. (1987). Why am I telling you this? Self-disclosure in a goal-based model of personality. In V. J. Derlega & J. H. Berg (Eds.), *Self-disclosure: Theory, research, and therapy* (pp. 35–58). New York: Plenum Press.

Minuchin, S. (1974). *Families and family therapy.* Cambridge, MA: Harvard University Press.

Mischel, W. (1966). A social learning view of sex differences in behavior. In E. E. Maccoby (Ed.), *Development of sex differences* (pp. 56–81). Stanford, CA: Stanford University Press.

Mittal, B., & Balasubramanian, S. K. (1987). testing the dimensionality of the self-consciousness scales. *Journal of Personality Assessment, 51,* 53–68.

Mongrain, M., & Zuroff, D. (1994). Ambivalence over emotional expression and negative life events: Mediators of depressive symptoms in dependent and self-critical individuals. *Personality and Individual Differences, 16,* 447–458.

Monsour, M. (1988). *Cross-sex friendships in a changing society: A comparative analysis of cross-sex friendships, same-sex friendships, and romantic relationships.* Unpublished dissertation, University of Illinois, Champaign, IL.

Monsour, M. (1992). Meanings of intimacy in cross- and same-sex friendships. *Journal of Social and Personal Relationships, 9,* 277–295.

Montgomery, B. M. (1988). Quality communication in personal relationships. In S. Duck (Ed.), *Handbook of personal relationships: Theory, research, and interventions* (pp. 343–359). London: Wiley.

Moon, J. R., & Eisler, R. M. (1983). Anger control: An experimental comparison of three behavioral treatments. *Behavior Therapy, 14,* 493–505.

Moore, M. M. (1985). Nonverbal courtship patterns in women: Context and consequences. *Ethology and Sociobiology, 6,* 237–247.

Moore, M. M. (1995). Courtship signaling and adolescents: "Girls just wanna have fun"? *Journal of Sex Research, 32,* 319–328.

Moore, M. M., & Butler, D. L. (1989). Predictive aspects of nonverbal courtship behavior in women. *Semiotica, 76,* 205–215.

Morris, D. (1971). *Intimate behavior.* New York: Random House.

Mosher, D. L. (1965). Approval motive and acceptance of "fake" personality test interpretations which differ in favorability. *Psychological Reports, 17,* 395–402.

Muehlenhard, C. L. (1988). "Nice women" don't say yes and "real men" don't say no: How miscommunication and the double standard can cause sexual problems. *Women and Therapy, 7,* 95–108.

Muehlenhard, C. L., & Hollabaugh, L. C. (1988). Do women sometimes say no when they mean yes? The prevalence and correlates of women's token resistance to sex. *Journal of Personality and Social Psychology, 54,* 872–879.

Mullen, B., & Suls, J. (1982). "Know thyself": Stressful life events and the ameliorative effects of private self-consciousness. *Journal of Experimental Social Psychology, 18,* 43–55.

Muran, J. C., & Safran, J. D. (1993). Emotional and interpersonal considerations in cognitive therapy. In K. T. Kuehlwein & H. Rosen (Eds.), *Cognitive therapies in action: Evolving innovative practice* (pp. 185–212). San Francisco: Jossey-Bass.

Murnen, S. K., Perot, A., & Byrne, D. (1989). Coping with unwanted sexual activity: Normative responses, situational determinants, and individual differences. *Journal of Sex Research, 26,* 85–106.

Murray, E. J. (1985). Coping and anger. In T. M. Field, P. M. McCabe, & N. Schneiderman (Eds.), *Stress and coping* (pp. 243–261). Hillsdale, NJ: Erlbaum.

Murray, E. J., Lamnin, A. D., & Carver, C. S. (1989). Emotional expression in written essays and psychotherapy. *Journal of Social and Clinical Psychology, 8,* 414–429.

Murray, H. A. (1938). *Explorations in personality.* New York: Oxford University Press.

Murray, L. (1992). The impact of postnatal depression on infant development. *Journal of Child Psychology and Psychiatry, 33,* 543–561.

Nasby, W. (1989). Private self-consciousness, self-awareness, and the reliability of self-reports. *Journal of Personality and Social Psychology, 56,* 950–957.

Neimeyer, R. (1993a). Constructivist psychotherapy. In K. T. Kuehlwein & H. Rosen (Eds.), *Cognitive therapies in action: Evolving innovative practice* (pp. 268–300). San Francisco: Jossey-Bass.

Neimeyer, R. (1993b). An appraisal of constructivist psychotherapies. *Journal of Consulting and Clinical Psychology, 2,* 221–234.

Nemiah, J. C. (1957). The psychiatrist and rehabilitation. *Archives of Physical Medicine and Rehabilitation, 38,* 143–147.

Nemiah, J. C. (1978). Alexithymia and psychosomatic illness. *Journal of Continuing Education in Psychiatry, 39,* 25–37.

Nemiah, J. C., Freyberger, H., & Sifneos, P. E. (1976). Alexithymia: A view of the psychosomatic process. In O. Hill (Ed.), *Modern trends in psychosomatic medicine* (Vol. 3, pp. 430–439). London: Butterworths.

Nemiah, J. C., & Sifneos, P. E. (1970). Psychosomatic illness: A problem of communication. *Psychotherapy and Psychosomatics, 18,* 154–160.

Newton, D. A., & Burgoon, J. K. (1990). Nonverbal conflict behaviors: Functions, strategies, and tactics. In D. D. Cahn (Ed.), *Intimates in conflict: A communication perspective* (pp. 77–104). Hillsdale, NJ: Erlbaum.

Newton, T. L., & Contrada, R. J. (1992). Repressive coping and verbal-autonomic response dissociation: The influence of social context. *Journal of Personality and Social Psychology, 62,* 159–167.

Newton, T. L., Haviland, J. M., & Contrada, R. J. (1996). The face of repressive coping: Context and the display of hostile expressions and social smiles. *Journal of Nonverbal Behavior, 20,* 3–22.

Nguyen, T., Heslin, R., & Nguyen, M. (1976). The meanings of touch: Sex and marital status differences. *Representative Research in Social Psychology, 7,* 13–18.

Nichols, M. P., & Efran, J. S. (1985). Catharsis in psychotherapy: A new perspective. *Psychotherapy, 22,* 46–58.

Nichols, M. P., & Zax, M. (1977). *Catharsis in psychotherapy.* New York: Gardner Press.

Nielsen, L. E., & Fleck, J. R. (1981). Defensive repressors and empathic impairment. *Psychological Reports, 48,* 615–624.

Nix, G., Watson, C., Pyszczynski, T., & Greenberg, J. (1995). Reducing depressive affect through external focus of attention. *Journal of Social and Clinical Psychology, 14,* 36–52.

Nolen-Hoeksema, S. (1991). Responses to depression and their effects on the duration of depressive episodes. *Journal of Abnormal Psychology, 100,* 569–582.

Nolen-Hoeksema, S., & Morrow, J. (1993). Effects of rumination and distraction on naturally occurring depressed mood. *Cognition and Emotion, 7,* 561–570.

Nolen-Hoeksema, S., Morrow, J., & Fredrickson, B. L. (1993). Response styles and duration of depressed moods. *Journal of Abnormal Psychology, 67,* 92–104.

Noller, P. (1978). Sex differences in the socialization of affectionate expression. *Developmental Psychology, 14,* 317–319.

Noller, P. (1984). *Nonverbal communication and marital interaction.* New York: Pergamon Press.

Noller, P., & Venardos, C. (1986). Communication awareness in married couples. *Journal of Personal and Social Relationships, 3,* 31–42.

Notarius, C. I., Benson, P. R., Sloane, D., Vanzetti, N. A., & Hornyak, L. M. (1989). Exploring the interface between perception and behavior: An analysis of marital interaction in distressed and nondistresssed couples. *Behavioral Assessment, 11,* 39–64.

Notarius, C. I., & Johnson, J. S. (1982). Emotional expression in husbands and wives. *Journal of Marriage and the Family, 44,* 483–489.

Notarius, C. I., & Levenson, R. W. (1979). Expressive tendencies and physiological response to stress. *Journal of Personality and Social Psychology, 37,* 1204–1210.

Notarius, C. I., & Vanzetti, N. A. (1983). Marital agendas protocol. In E. Filsinger (Ed.), *A sourcebook of marital and family assessment* (pp. 209–227). Beverly Hills, CA: Sage.

Novaco, R. W. (1980). Training of probation counselors for anger problems. *Journal of Counseling Psychology, 27,* 385–390.

Oatley, K., & Johnson-Laird, P. N. (1987). Towards a cognitive theory of emotions. *Cognition and Emotion, 1,* 29–50.

O'Brien, C. P. (1981). Commentary. *Medical Aspects of Human Sexuality, 15,* 117.

Ogden, J. A., & Von Sturmer, G. (1984). Emotional strategies and their relationship to complaints of psychosomatic and neurotic symptoms. *Journal of Clinical Psychology, 40,* 772–779.

O'Leary, K. D., & Beach, S. R. H. (1990). Marital therapy: A viable treatment for depression and marital discord. *American Journal of Psychiatry, 147,* 183–186.

Oliver, M. B., & Hyde, J. S. (1993). Gender differences in sexuality: A meta-analysis. *Psychological Bulletin, 114,* 29–51.

Oliver, M. B., & Sedikides, C. (1992). Effects of sexual permissiveness on desirability of partner as a function of low and high commitment to relationship. *Social Psychology Quarterly, 55,* 321–333.

Orbuch, T. L., Vernoff, J., & Holmberg, D. (1993). Becoming a married couple: The emergence of meaning in the first years of marriage. *Journal of Marriage and the Family, 55,* 815–826.

Orenstein, P. (1997, June 29). Thirty-five and mortal: A breast cancer diary. *New York Times Magazine,* pp. 28–52.

O'Sullivan, L. F., & Byers, E. S. (1993). Eroding stereotypes: College women's attempts to influence reluctant male sexual partners. *Journal of Sex Research, 30,* 270–282.

Owen, W. F. (1987). The verbal expression of love by women and men as a critical communication event in personal relationships. *Women's Studies in Communication, 10,* 15–24.

Paez, D., Basabe, N., Valdoseda, M., Velasco, C., & Iraurgi, I. (1995). Confrontation: Inhibition, alexithymia, and health. In J. W. Pennebaker (Ed.), *Emotion, disclosure, and health* (pp. 195–222). Washington, DC: American Psychological Association.

Papero, D. V. (1995). Bowen family systems and marriage. In N. S. Jacobson & A. S. Gurman (Eds.), *Clinical handbook of couple therapy* (pp. 11-31). New York: Guilford Press.

Parker, G., & Brown, L. (1982). Coping behaviors that mediate between life events and depression. *Archives of General Psychology, 39,* 1386–1391.

Patel, V. (1993). Crying behavior and psychiatric disorder in adults: A review. *Comprehensive Psychiatry, 34,* 206–211.

Patterson, M. L. (1983). *Nonverbal behavior: A functional perspective.* New York: Springer-Verlag.

Patterson, M. L. (1988). Functions of nonverbal behavior in close relationships. In S. Duck (Ed.), *Handbook of personal relationships: Theory, research, and interventions* (pp. 41–56). London: Wiley.

Patterson, M. L. (1991). A functional approach to nonverbal exchange. In R. S. Feldman & B. Rimé, (Eds.), *Fundamentals of nonverbal behavior* (pp. 458–495). Cambridge, UK: Cambridge University Press.

Pattison, E. M. (1977). *The experience of dying.* Englewood Cliffs, NJ: Prentice-Hall.

Pennebaker, J. W. (1985). Traumatic experience and psychosomatic disease: Exploring the roles of behavioural inhibition, obsession, and confiding. *Canadian Psychology, 26,* 82–95.

Pennebaker, J. W. (1990). *Opening up: The healing power of confiding in others.* New York: Morrow.

Pennebaker, J. W. (1992). Inhibition as the linchpin of health. In H. S. Friedman (Ed.), *Hostility, coping, and health* (pp. 127–139). Washington, DC: American Psychological Association.

Pennebaker, J. W. (1993a). Overcoming inhibition: Rethinking the roles of personality, cognition, and social behaviour. In H. C. Traue & J. W. Pennebaker (Eds.), *Emotion, inhibition, and health* (pp. 100–115). Seattle, WA: Hogrefe & Huber.

Pennebaker, J. W. (1993b). Putting stress into words: Health, linguistic, and therapeutic implications. *Behaviour Research and Therapy, 31,* 539–548.

Pennebaker, J. W. (1993c). Social mechanisms of constraint. In D. M. Wegner & J. W. Pennebaker (Eds.), *Handbook of mental control* (pp. 200–219). Englewood Cliffs, NJ: Prentice-Hall.

Pennebaker, J. W. (1995). *Emotion, disclosure, and health.* Washington, DC: American Psychological Association.

Pennebaker, J. W., Barger, S. D., & Tiebout, J. (1989). Disclosure of traumas and health among Holocaust survivors. *Psychosomatic Medicine, 51,* 577–589.

Pennebaker, J. W., & Beall, S. K. (1986). Confronting a traumatic event: Toward an understanding of inhibition and disease. *Journal of Abnormal Psychology, 95,* 274–281.

Pennebaker, J. W., Colder, M., & Sharp, L. K. (1990). Accelerating the coping process. *Journal of Personality and Social Psychology, 58,* 528–537.

Pennebaker, J. W., & Francis, M. E. (1996). Cognitive, emotional, and language processes in disclosure: Physical health and adjustment. *Cognition and Emotion, 10,* 601–626.

Pennebaker, J. W., Hughes, C. F., & O'Heeron, R. C. (1987). The psychophysiology of confession: Linking inhibitory and psychosomatic processes. *Journal of Personality and Social Psychology, 52,* 781–793.

Pennebaker, J. W., Kiecolt-Glaser, J. K., & Glaser, R. (1988). Disclosure of traumas and immune function: Health implications for psychotherapy. *Journal of Consulting and Clinical Psychology, 56,* 239–245.

Pennebaker, J. W., Mayne, T. J., & Francis, M. E. (1997). Linguistic predictors of adaptive bereavement. *Journal of Personality and Social Psychology, 72,* 863–871.

Pennebaker, J. W., & Roberts, T. (1992). Toward a his and hers theory of emotion: Gender differences in visceral perception. *Journal of Social and Clinical Psychology, 11,* 199–212.

Pennebaker, J. W., & Susman, J. R. (1988). Disclosure of traumas and psychosomatic processes. *Social Science and Medicine, 26,* 327–332.

Peplau, L., Rubin, Z., & Hill, C. (1977). Sexual intimacy in dating relationships. *Journal of Social Issues, 33,* 86–109.

Perls, F. (1969). *Ego, hunger and aggression.* New York: Random House.

Perls, F. (1973). *The Gestalt approach and eyewitness to therapy.* New York: Bantam Books.

Perper, T. (1985). *Sex signals: The biology of love.* Philadelphia: ISI Press.

Perper, T., & Weis, D. L. (1987). Proceptive and rejective strategies of U.S. and Canadian college women. *Journal of Sex Research, 23,* 455–480.

Person, J., & Miranda, J. (1991). Treating dysfunctional beliefs: Implications for the mood-state hypothesis. *Journal of Cognitive Psychotherapy: An International Quarterly, 5,* 15–25.

Pervin, L. A. (Ed.). (1989). *Goal concepts in personality and social psychology.* Hillsdale, NJ: Erlbaum.

Petrie, A. (1967). *Individuality in pain and suffering.* Chicago: University of Chicago Press.

Petrie, K. J., Booth, R. J., Pennebaker, J. W., Davison, K. P., & Thomas, M. G. (1995). Disclosure of trauma and immune response to a Hepatitis B vaccination program. *Journal of Consulting and Clinical Psychology, 63,* 787–792.

Petronio, S. (1991). Communication boundary management: A theoretical model of managing disclosure of private information between marital couples. *Communication Theory, 1,* 311–335.

Pettingale, K. W. (1985). Towards a psychobiological model of cancer: Biological considerations. *Social Science and Medicine, 20,* 779–787.

Piening, S. (1984). Family stress in diabetic renal failure. *Health and Social Work, 9,* 134–141.

Pierce, R. (1994). Helping couples make authentic emotional contact. In S. M. Johnson & L. S. Greenberg (Eds.), *The heart of the matter: Perspectives on emotion in marital therapy* (pp. 75–107). New York: Brunner/Mazel.

Pilkington, C. J., & Richardson, D. R. (1988). Perceptions of risk in intimacy. *Journal of Social and Personal Relationships, 5,* 503–508.

Polster, E., & Polster, M. (1973). *Gestalt therapy integrated.* New York: Random House.

Porter, B., & O'Leary, K. D. (1980). Marital discord and childhood behavior problems. *Journal of Abnormal Child Psychology, 8,* 287–295.

Porter, R. E., & Samovar, L. A. (1998). Cultural influences on emotional expression: Implications for intercultural communication. In P. A. Andersen & L. K. Guerrero (Eds.), *Handbook of communication and emotion: Research, theory, applications, and contexts* (pp. 451–472). San Diego, CA: Academic Press.

Prager, K. J. (1986). Intimacy status: Its relationship to locus of control, self-disclosure, and anxiety in adults. *Personality and Social Psychology Bulletin, 12,* 91–110.

Putallaz, M., & Gottman, J. M. (1981). An interactional model of children's entry into peer groups. *Child Development, 52,* 986–994.

Rabavilas, A. D. (1987). Electrodermal activity in low and high alexithymia neurotic patients. *Psychotherapy and Psychosomatics, 47,* 101–194.

Rachman, S., & Hodgson, R. (1974). Synchrony and desynchrony in fear and avoidance. *Behaviour Research and Therapy, 12,* 311–318.

Reis, H. T., Senchak, M., & Solomon, B. (1985). Sex differences in the intimacy of social interaction: Further examination of potential explanations. *Journal of Personality and Social Psychology, 48,* 1204–1217.

Reis, H. T., & Shaver, P. (1988). Intimacy as an interpersonal process. In S. Duck (Ed.), *Handbook of personal relationships: Theory, relationships, and interventions* (pp. 367–389). London: Wiley.

Reiss, I. L. (1989). Society and sexuality: A sociological explanation. In K. McKinney & S. Sprecher (Eds.), *Human sexuality: The societal and interpersonal context* (pp. 3–29). Norwood, NJ: Ablex.

Remoff, H. T. (1984). *Sexual choice: A woman's decision.* New York: Dutton-Lewis.

Rennie, D. L. (1993). Qualitative analysis of the client's experience of psychotherapy: The unfolding of reflexivity. In S. G. Toukmanian & D. L. Rennie (Eds.), *Psychotherapy process research: Paradigmatic and narrative approaches* (pp. 211–233). Newbury Park, CA: Sage.

Repetti, R. L. (1992). Social withdrawal as a short-term coping response to daily stressors. In H. S. Friedman (Ed.), *Hostility, coping, and health* (pp. 151–165). Washington, DC: American Psychological Association.

Revenson, T., & Majerovitz, D. (1990). Spouse's support provision to chronically ill patients. *Journal of Personal Relationships, 7,* 575–586.

Rice, L. N. (1974). The evocative function of the therapist. In D. Wexler & L. N. Rice (Eds.), *Innovations in client-centered therapy* (pp. 289–311). New York: Wiley.

Rice, L. N., & Kerr, G. (1986). Measures of client and therapist vocal quality. In L. S. Greenberg & W. M. Pinsof (Eds.), *The psychotherapeutic process: A research handbook* (pp. 73–105). New York: Guilford Press.

Rice, L. N., Koke, C., Greenberg, L. S., & Wagstaff, A. (1979). *Manual for client vocal quality* (Vol. I). Toronto, Ontario, Canada: Counseling and Development Centre, York University.

Rice, L. N., & Saperia, E. (1984). A task analysis of the resolution of problematic reaction. In L. N. Rice & L. S. Greenberg (Eds.), *Patterns of change: Intensive analysis of psychotherapy process* (pp. 29–66). New York: Guilford Press.

Rice, L. N., Watson, J. C., & Greenberg, L. S. (1993). *A measure of clients' expressive stance.* Toronto, Ontario, Canada: York University.

Rimé, B., Mesquita, B., Philippot, P., & Boca, S. (1991). Beyond the emotional event: Six studies on the social sharing of emotion. *Cognition and Emotion, 5,* 435–465.

Rinn, W. E. (1991). Neuropsychology of facial expression. In R. S. Feldman & B. Rimé, (Eds.), *Fundamentals of nonverbal behavior* (pp. 3–70). New York: Cambridge University Press.

Rippere, V. (1977). "What's the thing to do when you're feeling depressed?": A pilot study. *Behaviour Research and Therapy, 15,* 185–191.

Robins, C. J., & Hayes, A. M. (1993). An appraisal of cognitive therapy. *Journal of Consulting and Clinical Psychology, 2,* 205–214.

Robinson, R. J., & Pennebaker, J. W. (1991). Emotion and health: Towards an integrative approach. In K. T. Strongman (Ed.), *International review of studies on emotion* (Vol. 1, pp. 247–267). New York: Wiley.

Roche, J. P. (1986). Premarital sex: Attitudes and behavior by dating stage. *Adolescence, 21,* 107–121.

Roemer, L., & Borkovec, T. (1994). Effects about expressing thoughts about emotional material. *Journal of Abnormal Psychology, 103,* 467–474.

Rogers, C. (1951). *Person-centered therapy.* Boston: Houghton-Mifflin.

Rogers, C. (1965). *Client-centered therapy: Its current practice, implications, and theory.* Boston: Houghton-Mifflin.

Rogers, D., & Jamieson, J. (1988). Individual differences in delayed heart-rate recovery following stress: The role of extraversion, neuroticism, and emotional control. *Personality and Individual Differences, 9,* 721–726.

Rogers, D., & Nesshoever, W. (1987). The construction and preliminary validation of a scale for measuring emotional control. *Personality and Individual Differences, 8,* 527–534.

Roseman, I. J., Wiest, C., & Swartz, T. S. (1994). Phenomenology, behaviors, and goals differentiate discrete emotions. *Journal of Personality and Social Psychology, 67,* 206–221.

Rosen, H. (1993). Developing themes in the field of cognitive psychotherapy. In K. T. Kuehlwein & H. Rosen (Eds.), *Cognitive therapies in action: Evolving innovative practice* (pp. 403–434). San Francisco: Jossey-Bass.

Rosen, H. (1996). Meaning-making narratives: Foundations of constructivist and social-constructionist psychotherapies. In H. Rosen & K. T. Kuehlwein (Eds.), *Con-*

structing realities: Meaning-making perspectives for psychotherapists (pp. 3–51). San Francisco: Jossey-Bass.

Rosen, H. & Kuehlwein, K. T. (Eds.). (1996). *Constructing realities: Meaning-making perspectives for psychotherapists.* San Francisco: Jossey-Bass.

Rosenfeld, L. B. (1979). Self-disclosure avoidance: Why am I afraid to tell you who I am? *Communication Monographs, 46,* 63–74.

Rosenthal, T. L. (1993). To soothe the savage breast. *Behaviour Research and Therapy, 31,* 439–462.

Ross, C. E., & Mirowsky, J. (1984). Men who cry. *Social Psychology Quarterly, 49,* 1427–1433.

Rothbart, M. K. (1994). Broad dimensions of temperament and personality. In P. Ekman & R. J. Davidson (Eds.), *The nature of emotion: Fundamental questions* (pp. 337–341). New York: Oxford University Press.

Rothbart, M. K., & Derryberry, D. (1981). Development of individual differences in temperament. In M. E. Lamb & A. L. Brown (Eds.), *Advances in developmental psychology* (Vol. 1, pp. 37–86). Hillsdale, NJ: Erlbaum.

Rothbart, M. K., & Posner, M. I. (1985). Temperament and the development of self-regulation. In L. C. Hartlage & C. F. Telzrow (Eds.), *The neuropsychology of individual differences* (pp. 93–123). New York: Plenum Press.

Rubin, L. B. (1990). *Erotic wars: What happened to the sexual revolution?* New York: Harper Perennial.

Rubin, Z. (1973). *Liking and loving.* New York: Holt, Rinehart & Winston.

Rubin, Z., Hill, C. T., Peplau, L. A., & Dunkel-Schetter, C. (1980). Self-disclosure in dating couples: Sex roles and the ethic of openness. *Journal of Marriage and the Family, 42,* 305–317.

Ruckdeschel, K., & Hazan, C. (1994). From symptom to signal: An attachment view of emotion in marital therapy. In S. M. Johnson & L. S. Greenberg (Eds.), *The heart of the matter: Perspectives on emotion in marital therapy* (pp. 46–74). New York: Brunner/Mazel.

Rusting, C. L., & Nolen-Hoeksema, S. (1998). Regulating responses to anger: Effects of rumination and distraction on angry mood. *Journal of Personality and Social Psychology, 74,* 790–803.

Saarni, C. (1993). Socialization of emotion. In M. Lewis & J. M. Haviland (Eds.), *Handbook of emotions* (pp. 435–446). New York: Guilford Press.

Saarni, C., & Crowley, M. (1990). *The development of emotion regulation: Effects on emotional state and expression.* In E. A. Blechman (Ed.), *Emotions and the family: For better or for worse* (pp. 53–73). Hillsdale, NJ: Erlbaum.

Sachse, R. (1996). Goal-oriented client-centered psychotherapy of psychosomatic disorders. In L. S. Greenberg, J. C. Watson, & G. Lietaer (Eds.), *Handbook of experiential psychotherapy* (pp. 295–327). New York: Guilford Press.

Sackeim, H. A., & Gur, R. C. (1979). Self-deception and self-reported psychopathology. *Journal of Consulting and Clinical Psychology, 47,* 213–215.

Sadoff, R. (1966). On the nature of crying and weeping. *Psychiatric Quarterly, 40,* 490–503.

Safran, J. D. (1984). Assessing the cognitive-interpersonal cycle. *Cognitive Therapy and Research, 8,* 333–348.

Safran, J. D. (1990a). Towards a refinement of cognitive therapy in light of interpersonal theory: 1. Theory. *Clinical Psychology Review, 10,* 87–105.

Safran, J. D. (1990b). Towards a refinement of cognitive therapy in light of interpersonal theory: 2. Practice. *Clinical Psychology Review, 10,* 107–122.

Safran, J. D., & Greenberg, L. S. (1982). Eliciting hot-cognitions in cognitive therapy. *Canadian Psychology, 23,* 83–87.

Safran, J. D., & Greenberg, L. S. (1986). Hot cognition and psychotherapy in process: An information processing ecological perspective. In P. C. Kendall (Ed.), *Advances in cognitive-behavioral research and therapy* (Vol. 5, pp. 143–177). San Diego, CA: Academic Press.

Safran, J. D., & Greenberg, L. S. (1989). The treatment of anxiety and depression: The process of affective change. In P. C. Kendall & D. Watson (Eds.), *Anxiety and depression: Distinctive and overlapping features* (pp. 455–489). San Diego, CA: Academic Press.

Safran, J. D., & Greenberg, L. S. (Eds.). (1991). *Emotion, psychotherapy, and change.* New York: Guilford Press.

Safran, J. D., & Muran, J. C. (1995). Resolving therapeutic alliance ruptures: Diversity and integration. In *Session: Psychotherapy in Practice, 1,* 81–92.

Safran, J. D., & Segal, Z. V. (1990). *Interpersonal process in cognitive therapy.* New York: Basic Books.

Safran, J. D., Vallis, T. M., Segal, Z. V., & Shaw, B. F. (1986). Assessment of core cognitive processes in cognitive therapy. *Cognitive Therapy and Research, 10,* 509–526.

Salovey, P., Hsee, C. K., & Mayer, J. D. (1993). Emotional intelligence and the self-regulation of affect. In D. M. Wegner & J. W. Pennebaker (Eds.), *Handbook of mental control* (pp. 258–277). Englewood Cliffs, NJ: Prentice-Hall.

Salovey, P., & Mayer, J. D. (1990). Emotional intelligence. *Imagination, Cognition, and Personality, 9,* 185–211.

Salovey, P., Mayer, J. D., Goldman, S. L., Turvey, C., & Palfai, T. P. (1995). Emotional attention, clarity, and repair: Exploring emotional intelligence using the Trait Meta-Mood Scale. In J. W. Pennebaker (Ed.), *Emotion, disclosure, and health* (pp. 125–154). Washington, DC: American Psychological Association.

Salovey, P., & Turk, D. C. (1991). Clinical judgment and decision-making. In C. R. Snyder & D. R. Forsyth (Eds.), *Handbook of social and clinical psychology: The health perspective* (pp. 416–437). New York: Pergamon Press.

Sappington, A. A. (1990). The independent manipulation of intellectually and emotionally based beliefs. *Journal of Research in Personality, 24,* 487–509.

Sappington, A. A., & Russell, J. C. (1979). Self-efficacy and meeting: Candidates for a uniform theory of behavior. *Personality and Social Psychology Bulletin, 2,* 327.

Sarason, I. G., Sarason, B. R., & Pierce, G. R. (1990). Social support: The search for theory. *Journal of Social and Clinical Psychology, 9,* 133–147.

Scarr, S., & McCartney, K. (1983). How people make their own environments: A theory of genotype → environment effects. *Child Development, 54,* 424–435.

Schedler, J., Mayman, M., & Manis, M. (1993). The illusion of mental health. *American Psychologist, 48,* 1117–1131.

Scheff, T. J. (1979). *Catharsis in healing, ritual, and drama.* Berkeley: University of California Press.

Scheflen, A. E. (1974). *How behavior means.* Garden City, NY: Doubleday.

Scherer, K. R., & Ekman, P. (1982). *Handbook of research in nonverbal behavior.* Cambridge, UK: Cambridge University Press.

Schuerger, J. M., Zarrella, K. L., & Hotz, A. S. (1989). Factors that influence the temporal stability of personality by questionnaire. *Journal of Personality and Social Psychology, 56,* 777–783.

Schwartz, G. E. (1983). Disregulation theory and disease: Applications to the repression/cerebral disconnection/cardiovascular disorder hypothesis. *International Review of Applied Psychology, 32,* 95–118.

Schwartz, G. E. (1990). Psychobiology of repression and health: A systems approach. In J. Singer (Ed.), *Repression and dissociation: Implications for personality theory, psychopathology, and health* (pp. 405–434). Chicago: University of Chicago Press.

Schwartz, J. C., & Shaver, P. (1987). Emotions and emotion knowledge in interpersonal relations. In W. H. Jones & D. Perlman (Eds.), *Advances in personal relationships* (Vol. 1, pp. 197–241). Greenwich, CT: JAI Press.

Schwarz, N. (1990). Feelings as information: Informational and motivational functions of affective states. In E. T. Higgins & R. M. Sorrentino (Eds.), *Handbook of motivation and cognition: Foundations of social behavior* (Vol. 2, pp. 527–561). New York: Guilford Press.

Schwarz, N., & Clore, G. L. (1988). How do I feel about it? The informative functions of affective states. In K. Fiedler & J. Forgas (Eds.), *Affect, cognition, and social behavior* (pp. 44–62). Toronto, Ontario, Canada: Hogrefe International.

Segrin, C. (1998). Interpersonal communication problems associated with depression and loneliness. In P. A. Andersen & L. K. Guerrero (Eds.), *Handbook of communication and emotion: Research, theory, applications, and contexts* (pp. 215–242). San Diego, CA: Academic Press.

Segrin, C., & Abramson, L. Y. (1994). Negative reactions to depressive behaviors: A communication theories analysis. *Journal of Abnormal Psychology, 103,* 655–668.

Shaffer, D. R., & Ogden, J. K. (1986). On sex differences in self-disclosure during the acquaintance process: The role of anticipated future interaction. *Journal of Personality and Social Psychology, 51,* 92–101.

Shaffer, D. R., Smith, J. E., & Tomarelli, M. (1982). Self-monitoring as a determinant of self-disclosure reciprocity during the acquaintance process. *Journal of Personality and Social Psychology, 43,* 163–175.

Shaver, P. R., & Hazan, C. (1994). Attachment as an organizational framework for research in close relationships. *Psychological Inquiry, 5,* 1–22.

Shields, S. A. (1987). Women, men, and the dilemma of emotion. In P. Shaver & C. Hendrick (Eds.), *Review of personality and social psychology: Vol. 7. Sex and gender* (pp. 229–250). Beverly Hills, CA: Sage.

Shimanoff, S. B. (1983). The role of gender in linguistic references to emotive states. *Communication Quarterly, 30,* 174–179.

Shimanoff, S. B. (1987). Types of emotional disclosures and request compliance between spouses. *Communication Monographs, 54,* 85–100.

Shotland, R. L., & Craig, J. M. (1988). Can men and women differentiate between friendly and sexually interested behavior? *Social Psychology Quarterly, 51,* 66–73.

Shuchter, S. R., & Zisook, S. (1993). The course of normal grief. In M. S. Stroebe, W. Stroebe, & R. O. Hansson (Eds.), *Handbook of bereavement: Theory, research, and intervention* (pp. 23–43). Cambridge, UK: Cambridge University Press.

Siegel, B. (1986). *Love, medicine, and miracles.* New York: Harper & Row.

Siegel, B. (1989). *Peace, love, and healing.* New York: Harper & Row.

Siegel, S. J., & Alloy, L. B. (1990). Interpersonal perceptions and consequences of depressive–significant other relationships: A naturalistic study of college roommates. *Journal for Abnormal Psychology, 99,* 361–373.

Siegman, A. W. (1992, July). *The role of expressive vocal behavior in negative emotions: Implications for stress management.* Paper presented at the XXV International Congress of Psychology, Brussels, Belgium.

Siegman, A. W. (1993). Paraverbal correlates of stress: Implications for stress identification and stress management. In L. Goldberger & S. Breznitz (Eds.), *Handbook of stress: Theoretical and clinical aspects* (2nd ed., pp. 274–299). New York: Free Press.

Siegman, A. W. (1994). Cardiovascular consequences of expressing and repressing anger. In A. W. Siegman & T. W. Smith (Eds.), *Anger, hostility, and the heart* (pp. 173–197). Hillsdale, NJ: Erlbaum.

Siegman, A. W., Anderson, R. W., & Berger, T. (1990). The angry voice: Its effects on the experience of anger and cardiovascular reactivity. *Psychosomatic Medicine, 52,* 631–643.

Siegman, A. W., & Smith, T. W. (Eds.). *(1994). Anger, hostility, and the heart.* Hillsdale, NJ: Erlbaum.

Sifneos, P. E. (1972). *Short-term psychotherapy and emotional crisis.* Cambridge, MA: Harvard University Press.

Sifneos, P. E. (1973). The prevalence of "alexithymic" characteristics in psychosomatic patients. *Psychotherapy and Psychosomatics, 22,* 255–262.

Sifneos, P. E. (1991). Affect, emotional conflict, and deficit: An overview. *Psychotherapy and Psychosomatics, 56,* 116–122.

Sillars, A. L., Pike, G. R., Jones, T. S., & Murphy, M. A. (1984). Communication and understanding in marriage. *Human Communication Research, 10,* 317–350.

Silver, R. L., Boon, C., & Stones, M. H. (1983). Searching for meaning in misfortune: Making sense of incest. *Journal of Social Issues, 39,* 81–102.

Silver, R. L., & Wortman, C. B. (1980). Coping with undesirable life events. In J. Garber & M. E. P. Seligman (Eds.), *Human helplessness: Theory and applications* (pp. 279–340). New York: Academic Press.

Simon, W., & Gagnon, J. H. (1987). A sexual scripts approach. In J. H. Geer & W. O'Donohue (Eds.), *Theories of human sexuality* (pp. 363–383). New York: Plenum Press.

Simpson, J. A. (1990). Influence of attachment styles on romantic relationships. *Journal of Personality and Social Psychology, 59,* 971–980.

Simpson, J. A., & Rholes, W. S. (1994). Stress and secure base relationships in adulthood. In K. Bartholomew & D. Perlman (Eds.), *Advances in personal relationships: Vol. 5. Attachment processes in adulthood* (pp. 181–204). Bristol, PA: Kingsley.

Simpson, J. A., Rholes, W. S., & Nelligan, J. S. (1992). Support-seeking and support-giving within couples in an anxiety-provoking situation: The role of attachment styles. *Journal of Personality and Social Psychology, 62,* 434–446.

Singer, J. A., & Salovey, P. (1993). *The remembered self.* New York: Free Press.

Singer, J. A., & Salovey, P. (1996). Motivated memory: Self-defining memories, goals, and affect regulation. In L. L. Martin & A. Tesser (Eds.), *Striving and feeling: Interactions among goals, affect, and self-regulation* (pp. 229–250). Mahwah, NJ: Erlbaum.

Smith, T. W. (1992). Hostility and health: Current status of a psychosomatic hypotheses. *Health Psychology, 11,* 139–150.

Smith, T. W., & Pope, M. K. (1990). Cynical hostility as a health risk: Current status and future directions. *Journal of Social Behavior and Personality, 5,* 77–88.

Smyth, J. M. (1998). Written emotional expression: Effect sizes, outcome types, and moderating variables. *Journal of Consulting and Clinical Psychology, 66,* 174–184.

Snell, W. E. (1986). The Masculine Role Inventory: Components and correlates. *Sex Roles, 15,* 443–455.

Snyder, M. (1974). Self-monitoring of expressive behavior. *Journal of Personality and Social Psychology, 30,* 526–537.

Snyder, M., Tanke, E. D., & Berscheid, E. (1977). Social perception and interpersonal behavior: On the self-fulfilling nature of social stereotypes. *Journal of Personality and Social Psychology, 35,* 656–666.

Sommers, S. (1981). Emotionality reconsidered: The role of cognition in emotional responsiveness. *Journal of Personality and Social Psychology, 41,* 553–561.

Spiegel, D., Bloom, J. R., Kraemer, H. C., & Gottheil, E. (1989). Effects of psychosocial treatment on survival of patients with metastatic breast cancer. *Lancet, 2,* 888–891.

Spiegel, D., Bloom, J., & Yalom, I. (1981). Group support for patients with metastatic cancer: A prospective randomized outcome study. *Archives of General Psychiatry, 38,* 527–533.

Spitz, C., Gold, A., & Adams, D. (1975). Cognitive and hormonal factors affecting coital frequency. *Archives of Sexual Behavior, 4,* 249–264.

Sprague, J., & Quadagno, D. (1989). Gender and sexual motivation: An exploration of two assumptions. *Journal of Psychology and Human Sexuality, 2,* 57–76.

Sprecher, S., & McKinney, K. (1993). *Sexuality.* Newbury Park, CA: Sage.

Sprecher, S., & Metts, S. (1989). Development of the "Romantic Beliefs Scale" and examination of the effects of gender and gender-role orientation. *Journal of Social and Personal Relationships, 6,* 387–411.

Stafford, L., & Canary, D. J. (1991). Maintenance strategies and romantic relationship type, gender, and relational characteristics. *Journal of Social and Personal Relationships, 6,* 413–434.

Stanton, A. L., Danoff-Burg, S., Cameron, C. L., & Ellis, A. P. (1994). Coping through emotional approach: Problems of conceptualization and confounding. *Journal of Personality and Social Psychology, 66,* 350–362.

Stearns, P. N. (1993). History of emotions: The issue of change. In M. Lewis & J. M. Haviland (Eds.), *Handbook of emotions* (pp. 17–28). New York: Guilford Press.

Steinmetz, S. K. (1977). *The cycle of violence.* New York: Praeger.

Stern, J. J., & Pascale, L. (1979). Psychosocial adaptation post-myocardial infarction: The spouse's dilemma. *Journal of Psychosomatic Research, 23,* 83–87.

Sternberg, R. J. (1986). A triangular theory of love. *Psychological Review, 93,* 119–135.

Stiles, W. B. (1984). Counseling session impact as viewed by novice counselor and new clients. *Journal of Counseling Psychology, 31,* 3–12.

Stiles, W. B. (1987). "I have to talk to somebody." A fever model of disclosure. In V. J. Derlega & J. H. Berg (Eds.), *Self-disclosure: Theory, research, and therapy* (pp. 257–282). New York: Plenum Press.

Stiles, W. B. (1995). Disclosure as a speech act: Is it psychotherapeutic to disclose? In J. W. Pennebaker (Ed.), *Emotion, disclosure, and health* (pp. 71–91). Washington, DC: American Psychological Association.

Stokes, J. P. (1987). The relation of loneliness and self-disclosure. In V. J. Derlega & J. H. Berg (Eds.), *Self-disclosure: Theory, research, and therapy* (pp. 175–201). New York: Plenum Press.

Stokes, J. P., Childs, L., & Fuehrer, A. (1981). Gender and sex roles as predictors of self-disclosure. *Journal of Counseling Psychology, 28,* 510–514.

Strachan, A. M., Leff, J. P., Goldstein, M. J., Doane, J. A., & Burtt, C. (1986). Emotional attitudes and direct communication in the families of schizophrenics: A cross-national replication. *British Journal of Psychiatry, 149,* 279–287.

Straton, D. (1990). Catharsis reconsidered. *Australian and New Zealand Journal of Psychiatry, 124,* 543–551.

Strelau, J. (1987). Personality dimensions based on arousal theories: Search for integration. In J. Strelau & H. J. Eysenck (Eds.), *Personality dimensions and arousal* (pp. 269–286). New York: Plenum Press.

Stretton, M. S., & Salovey, P. (1997). Cognitive and affective components of hypochondriacal concerns. In W. F. Flack & J. D. Laird (Eds.), *Emotions in psychopathology: Theory and research* (pp. 265–279). New York: Oxford University Press.

Suls, J., & Fletcher, B. (1985). The relative efficacy of avoidant and nonavoidant coping strategies: A meta-analysis. *Health Psychology, 4,* 249–288.

Surra, C. A., Batchelder, M. L., & Hughes, D. K. (1995). Accounts and the demystification of courtship. In M. A. Fitzpatrick & A. L. Vangelisti (Eds.), *Explaining family interactions* (pp. 112–141). Thousand Oaks, CA: Sage.

Surra, C. A., & Hughes, D. K. (1997). Commitment processes in the development of premarital relationships. *Journal of Marriage and the Family, 59,* 5–21.

Swiller, H. I. (1988). Alexithymia: Treatment utilizing combined individual and group psychotherapy. *International Journal of Group Psychotherapy, 38,* 47–61.

Tait, R., & Silver, R. C. (1989). Coming to terms with major negative life events. In J. S. Uleman & J. A. Bargh (Eds.), *Unintended thought* (pp. 351–382). New York: Guilford Press.

Tavris, C. (1984). On the wisdom of counting to ten: Personal and social dangers of anger expression. In P. Shaver (Ed.), *Review of personality and social psychology: Vol. 5. Emotions, relationships, and health* (pp. 170–191). Beverly Hills, CA: Sage.

Tavris, C. (1989). *Anger: The misunderstood emotion* (rev. ed.). New York: Simon & Schuster.

Tavris, C., & Sadd, S. (1978). *The Redbook report on female sexuality.* New York: Dell.

Taylor, G. J. (1984). Psychotherapy with the boring patient. *Canadian Journal of Psychiatry, 29,* 217–222.

Taylor, G. J., Bagby, R. M., & Parker, J. D. A. (1991). The alexithymia construct: A potential paradigm for psychosomatic medicine. *Psychosomatics, 32,* 153–164.

Taylor, G. J., Bagby, R. M., & Parker, J. D. A. (1992). The Revised Toronto Alexithymia Scale: Some reliability, validity, and normative data. *Psychotherapy and Psychosomatics, 57,* 34–41.

Taylor, G. J., Parker, J. D. A., Bagby, R. M., & Acklin, M. W. (1992). Alexithymia and somatic complaints in psychiatric out-patients. *Journal of Psychosomatic Research, 36,* 417–424.

Taylor, G. J., Ryan, D., & Bagby, R. M. (1985). Toward the development of a new self-report alexithymia scale. *Psychotherapy and Psychosomatics, 44,* 191–199.

Tellegen, A. (1985). Structures of mood and personality and their relevance to assessing anxiety, with an emphasis on self-report. In A. H. Tuma & J. D. Maser (Eds.), *Anxiety and the anxiety disorders* (pp. 681–706). Hillsdale, NJ: Erlbaum.

Temoshok, L. (1987). Personality, coping style, emotion, and cancer: Towards an integrative model. *Cancer Surveys, 6,* 545–567.

Temoshok, L. (1990). On attempting to articulate the biopsychosocial model: Psychological–psychophysiological homeostasis. In H. S. Friedman (Ed.), *Personality and disease* (pp. 203–225). New York: Wiley.

Temoshok, L. (1993). Emotions and health outcomes: Some theoretical and methodological considerations. In H. C. Traue & J. W. Pennebaker (Eds.), *Emotion, inhibition, and health* (pp. 247–256). Seattle, WA: Hogrefe & Huber.

Thibaut, J. W., & Kelley, H. H. (1959). *The social psychology of groups.* New York: Wiley.

Thoits, P. A. (1985). Self-labeling processes in mental illness: The role of emotional deviance. *American Journal of Sociology, 91,* 221–249.

Thomas, A., & Chess, S. (1977). *Temperament and development.* New York: Brunner/Mazel.

Thomas, A. M., & Forehand, R. (1991). The relationship between parental depressive mood and early adolescent parenting. *Journal of Family Psychology, 4,* 260–271.

Thomas, G., Fletcher, G. J. O., & Lange, C. (1997). On-line empathic accuracy in marital interaction. *Journal of Personality and Social Psychology, 72,* 839–850.

Thompson, E. H., & Doll, W. (1982). The burden of families coping with the mentally ill: An invisible crisis. *Family Relations, 31,* 379–388.

Thompson, R. A. (1991). Emotional regulation and emotional development. *Educational Psychology Review, 3,* 269–307.

Thoresen, C. E., & Powell, L. H. (1992). Type A behavior pattern: New perspectives on theory, assessment, and intervention. *Journal of Consulting and Clinical Psychology, 60,* 595–604.

Thorne, B. (1993). *Gender play: Girls and boys in school.* New Brunswick, NJ: Rutgers University Press.

Thurman, C. W. (1985a). Effectiveness of cognitive-behavioral treatments in reducing Type A behavior among university faculty. *Journal of Counseling Psychology, 32,* 74–83.

Thurman, C. W. (1985b). Effectiveness of cognitive-behavioral treatments in reducing Type A behavior among university faculty—One year later. *Journal of Counseling Psychology, 32,* 445–448.

Tice, D. M. (1990, June). *Self-regulation of mood: Some self-report data.* Paper presented at the Nagshead Conference on Self-Control of Thought and Emotion, Nagshead, NC.

Tice, D. M., & Baumeister, R. F. (1993). Controlling anger: Self-induced emotion change. In D. M. Wegner & J. W. Pennebaker (Eds.), *Handbook of mental control* (pp. 393–409). Englewood Cliffs, NJ: Prentice Hall.

Tickle-Degnen, L., & Rosenthal, R. (1990). The nature of rapport and its nonverbal correlates. *Psychological Inquiry, 1,* 285–293.

Tolhuizen, J. H. (1989). Communication strategies for intensifying dating relationships: Identification, use and structure. *Journal of Social and Personal Relationships, 6,* 413–434.

Traue, H. C. (1989). Behavioral inhibition in stress disorders and myogenic pain. In C. Bischoff, H. C. Traue, & H. Zenz (Eds.), *Clinical perspective on headache and low back pain* (pp. 29–46). Toronto, Ontario, Canada: Hogrefe & Huber.

Tronick, E. Z., & Gianino, A. F., Jr. (1986). The transmission of maternal disturbance to the infant. In E. Z. Tronick & T. Field (Eds.), *New directions for child development: Vol. 34. Maternal depression and infant disturbance* (pp. 5–11). San Francisco: Jossey-Bass.

Tublin, S. K., Bartholomew, K., & Weinberger, D. A. (1987, August). *Peer perceptions of preadolescent boys with repressive coping styles.* Paper presented at the annual meeting of the American Psychological Association, New York.

Tucker, J. S., & Friedman, H. S. (1996). Emotion, personality, and health. In C. Magai & S. H. McFadden (Eds.), *Handbook of emotion, adult development, and aging* (pp. 307–326). San Diego, CA: Academic Press.

Tucker, R. K., Marvin, M. G., & Vivian, B. (1991). What constitutes a romantic act? An empirical study. *Psychological Reports, 69,* 651–654.

Tucker, R. K., Vivian, B., & Marvin, M. G. (1992). Operationalizing the *romance* construct in an adult sample. *Psychological Reports, 71,* 115–120.

Tucker, R. K., & Yuhas Byers, P. (1992). *Keeping the romance in love.* Unpublished manuscript, Bowling Green State University, Bowling Green, OH.

Turner, R. G. (1978). Effects of differential request procedures and self-consciousness on trait attributions. *Journal of Research in Personality, 12,* 431–438.

Turvey, C., & Salovey, P. (1993). Measures of repression: Converging on the same construct? *Imagination, Cognition, and Personality, 13,* 279–289.

van der Kolk, B. (1987). *Psychological trauma.* Washington, DC: American Psychiatric Press.

Vaughn, C. E., & Leff, J. P. (1976a). The influence of family and social factors on the course of psychiatric illness: A comparison of schizophrenic and depressed neurotic patients. *British Journal of Psychiatry, 129,* 125–137.

Vaughn, C. E., & Leff, J. P. (1976b). The measurement of expressed emotion in the families of psychiatric patients. *British Journal of Clinical Psychology, 15,* 157–165.

Vingerhoets, A. J. J. M., Van Den Berg, M. P., Kortekaas, R. T., Van Heck, G. L., & Croon, M. A. (1993). Weeping: Associations with personality, coping, and subjective health status. *Personality and Individual Differences, 14,* 185–190.

Waters, E., Crowell, J., Treboux, D., Merrick, S., & Albersheim, L. (1995, March). *Attachment security from infancy to early adulthood: A 20-year longitudinal study.* Paper presented at the biennial meeting of the Society for Research in Child Development, Indianapolis, IN.

Watson, D. (in press). *Mood and temperament.* New York: Guilford Press.

Watson, D., & Clark, L. A. (1984). Negative affectivity: The disposition to experience aversive emotional states. *Psychological Bulletin, 96,* 465–490.

Watson, D., & Pennebaker, J. W. (1989). Health complaints, stress, and distress: Exploring the central role of negative affectivity. *Psychological Review, 96,* 234–254.

Watson, J. C. (1997). *Manifesting clients' agency in process–experiential therapy.* Paper presented at the 13th annual meeting of the Society for Psychotherapy Integration, Toronto, Ontario, Canada.

Watson, J. C. (in press). Re-exploring empathy: Reflections and conjectures. In D. Cain (Ed.), *Handbook of humanistic psychotherapy*. Washington: APA Books.

Watson, J. C., Goldman, R., & Greenberg, L. S. (1996). Change processes in experiential therapy. In R. Hutterer, G. Pawlowsky, P. Schmid, & R. Stipsits (Eds.), *Client-centered and experiential psychotherapy: A paradigm in motion* (pp. 35–46). Vienna: Peter Lang.

Watson, J. C., Goldman, R., & Vanaerschot, G. (1998). Empathic: A postmodern way of being. In L. S. Greenberg, J. C. Watson, & G. Lietaer (Eds.), *Handbook of experiential psychotherapy* (pp. 61–81). New York: Guilford Press.

Watson, J. C., & Greenberg, L. S. (1994). The alliance in experiential therapy: Enacting the relationship conditions. In A. Horvath & L. Greenberg (Eds.), *The working alliance: Theory, research and practice* (pp. 153ÿ2D172). New York: Wiley.

Watson, J. C., & Greenberg, L. S. (1995). Alliance ruptures and repairs in experiential therapy. *In Session: Psychotherapy in Practice, 1,* 19–31.

Watson, J. C., & Greenberg, L. S. (1996a). Emotion and cognition in experiential therapy: A dialectical–constructivist position. In H. Rosen & K. T. Kuehlwein (Eds.), *Constructing realities: Meaning-making perspectives for psychotherapists* (pp. 253–274). San Francisco: Jossey-Bass.

Watson, J. C., & Greenberg, L. S. (1996b). Pathways to change in the psychotherapy of depression: Relating process to session change and outcome. *Psychotherapy Research, 33,* 262ÿ2D274.

Watson, J. C., & Greenberg, L. S. (1998). The therapeutic alliance in short-term humanistic and experiential therapies. In J. Safran & C. Muran (Eds.), *The therapeutic alliance in brief psychotherapy* (pp. 123–146). Washington: APA Books.

Watson, J. C., & Rennie, D. L. (1994). Qualitative analysis of clients' subjective experience of significant moments during the exploration of problematic reactions. *Journal of Counseling Psychology, 41,* 500–509.

Weary, G., Gleicher, F., & Marsh, K. L. (Eds.). *(1993). Control motivation and social cognition.* New York: Springer-Verlag.

Weber, A. L., Harvey, J. H., & Stanley, M. A. (1987). The nature and motivations of accounts for failed relationships. In R. Burnett, P. McGhee, & D. Clarke (Eds.), *Accounting for relationships: Explanation, representation, and knowledge* (pp. 114–133). London: Methuen.

Wegner, D. M., & Gold, D. B. (1995). Fanning old flames: Emotional and cognitive effects of suppressing thoughts of a past relationship. *Journal of Personality and Social Psychology, 68,* 782–792.

Wegner, D. M., Schneider, D. J., Carter, S., III, & White, T. (1987). Paradoxical effects of thought suppression. *Journal of Personality and Social Psychology, 53,* 3–13.

Wegner, D. M., & Zanakos, S. (1994). Chronic thought suppression. *Journal of Personality, 62,* 615–640.

Wehmer, F., Brejnak, C., Lumley, M., & Stettner, L. (1995). Alexithymia and physiological reactivity to emotion-provoking visual scenes. *Journal of Nervous and Mental Disease, 183,* 351–357.

Weinberger, D. A. (1990). The construct validity of repressive coping. In J. L. Singer (Ed.), *Repression and dissociation: Implications for personality theory, psychopathology, and health.* Chicago: University of Chicago Press.

Weinberger, D. A. (1991). *Social-emotional adjustment in older children and adults: I. Psychometric properties of the Weinberger Adjustment Inventory.* Unpublished manuscript, Stanford University, Stanford, CA.

Weinberger, D. A., & Davidson, M. N. (1994). Styles of inhibiting emotional expression: Distinguishing repressive coping from impression management. *Journal of Personality, 62,* 587–613.

Weinberger, D. A., & Schwartz, G. E. (1990). Distress and restraint as superordinate dimensions of self-reported adjustment: A typological perspective. *Journal of Personality, 58,* 381–417.

Weinberger, D. A., Schwartz, G. E., & Davidson, R. J. (1979). Low-anxious, high-anxious, and repressive coping styles: Psychometric patterns and behavioral and physiological responses to stress. *Journal of Abnormal Psychology, 88,* 369–380.

Wheeler, L., Reis, H., & Nezlek, J. (1983). Loneliness, social interactions, and sex roles. *Journal of Personality and Social Psychology, 45,* 943–953.

Wile, D. (1994). The ego-analytic approach to emotion in couples therapy. In S. M. Johnson & L. S. Greenberg (Eds.), *The heart of the matter: Perspectives on emotion in marital therapy* (pp. 27–45). New York: Brunner/Mazel.

Wile, D. (1995). The ego-analytic approach to couple therapy. In N. S. Jacobson & A. S. Gurman (Eds.), *Clinical handbook of couple therapy* (pp. 91–120). New York: Guilford Press.

Wilfong, E. W., Saylor, C., & Elksnin, N. (1991). Influences on responsiveness: Interactions between mothers and their premature infants. *Infant Mental Health Journal, 12,* 31–40.

Wills, T. A. (1985). Supportive functions of interpersonal relationships. In S. Cohen & S. L. Syme (Eds.), *Social support and health* (pp. 61–82). Orlando, FL: Academic Press.

Wills, T. A. (1990). Social support and the family. In E. A. Blechman (Ed.), *Emotions and the family: For better or for worse* (pp. 75–98). Hillsdale, NJ: Erlbaum.

Winn, L. (1994). *Post-traumatic stress disorder and drama therapy: Treatment and risk reduction.* London: Jessica Kingley.

Wood, J. V., Saltzberg, J. A., Neale, J. M., Stone, A. A., & Rachmiel, T. B. (1990). Self-focused attention, coping responses, and distressed mood in everyday life. *Journal of Personality and Social Psychology, 58,* 1027–1036.

Woody, E. Z., & Costanzo, P. R. (1990). Does marital agony precede marital ecstasy?: A comment on Gottman & Krokoff's "Marital interaction and satisfaction: A longitudinal view." *Journal of Consulting and Clinical Psychology, 58,* 499–501.

Wortman, C. B., Adesman, P., Herman, E., and Greenberg, R. (1976). Self-disclosure: An attributional perspective. *Journal of Personality and Social Psychology, 33,* 184–191.

Wortman, C. B., & Dunkel-Schetter, C. (1979). Interpersonal relationships and cancer: A theoretical analysis. *Journal of Social Issues, 35,* 120–156.

Wortman, C. B., Kessler, R., Bolger, N., & House, J. (1991). *The time course of adjustment to widowhood: Evidence from a national probability sample.* Unpublished manuscript.

Wortman, C. B., Sheedy, C., Gluhoski, V., & Kessler, R. (1992). Stress, coping, and health: Conceptual issues and directions for future research. In H. S. Friedman (Ed.), *Hostility, coping, and health* (pp. 227–256). Washington, DC: American Psychological Association.

Wortman, C. B., & Silver, R. C. (1987). Coping with irrevocable loss. In G. R. VandenBos & B. K. Bryant (Eds.), *Cataclysms, crises, and catastrophes: Psychology in action* (pp. 189–235). Washington, DC: American Psychological Association.

Wortman, C. B., & Silver, R. C. (1989). The myths of coping with loss. *Journal of Consulting and Clinical Psychology, 57,* 349–357.

Wortman, C. B., & Silver, R. C. (1990). Successful mastery of bereavement and widowhood: A life course perspective. In P. B. Baltes & M. M. Baltes (Eds.), *Successful aging: Perspectives from the behavioral sciences* (pp. 225–264). New York: Cambridge University Press.

Wortman, C. B., Silver, R. C., & Kessler, R. C. (1992). The meaning of loss and adjustment to bereavement. In M. S. Stroebe, W. Stroebe, & R. O. Hansson (Eds.), *Handbook of bereavement* (pp. 349–366). New York: Cambridge University Press.

Yontef, G.M. (1991). *Awareness, dialogue and process: Essays on Gestalt therapy.* New York: Gestalt Journal Press.

Yontef, G. M. (1995). Gestalt therapy. In A. S. Gurman & S. B. Messer (Eds.), *Essential psychotherapies: Theory and practice* (pp. 261–303). New York: Guilford Press.

Yontef, G. M., & Simkin, J. S. (1989). Gestalt therapy. In R. J. Corsini & D. Wedding (Eds.), *Current psychotherapies* (pp. 323–361). Itasca, IL: Peacock.

Zahava, S., Mikulincer, M., & Arad, R. (1991). Monitoring and blunting: Implications for combat-related post-traumatic stress disorder. *Journal of Traumatic Stress, 4,* 209–221.

Zajonc, R. B. (1980). Feeling and thinking: Preferences need no inference. *American Psychologist, 35,* 151–175.

Zajonc, R. B. (1984). On the primacy of affect. *American Psychologist, 39,* 117–123.

Zeigarnik, B. (1938). Ueber das Behalten von erledigten und unerledigten Handlungen. *Psychologische Forschung, 9,* 1–85.

Zeiss, A. M., Lewinsohn, P. M., & Muñoz, R. F. (1979). Nonspecific improvements effects in depression using interpersonal skills training, pleasant events schedules, or cognitive training. *Journal of Consulting and Clinical Psychology, 47,* 427–439.

Zillmann, D. (1993). Mental control of angry aggression. In D. Wegner & J. W. Pennebaker (Eds.), *Handbook of mental control* (pp. 370–392). Englewood Cliffs, NJ: Prentice-Hall.

Zivin, G. (1982). Watching the sands shift: Conceptualizing development of nonverbal mastery. In R. S. Feldman (Ed.), *Development of nonverbal behavior in children* (pp. 63–98). New York: Springer-Verlag.

Zuckerman, M. (1995). Good and bad humors: Biochemical bases of personality and its disorders. *Psychological Science, 6,* 325–332.

Zuckerman, M., Lipets, M., Koivumaki, J., & Rosenthal, R. (1975). Encoding and decoding nonverbal cues of emotion. *Journal of Personality and Social Psychology, 32,* 1968–1976.

Index